MW00604584

Practical Considerations for
School-Based
Occupational
Therapists

By **Lynne Pape**, MEd, OTR/L, and **Kelly Ryba**, OTR/L

Foreword by **Jane Case-Smith**, EdD, OTR/L, FAOTA

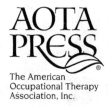

AOTA PRESS

The American
Occupational Therapy
Association, Inc.

Vision Statement
AOTA advances occupational therapy as the preeminent profession in promoting the health, productivity, and quality of life of individuals and society through the therapeutic application of occupation.

Mission Statement
The American Occupational Therapy Association advances the quality, availability, use, and support of occupational therapy through standard-setting, advocacy, education, and research on behalf of its members and the public.

AOTA Staff
Frederick P. Somers, *Executive Director*
Christopher M. Bluhm, *Chief Operating Officer*
Audrey Rothstein, *Group Leader, Communications*
Chris Davis, *Managing Editor, AOTA Press*
Barbara Dickson, *Production Editor*
Robert A. Sacheli, *Manager, Creative Services*
Sarah E. Ely, *Book Production Coordinator*
Marge Wasson, *Marketing Manager*

The American Occupational Therapy Association, Inc.
4720 Montgomery Lane
Bethesda, MD 20814
Phone: 301-652-AOTA (2682)
TDD: 800-377-8555
Fax: 301-652-7711
www.aota.org
To order: 1-877-404-AOTA (2682)

ISBN: 1-56900-196-0

Library of Congress Control Number: 2004115390

Design by Sarah E. Ely
Composition by Electronic Quill, Silver Spring, MD
Printed by Automated Graphic Systems, White Plains, MD

Contents

List of Tables, Figures, Exhibits, and Appendixes

Also available on the enclosed CD-ROM.

Foreword

School-based practice offers both tremendous challenges and rewards to occupational therapists and occupational therapy assistants. Challenges include the need for school-based therapists to continually update discipline skills, stay current with best practice models of service delivery, and understand the application of federal laws and regulations. Rewards include the satisfaction of contributing to children's learning and development and participating on a professional team that effectively supports children's success in school. This book helps therapists meet the challenges and reap the rewards of school-based practice.

Authors Lynne Pape, MEd, OTR/L, and Kelly Ryba, OTR/L, offer invaluable resources to school-based occupational therapists that will enhance their services to children and maximize their success in the public education system. The book provides extensive, up-to-date information about therapy approaches, service delivery models, and legal mandates, and it explains step-by-step methods for applying this essential information to daily school-based practice. The book is particularly helpful to occupational therapists who are new to the schools or ones practicing in isolated settings without a network of other occupational therapists.

Pape and Ryba have written chapters based on their own experiences in schools and their tried-and-true strategies for best practice service delivery. They explain how occupational therapists can most effectively function in all aspects of the public school system and can optimally contribute to the education of children with special needs. Included are strategies to both coach and support teachers so that students' learning is optimal.

This book is essential reading. Chapters are easy to read and well organized, each providing helpful resources that will aide in providing efficient best practice services. The forms and examples can help organize data, explain occupational therapy services, document evaluation results for purposes of intervention planning, and record a student's progress on educational goals. These resources translate legislative mandates for documentation and reporting into easy-to-use formats and well-explained procedures. This book will enable therapists to effectively help students with individualized education programs learn and function in school and to lead the interdisciplinary teams who plan and provide special education services.

Jane Case-Smith, EdD, OTR/L, FAOTA
Professor, School of Allied Medical
  Professions, Ohio State University
Columbus

Introduction

Occupational therapists and occupational therapy assistants working in school-based settings must remain current and knowledgeable on a wide range of topics that can affect a student's educational performance, including sensory–motor, gross motor, fine motor, visual–motor, visual–perceptual, and activities of daily living (ADL) skills. We have found that, through our own experiences, therapists in school-based practice often work in isolation or have limited contact with other school-based therapists. They frequently have limited to no supervision from an experienced occupational therapist or director who is knowledgeable in school-based occupational therapy issues and federal and state educational procedures. This results in therapists not having the opportunity to collaborate with other occupational therapy professionals working in the same practice arena to gain additional evaluation or intervention ideas or to discuss current trends in the literature or practice. Through conversations with occupational therapists and occupational therapy assistants in our state, we feel that therapists need continued access to resources that can be used in their daily practice.

We wrote this book to provide an overall framework and reference for occupational therapists and occupational therapy assistants in school-based practice. The book primarily focuses on preschool and elementary-age children, with the intent that the overall principles and strategies could be applied to students across grade levels. Resources for specific topics and practical information and suggestions are provided that can be used in

everyday practice. We offer scenarios and situations that we are currently facing where we live in hopes that others also can learn from these experiences.

Chapters are organized by specific topic areas to help readers access the information that they need efficiently. In Chapter 1, we provide an overview of the roles of occupational therapists and occupational therapy assistants working in school-based settings. A synopsis of the Individuals With Disabilities Education Act is provided as a resource for therapists who are unfamiliar with this legislation. We detail the importance of establishing a referral procedure within a therapist's individual school district, discuss evaluation approaches, describe how to write educationally based assessments, and examine considerations for evaluating students at varying cognitive and developmental levels. Finally, we discuss the important roles that occupational therapists and occupational therapy assistants can play as members of a student's educational team, including the need to be an active part of the development of a student's individualized educational program (IEP).

In Chapter 2 on documentation and data collection, we describe the components of a student's IEP, including how to write a comprehensive present level of performance and how to write measurable and educationally relevant annual goals and short-term objectives or benchmarks. We discuss data collection procedures and provide examples for various intervention areas supported by occupational therapists, including self-care skills, scissor skills, prewriting, and handwriting.

Examples outline how to collect and report numerical data, describe what relevant narrative information to include within a daily documentation note, and describe how to average data at the end of a grading period to report in a progress note to parents.

In Chapter 3 on dyspraxia, we describe the characteristics of a student with motor planning problems by age group (e.g., toddler, preschool, and school age). Methods for evaluating a student with dyspraxia are discussed, including considerations when completing observations and when interviewing parents and teachers, and descriptions of formal assessments for gross motor skills, visual–motor skills, visual–perceptual skills, handwriting, and self-care are provided. We have developed questionnaires that can be used during the evaluation process to gain additional information on the student's birth and developmental history and overall performance within the classroom setting and at home. Intervention strategies and suggested modifications and accommodations that can be used in the classroom are also illustrated.

Chapter 4 on ADL skills provides detailed information and task analysis for specific skills for dressing, feeding, and managing the school environment. Considerations for evaluation and providing intervention to students with ADL skills deficits are provided. The Self-Care Functional Checklist can be used during the interview or observation process to gain additional information about a student's level of independence with his or her self-help skills and ADLs. Sample goals and objectives are also included that can be used for a student's IEP.

In Chapter 5 on hand skills, we provide comprehensive information on developmental milestones and the acquisition of fine motor skills; describe the hand skills components needed to complete selected fine motor tasks; and detail the fine motor components needed for managing specific classroom tasks, includ-

ing tool use, bilateral hand skills, and hand separation for effective pencil grips and scissors' use. Intervention strategies for the development of hand skills are provided. Samples of goals and objectives are also included.

Chapter 6 on handwriting discusses the perceptual, motor, and cognitive components that affect a student's writing abilities and also how to develop a process to deal with handwriting issues. Prerequisite skills for handwriting are delineated. Considerations for evaluation are examined for students with varying developmental and cognitive ability levels. Formal and informal evaluation techniques are mentioned. The Handwriting Teacher Questionnaire can be used by occupational therapists during the evaluation process to gain additional information about a student's overall academic and handwriting skills. Intervention strategies and handwriting curricula are discussed. Use of assistive technology for functional written communication is outlined, and specific short-term objectives are included that can be used on a student's IEP.

Chapter 7 on preschool children describes the various roles of occupational therapists in the preschool environment, including those as a direct service provider, consultant, or collaborator. Considerations when evaluating preschool students in fine motor, self-help, and sensory–motor skills are provided. We have developed the Preschool Functional Educational Checklist to help gain additional information during the observation and interview process about a student's behavior, fine motor, visual–motor, gross motor, and sensory–motor skills. Different service delivery models are discussed, including direct service options versus providing consultation or collaboration with classroom teachers. Considerations for intervention strategies are provided for development of fine motor skills, self-help skills, and sensory–motor interventions and accommodations in a preschool setting.

In Chapter 8 on sensory issues, we give an overview of the major sensory systems (e.g., tactile, proprioceptive, and vestibular) and neurological background information. Evaluation methods are described, including considerations when conducting an interview with a student's parents and teaching staff, observing a student at his or her home or in school, and using more formal assessment tools. We describe methods to support a student's sensory–motor issues, including advocating for sensory–motor activities to be incorporated within a classroom setting for all students, developing activities and modifications that can occur for the student in the classroom, or developing activities and modifications that occur outside of the classroom (e.g., a sensory–motor room). Development of sensory–motor plans that meet a student's individualized sensory needs are described. We provide examples of how to take data to determine the effectiveness of intervention strategies on a student's performance. Intervention strategies and activities specific to the major sensory systems also are provided.

We hope that, after reading this book, readers take away practical information that can be applied and used in everyday practice when evaluating students, providing intervention, and documenting occupational therapy services.

Lynne Pape, MEd, OTR/L
President, North Coast Therapy
*   Associates, Inc., LLC*
Strongsville, Ohio

Kelly Ryba, OTR/L
Vice President, North Coast Therapy
*   Associates, Inc., LLC*
Strongsville, Ohio

Acknowledgments

We acknowledge the school districts with which North Coast Therapy contracts and thank them for supporting our philosophy and approach to providing therapy services in an educational setting. We also thank all of the occupational therapists who work for North Coast Therapy. It is their desire and drive to continually improve the quality of services that motivates us to continue to support their efforts. Without the high caliber of staff, North Coast Therapy would not be able to maintain the positive relationships with all of our school districts. We express our gratitude to Sharon Galvan, North Coast administrative assistant, and to our "peer reviewers" for their comments and feedback.

Above all, we thank our family, friends and, most importantly, our husbands, Dave and Cameron; without their ongoing support and encouragement, this project could not have been possible.

Kelly Ryba, OTR/L
Lynne Pape, MEd, OTR/L

Roles of Occupational Therapy in the School Setting

The roles of occupational therapy as a related service in the school setting have evolved over the years. The definitions of a related service as well as occupational therapy are provided in federal law, but the criteria for when a child should receive occupational therapy services depends on a team process.

Both federal and state special education and early intervention laws mandate the provision of occupational therapy services for eligible children. Guidelines have been developed to help occupational therapists understand their roles and responsibilities when working in schools. These guidelines are typically based on the federal law, which is the primary policy that affects the education of children with disabilities. In addition, it is critical that therapists providing services in schools be familiar with their own state and local laws, regulations, and procedures for implementation.

As it is sometimes difficult for occupational therapists to understand the Individuals With Disabilities Education Act (IDEA) requirements, this chapter gives an overview of the history of IDEA, which provides for a free appropriate public education for students with disabilities. A description of IDEA's primary components is presented as they affect the provision of occupational therapy services in schools, including the definition of related services, occupational therapy as a related service, the evaluation process, and the individualized educational program (IEP). It is not the intent of this chapter to provide a definitive interpretation of IDEA but instead to help therapists understand the

provisions that affect occupational therapy practice in schools.

Procedures for referral for an occupational therapy assessment, as well as the occupational therapy evaluation process, are discussed. Determining the need for occupational therapy services is also discussed as a part of the evaluation and IEP processes. Methods of appropriately providing occupational therapy services are presented. The occupational therapist's collaborative role as a member of the team is stressed as it relates to student achievement and the accomplishment of student goals and objectives.

The roles of occupational therapy assistants in service provision and the responsibilities of occupational therapists for supervision and direction are presented, in addition to defining the responsibilities of each in schools. A comparison of service delivery in educational and medical settings is outlined to help readers understand the differences.

Occupational Therapy's Early Involvement in Educational Settings

Hanft and Place (1996) have outlined how occupational therapy became involved in educational settings in the United States. In 1935, federal grants created the Crippled Children's Services (CCS) under the Maternal and Child Health Program of the Social Security Act (Social Security Act of 1935, P.L. 74–271, Sections 701–710). Initially, occupational and physical therapy services were provided to children with orthopedic and neurological problems secondary to polio. Occupational therapists were hired by CCS clinics from 1940 through 1950 to work in the public schools to provide direct intervention to children with cerebral palsy, muscular dystrophy, polio, and other orthopedic handicaps.

During the 1960s and early 1970s, the educational needs of children with disabilities were not being met, and more than half of the children with disabilities did not receive appropriate educational services. It has been estimated that 1 million children with disabilities were excluded from the public school system or denied the opportunity to experience the educational process with their peers due to their disabilities (Hanft & Place, 1996). Because of the lack of adequate services, families were often forced to seek services outside the public school system at their own expense. Those students with significant motor disabilities who were able or allowed to attend school were serviced by therapists who provided direct therapy that replicated the rehabilitation medical-based model in which they were trained to provide in a hospital setting (Hanft & Place, 1996).

Two major Supreme Court decisions in early 1970s determined children with disabilities had a constitutional right to a public education (*Mills v. Board of Education of the District of Columbia,* 1972; *Pennsylvania Association for Retarded Children v. Commonwealth of Pennsylvania,* 1971). These decisions led Congress to enact the Education for the Handicapped Act (EHA) in 1975, which was amended as the Education for All Handicapped Children Act, also known as P.L. 94-142. This 1975 law is the precursor to IDEA.

Definitions of Terms Relating to IDEA

It is important for occupational therapists to understand the focus of IDEA. Therapists should also review their individual state special education and early intervention laws, rules, and regulations that specifically describe how services are to be provided in their state.

Following are brief definitions of selected terms used relative to IDEA (American Occupational Therapy Association [AOTA], 1997):

- *Federal regulations* are rules generated by administrative agencies to help implement laws. These rules interpret and translate the broad and nonspecific policies and procedures outlined in the law. The U.S. Department of Education generates regulations for IDEA.
- *Law* (also known as *Code*) is an act of Congress that has been signed by the president or passed by Congress over the president's veto. The Code is divided into subparts, and each subpart may have one or more sections.
- *State laws* about special education, along with state rules and regulations, are derived from federal law, rules, and regulations. It is important that readers obtain and read their state policies and procedures for implementation of IDEA. States have to follow the federal law but may provide expanded services.

History of IDEA

The U.S. Congress passed P.L. 94-142 in November 1975. This law guaranteed children with disabilities, ages 6 to 21 years, a free and appropriate education. The act included the following provisions:

- The concept of "zero reject" indicated that no child with a disability could be excluded because of the severity or nature of his or her disability;
- Children with disabilities were to be educated in the least restrictive environment with children who do not have disabilities to the maximum extent possible;
- A team of individuals, including the child's parents, would develop an IEP that would meet each child's unique needs;
- The provision of related services, including occupational therapy, was made "as

required to assist a handicapped child to benefit from special education"; and

- Parents would have the right to request a due process hearing if they disagreed with their child's placement or services (McEwen, 2000).

Since EHA was first passed, many changes have occurred pertaining to the provision of special education and related services, including occupational therapy, in school settings. In 1986, amendments to EHA added the early childhood component to the law (P.L. 94-457). In addition to mandating services for preschool children (ages 3–5 years) with disabilities in Part B §619, amendments also gave states the option of developing systems to serve infants and toddlers with disabilities and their families, in what is now Part C (formerly Part H). The individualized family service plan (IFSP) requirement was added at this time.

In 1990, the law was changed again, and the title of the law changed to the Individuals With Disabilities Education Act (P.L. 101-476). The name was changed to indicate the importance of using people-first language rather than identifying children by disability. At that time autism and traumatic brain injury were added as disability eligibility categories.

By 1991, services relevant to occupational therapy were added (P.L. 102-119). These included assistive technology and a requirement for state departments of education to develop and implement policies and procedures to ensure smooth transitions of children from the Part C early intervention system to Part B programs.

In 1997, Congress further amended IDEA (P.L. 105-17). Changes relevant to occupational therapy services included

- Addition of related services to transition services;
- Inclusion of related service personnel in IEP meetings, if appropriate;

- Focus of special education and related services on assisting children with disabilities to access and succeed in the general curriculum;
- Increased emphasis on educating students with disabilities with students without disabilities; and
- Increased expectations and education agency accountability for student outcomes.

The 1997 amendments also added a provision that general education teachers should participate in IEP meetings. This provision is intended to help integrate special and regular education. In addition, the expectation that related services personnel (occupational therapists) attend IEP meetings provides additional opportunities for teachers, parents, and therapists to communicate and develop consensus about the most appropriate educational program for the child (Case-Smith, 1998).

The final regulations for the 1997 amendments were published in the March 12, 1999 *Federal Register*. Part 300 of the regulations covers the Part B state grant program, which provides services for students ages 3 and older, while Part 303 covers the early intervention program for infants and toddlers and their families, ages birth through 2 years. In this chapter, only those regulations directly related to school-based occupational therapy services under Part B are included. Interested therapists can access the complete law and regulations on the U.S. Department of Education Web site at http://www.ed.gov/offices/OSERS/IDEA/index.html or from their individual school districts.

Components of IDEA

IDEA provides federal funds to help state and local governments establish and maintain special education programs for students with disabilities, in addition to providing related services to those students who require them to benefit from their educational program. The primary purpose of Part B of IDEA is to "ensure that all children with disabilities have available to them a free appropriate public education that includes special education and related services to meet their unique needs." Other purposes include the assurance that the rights of children with disabilities and their parents are protected; assistance to states, localities, educational service agencies, and federal agencies to provide for the education of all children with disabilities; and determination of the effectiveness of efforts to educate children with disabilities (§300.1(a)(b)(c)(d)). These purposes also apply to other state agencies that are involved in the education of children with disabilities and children and youth referred to or placed in private schools and facilities by that agency (§300.2(c)).

Free Appropriate Public Education

Each state is required to provide a free appropriate public education to every eligible child or youth (ages 3–21) with a disability. *Free appropriate public education* is defined in the regulations (§300.340–300.350) as special education and related services that

- Are provided at public expense under public supervision in direction and without charge;
- Meet the standards of the state education agency, including the requirements of this part of the law;
- Include preschool, elementary school, or secondary school education in the state; and
- Are provided in conformity with an IEP that meets the requirements of §300.340–300.350.

Student Eligibility

A student who is eligible for services under IDEA is defined as a child

- Who has been evaluated according to IDEA's evaluation requirements (specified at §300.530–300.536); and
- Who has been determined, through this

evaluation, to have one or more of the disabilities listed below; and
- Who, because of the disability, needs special education and related services to receive a free appropriate public education.

Disability Categories

Specific disability categories covered under IDEA (§300.7(a)(1)) are
- Autism
- Deaf-blindness
- Deafness
- Emotional disturbance
- Hearing impairments
- Mental retardation
- Multiple disabilities
- Orthopedic impairments
- Other health impairments
- Specific learning disability
- Speech or language impairments
- Traumatic brain injury
- Visual impairments, including blindness.

Special Education and Related Services

Special education is defined as (§300.26)
- Specially designed instruction, at no cost to the parents, to meet the unique needs of a child with a disability;
- Addressing the unique needs of the child that result from his or her disability; and
- Ensuring access of the child to the general curriculum, so that he or she can meet the educational standards within the jurisdiction of the public agency that apply to all children.

Special education and related services can be provided in several settings, including in the classroom, in the home, at hospitals and institutions, and in other settings (§300.26). In addition, state and local education agencies must ensure that a continuum of alternative placements is available to meet children's needs and that provisions for supplemental services (e.g., resource room, itinerant instruction) are provided in conjunction with regular class placement (§300.551(a)).

Unless the IEP of the child with a disability requires some other arrangement, the child is educated in the school that he or she would attend if he or she did not have a disability (§300.552(c)). Special education and related services must be provided in the least restrictive environment. Specifically, children with disabilities, including children in public or private institutions or other care facilities, are, to the maximum extent appropriate, educated with children who do not have disabilities. Furthermore, special classes, separate schooling, or other removal of children with disabilities from the regular education environment occur only when the nature or severity of the disability is such that education in regular classes with the use of supplemental aides and services cannot be achieved satisfactorily (§300.550(b)(2)).

Related services are defined as transportation and such developmental, corrective, and other supportive services that are required to help the child with a disability benefit from special education (§300.24) and include

- Speech-language pathology and audiology
- Psychological services
- Occupational and physical therapy
- Recreation, including therapeutic recreation
- Early identification and assessment of children and disabilities
- Counseling services, including rehabilitation counseling
- Orientation of mobility services
- Medical services for diagnostic or evaluation purposes only
- School health services
- Social work services
- Parent counseling and training.

The list of related services in the law and regulations could include other developmental, corrective, or support services, such as creative arts (e.g., music, dance, art), if they are required to help the child with a disability

benefit from special education (Kupper & Gutierrez, 2000).

Accessing Services

Under IDEA, a complete and individualized evaluation of the child's educational needs must be performed to determine eligibility for special education and related services (Clark & Coster, 1998). The parent may initiate a request for the evaluation by contacting the appropriate individual in the school district. The school district may also initiate a referral for evaluation. This evaluation, which may or may not include an occupational therapy assessment, is to be conducted at no cost to the family. The parent must give written informed permission before the school can begin the evaluation (Kupper & Gutierrez, 2000).

Initial Evaluation and Requirements

The public agency may evaluate a child based on a teacher's recommendation or observations or from the results of tests given to all children in a particular grade. The school district may recommend that a child receive screening or an assessment to determine if he or she has a disability and needs special education and related services.

When conducting the initial evaluation, each public agency has to ensure that a full and individualized evaluation is conducted for each child being considered for special education and related services

- To determine if the child is a "child with a disability" under §300.7, and
- To determine the educational needs of the child.

The evaluation is to be conducted in accordance with specific procedures, and the results are used by the child's IEP team to meet the requirements of §300.501–§300.536, listed below.

The evaluation involves a variety of assessment tools and strategies, including information provided by the parents, to gather relevant functional and developmental information. Furthermore, the district is not to use any single procedure as the sole criteria to determine whether a child has a disability. In addition, technically sound instruments are to be used to assess a student's cognitive and behavioral factors, in addition to physical or developmental factors.

The local educational agency must assess the child in all areas of suspected disability, including, if appropriate, health, vision, hearing, social and emotional status, general intelligence, academic performance, communicative status, and motor abilities. Furthermore, the evaluation is to be sufficiently comprehensive to identify all of the child's special education and related services needs, whether or not commonly linked to the disability category in which the child has been classified (§300.352, summarized below).

Tests and other evaluation materials shall
• Be selected and administered so they will not be culturally or racially discriminatory
• Be provided and administered in the child's native language or other mode of communication, unless it is not feasible to do so
• Be administered by trained personnel in accordance with instructions provided by the producer if a standardized test
• Provide relevant functional and developmental information, including information provided by the parents, to assist the team in determining the educational needs of the child based on the assessment tools and strategies.

Other data, including evaluations and information provided by the parents of the child, current classroom-based assessments, and observations by teachers and related service providers, will also be reviewed.

Determining Eligibility and Placement

When the evaluation is completed, the team, including the parents, must meet to discuss the results and determine whether the child has a disability and requires special education and related services (§300.7). Information obtained from all of the sources (i.e., testing, parent input, teacher recommendations) must be considered.

In interpreting evaluation data for the purpose of determining if a student is a child with a disability under IDEA §300.535, the team shall
• Draw on information from a variety of sources, including aptitude and achievement tests, parent input, teacher recommendations, physical condition, social or cultural background, and adaptive behavior
• Ensure that information obtained from all of the documented sources has been carefully considered
• Develop an IEP for the child in accordance with IDEA requirements if a determination is made that a child has a disability and needs special education and related services.

The IEP

Once it has been determined that a child has a disability and needs special education and related services, an IEP—the written document that identifies the student's specific educational needs and how they will be met— must be developed and implemented as soon as possible following the IEP meeting. IDEA does not specify a specific time frame for the development of the IEP; the law allows states and local districts to make that determination. The IEP must be in effect before a child can receive special education or related services and must be reviewed at least yearly (although the review can occur more frequently if necessary for a particular child).

The IEP is generated by a team and should reflect information obtained through the initial evaluation or reevaluation. Members of the team include the child's parents, at least one regular education teacher, at least one special education teacher, and a representative of the public agency (school district) who is qualified to supervise the specially designed instruction and who is knowledgeable about the curriculum and other resources within the district. Other individuals who may have knowledge or special expertise about the child, including related service personnel, may also be included on the team. The child, when appropriate, can be a member of the team.

The IEP team is responsible for determining if occupational therapy services are or are not needed for the child to meet his or her educational outcomes. For that reason, it is important for occupational therapists to attend IEP meetings, especially when occupational therapy services are being considered. Even if therapists cannot attend the meetings, they should still communicate relevant information to the team so that appropriate decisions can be made about the need for occupational therapy services.

The IEP is a legal contract that commits resources and services to address unique needs of individual students. IDEA specifies content but does not mandate a specific format. The IEP must include (§300.347)

- A statement of the child's present level of educational performance, including how the child's disability affects his or her involvement in and progress in the general curriculum (i.e., the same curriculum as for children without disabilities)—or as appropriate for a preschool child, how the disability effects his or her participation in appropriate activities

- A statement of measurable annual goals related to meeting the child's needs that result from his or her disability and to encourage the child to be involved in the general curriculum (i.e., the same curriculum as for children without disabilities)—or as appropriate for a preschool child, to participate in appropriate activities—and to

meet each of the child's other educational needs that result from his or her disability

- A statement of special education and related services and supplementary aids and services to be provided to the child, or on behalf of the child, and a statement of the program modification or supports for school personnel that will be provided for the child to allow him or her to advance appropriately toward attaining the annual goals, to be involved in progress in the general curriculum and to participate in extracurricular and other nonacademic activities, and to be educated and participate with other children with and without disabilities in the activities described

- An explanation of the extent, if any, to which the child will not participate with children without disabilities in the regular classroom and the activities described

- A statement of any individual modifications in the administration of state or districtwide assessments of student achievement that are needed for the child to participate in the assessment and, if the IEP team determines that the child will not participate, a statement of why the assessment is not appropriate for the child and then how he or she will be assessed

- The projected date for the beginning of the services and modifications described and statements of how the child's progress toward the annual goals will be measured, how the child's parents will be regularly informed (e.g., through report cards), the child's progress toward the annual goals, and the extent to which progress is sufficient to enable the child to achieve the goals by the end of the year

- A statement of the transition services required, which must be included for each student with a disability beginning at age 14 (or younger, if determined appropriate by the IEP team) and updated annually; for students beginning at age 16 (or younger, if determined appropriate by the IEP team), the statement must include any inter-agency responsibilities or needed linkages (McEwen, 2000).

Role of Occupational Therapy in the Evaluation Process

IDEA requires state education agencies to identify, locate, and evaluate all children with disabilities in the state, including those attending private schools, regardless of the severity of their disability, and also those who need special education and related services. As a part of that process, the local education agency may refer a child for an occupational therapy evaluation if he or she demonstrates dysfunction in the following performance areas:

- Self-help or adaptive skills, work, and productive activities;
- Leisure or play activities; and
- Performance components of sensory motor, cognitive, and psychosocial development that may affect the learning process (AOTA, 1999a).

Some states use pre-referral, which will become a requirement under the pending IDEA reauthorization, or problem-solving strategies before making a formal referral for an initial evaluation. Occupational therapy can provide input as a part of this process. The purpose of this process is to identify specific problems and provide intervention strategies or modifications to support the student's learning sooner rather than later. In those cases in which this approach does not positively affect the student's learning or behavior, the team may consider the need for an evaluation, at which time parent permission is required. It is important that therapists be familiar with their state guidelines in terms of the pre-referral process and the latitude to provide intervention before referral for initial evaluation.

Establishing a Referral Process for Occupational Therapy Evaluations

AOTA has developed a position in reference to *referral,* the practice of directing an initial request for service or changing the degree and direction of service (AOTA, 1999b).

The need for an occupational therapy assessment as a part of the initial evaluation is determined during the team planning process. Because occupational therapists might not be involved at this level, a procedure for initiating occupational therapy referrals should be established by each school district to help minimize confusion and clarify the reasons for and expectations of the referral. It has been the authors' experience that occupational therapists often identify the need for and initiate the development of the referral process and accompanying procedures and forms.

Occupational therapists can find themselves in an awkward position when a referral process does not exist. To resolve this, the procedure should define how a referral for an occupational therapy assessment is generated and who has the authority to initiate the request. When approached about evaluating a student, therapists must be able to explain to parents, teachers, psychologists, or administrators the procedure to initiate an occupational therapy evaluation.

Requesting Occupational Therapy Input in General Education

Teachers often approach occupational therapists with requests to "look at" students. The school district needs to determine if and how occupational therapy input can be provided, especially for students who do not have IEPs. If the district uses a pre-referral process, occupational therapy supports may be provided under that approach. Some districts have building intervention teams that meet regularly to discuss learning and behavioral concerns about general education students. Occupational therapists can be a resource to that team if occupational therapy–related concerns exist.

Suggestions and interventions to be tried with the student can be provided to the team. Typically, a follow-up meeting is held to discuss the impact of the interventions and to determine if it is necessary to initiate the referral process to conduct an initial evaluation to determine if the child is eligible for special education services. Occupational therapists need to be familiar with their state's laws, rules, and regulations in this area.

Creating a Referral Form

In addition to defining the process, a form should be created to help occupational therapists clarify the areas of concern. (See Appendix 1.1 for an example of a referral form.) As the authors are members of a contract agency providing occupational and physical therapy services to school districts, it is very important to us that we receive adequate information to help us determine the exact concern and information being sought to assist in defining the problem so that we know how to approach the evaluation.

To be able to track requests for occupational therapy evaluations as well as define the areas of concern, our agency developed a referral form with an accompanying procedure. The school district completes the form and sends it to our office so that it can be entered into our database for tracking purposes.

The completed packet is then forwarded to the occupational therapist who will perform the evaluation. Once a packet has been received, the therapist knows that he or she has been authorized to initiate the process and has permission to contact the appropriate staff to obtain more specific information.

Identifying Information. The following items are included on our evaluation form and are considered identifying information:

- Evaluation date
- Student's name, address, birthdate, and grade level
- Parents' names (important, especially if the mother has a different last name than the child) and phone number
- General education teacher and special education teacher, if applicable
- Special education disability classification, if applicable
- Building-level contact and person initiating the referral
- Source of referral, so that the therapist knows how the need for the referral was identified (e.g., the IEP team, parent, regular education teacher, special education teacher, psychologist, physician).

Type of Evaluation Requested. The type of student (e.g., preschool, school age) is identified on the form, along with the type of evaluation (e.g., initial evaluation, reevaluation, request for a student who is already receiving special education services but has occupational therapy–related concerns). Occupational therapists should be aware of their state guidelines regarding procedures for evaluating students for a related service if they already have been receiving special education services. For example, in Ohio, when a related service is being considered as an addition to an existing IEP, an entire reevaluation must be completed.

Miscellaneous Information. In addition to the above criteria, the form requests areas of concern. This section helps occupational therapists identify in what areas information is being sought as well as clearly define the referring question. Depending on the stage of the evaluation process during which the occupational therapy referral was initiated, it is also helpful for therapists to know the approximate date that the team will reconvene to share the results of the evaluation.

Signature of Special Education Administrator. As the authors are members of a contract agency, it is important to us that an administrator from the school district review the request for every occupational and physical therapy referral and then sign and date it, indicating that we have permission to initiate the evaluation. At times the administrators may ask for more information before signing the forms.

Documenting the Referral Process

In school-based and early intervention settings, the referral process covers many issues. After an occupational therapist receives a referral, he or she should document it and include the following:

- A copy of the referral form or, if no form is used, documentation of the source of referral
- A copy of the parent permission form or documentation of the date that the form was signed
- An indication that available information was reviewed to assist in determining if the referral was appropriate
- The expected completion date of the evaluation, if determined appropriate
- Documentation of the date that the evaluation results were shared with the team, including the parents, indicating which team members were present
- A summary of the team meeting, including the need for occupational therapy services if indicated by the team.

Beginning the Evaluation Process

Once the referral is received and parental consent obtained, the occupational therapist is ready to begin the occupational therapy evaluation process. It is important for therapists to understand specifically what information is being sought. If the referral indi-

cates only global areas of concern (e.g., "problems writing") rather than a specific problem, then the first step is for the therapist to clarify the team's concerns.

Standardized Assessments. Once the concern is identified, the occupational therapist will need to determine how to obtain relevant functional and developmental information. IDEA emphasizes using a variety of assessment tools and strategies (§300.532 2(b)). These may include standardized and nonstandardized methods. Waterman (1994) has indicated that, even though standardized tests are readily available and provide normative scores to assist in determining eligibility, they lack the ability to provide a comprehensive picture of how the child is performing within the educational setting in terms of relevant functional information. Scores achieved on standardized tests can sometimes indicate below-average skills while the teacher is indicating that the child is functioning in the classroom with minimal support.

If a standardized assessment is chosen, it will be important to support evaluation information with examples of how the results of specific test score items are affecting the child's ability to function in the school setting. Standardized assessments require further application and inferences by occupational therapists in an attempt to relate performance on the test to performance in the classroom.

Discipline-Specific Assessments. Using a discipline-specific approach to evaluation does not reflect the intent of IDEA. In this approach, the occupational therapist would conduct a separate assessment of the student's needs, possibly using a deficit-based model, in that if the child is unable to accomplish a task, occupational therapy services would be recommended. Individual discipline-specific goals and interventions would be developed and provided without considering the student's educational plan.

Occupational therapists need to move out of the deficit-based approach used in the past because, when deficits were found, treatment was indicated without considering if the specific deficits affected the student's ability to function in the educational setting (Clark & Coster, 1998).

Giangreco (1986) has suggested that the quasi-team (in which individual team members meet to discuss the student but pursue their own separate, specific discipline-reference goals) does not reflect collaboration as intended by IDEA. Put another way, under IDEA, clinical or educational diagnosis (e.g., cerebral palsy), low test scores (–2 standard deviations or developmental age equivalent lower than chronological age), or other indicator of limitations do not automatically qualify students for occupational therapy services. Rather, priorities and outcomes of the student's educational program are to be established collaboratively by the team before the need for specific services can be indicated.

Functional-Based Assessment. An occupational therapy evaluation should be done when problems with performance exist that affect a child's ability to function in school. The method of evaluation should be based on the specific needs of the child. A combination of techniques can be used in this process to gather critical information needed to assist the team in determining if the child has difficulty performing tasks that are necessary for him or her to function in the educational setting (Clark & Coster, 1998).

Dunn (1993) proposed several general considerations to help occupational therapists perform functional assessments. She recommended a contextual approach, which allows therapists to better identify what students need to do. A contextual approach provides a frame of reference for the collection of data. If a child were having difficulty completing a multistep art project, the therapist would observe him or her during art class to accurately identify what the child needs to do and what he or she is having problems with in the environment in which he or she has to perform the task or activity. It is necessary to not only focus on the content of the performance but also on the demands of the task rather than trying to identify what is wrong apart from the context.

Strategies that focus on the context of the performance and acknowledge that there are other resources can be used when providing intervention. A contextual approach to evaluation allows occupational therapists to identify, with input from teachers, what a child needs to be able to do in school and his or her strengths and weaknesses relative to the tasks, the setting, and expectations. These include

- *Promotion*—Creating a plan that promotes the typical development of the skill
- *Prevention–intervention*—Identifying risk factors and creating a plan to prevent the problem from occurring
- *Compensation*—Identifying the problem and providing an alternate way to address it (Dunn, 1993).

Dunn (1993) has suggested that, when deciding on the type of assessment to use, occupational therapists should apply the "so-what" criteria. Therapists should ask what will they know after administering a specific test and the relevance of that information in relation to a student's ability to function in the school environment. For example, so what if a student is able to put 20 pennies in a bottle within 15 seconds? Is this relevant to school functioning and success? If not, the therapist needs to consider another approach that will provide appropriate functional and academic information in relationship to the school setting. Therapists need to be strategic and systematic in their selection and use of assessments to accurately identify and address students' functional and educational needs, including using a variety of strategies and methods, as required by IDEA, to collect relevant information (e.g., interviews, observations in natural settings, tests).

Components of the Occupational Therapy Evaluation

There are several components in the occupational therapy evaluation process that can help identify the student's occupational needs, problems, and concerns.

Gathering Background Information

Occupational therapists can contact the referral source, the parent, classroom teacher and relevant school staff, and the student (as appropriate) to understand the concerns that affect occupational performance and reasons for referral. These include how the concern is perceived by others in school and at home and when the problem was first noticed or identified. Therapists should also review students' records and other relevant documentation, including previous performance information. It is also important to determine what, if any, interventions have been provided to improve engagement in occupations for those concerns. It is important to know what was done, for how long, the outcomes, and what the data reflected before and after intervention.

Reviewing Work Samples

It is necessary to review students' work samples to obtain information about how they completed the task and the type and amount of support needed to do so. It also may be helpful to compare students' work to their classmates to determine age or grade appropriateness of the samples.

Interviewing Parents and Relevant School Personnel

Occupational therapists should interview parents and classroom personnel to determine students' performance at school, at home, and in the community, as appropriate. Using a questionnaire or other tools to structure the interview can assist in discussing the same information with the teacher and parents.

Selecting the Appropriate Assessment Tool

This step is important to help identify relevant tasks the student is expected to complete throughout the school day. Checklists such as the Functional Education Checklist (developed by the authors; see Chapter 5) can help therapists obtain information about students' needs in school and at home, such as utensil use; writing skills as they relate to school assignments and homework; managing personal belongings; self-care and eating skills; and managing within the school environment, including gross motor skills.

Observing the Student in the Natural Environment

Because the setting is critical to successful completion of educational tasks, it is vital to observe students actually performing these tasks at the time they naturally occur during the day. Information about the setting as well as the task can be gathered at this time. Looking at the setting will provide additional information about how students perform and under what conditions. Occupational therapists can observe the direct results of the child's performance (e.g., cutting, dressing) rather than relying on criterion reference (standardized) tools.

One method, the ecological assessment, facilitates observation in a variety of environments. It can be used for analyzing expected school tasks and activities in different settings so that student strengths and needs are identified (Benner, 1992). For example, when observing preschool students with sensory needs, occupational therapists would look at a variety of locations including at school and at home.

Directly Assessing Identified Concerns

After identifying all areas of concern, further assessment may be needed to determine what is interfering with a student's performance. For privacy reasons, this assessment should be done at a separate time and location.

Dynamic assessment involves ongoing interaction between occupational therapists and students (Clark & Coster, 1998). Therapists may provide prompts, cues, or demonstrations. Interventions can also be incorporated to see if changes can be made immediately as a result of the input. For example, when cutting was observed as a part of a student's evaluation, the therapist saw that the child pronated the hand holding the scissors, which resulted in abduction of that arm so that the arm was positioned out away from the body. Prompting the child to hold his arm up against his trunk resulted in the hand being in a more neutral thumb-up position, improving his ability to cut.

Using a Problem-Solving Process in Occupational Therapy Evaluation

The purpose of the occupational therapy evaluation is to obtain relevant information to determine the need for intervention. Sometimes a problem-solving approach is used to identify and quickly address student needs. This approach requires and facilitates collaboration among school personnel. The goal is to identify the problem and develop an intervention plan, determine a desired outcome, and evaluate the effectiveness of the intervention. The evaluation is based on classroom expectations and has a direct relationship to the student's ability to function within the natural (school) setting (Clark & Coster, 1998).

Using Evaluation Information to Determine Needs

After the occupational therapy evaluation is completed, the results should be shared in a

timely manner with the team so they can make an appropriate decision about the need for occupational therapy services. This is a critical step, as the team is responsible for reviewing all of the evaluation data and deciding what services and supports a student might need. This process is very different than the deficit-based approach typically used in a medical-based setting. Therefore, it is important for occupational therapists to present their assessment information in a manner that helps the team make appropriate decisions about children's needs. Rather than just recommending occupational therapy services because a student cannot tie shoes or button small buttons, for example, the team should discuss the findings of the occupational therapy evaluation and decide their relevance to student success in that setting.

Using Evaluation Results

Once the occupational therapy evaluation is completed, therapists should compile the information into an appropriate format that describes students' needs and concerns and explains how they affect the ability to function in the school setting. This information is then shared with the team, which includes the parents, so that it can be included as part of a student's present levels of performance (PLOP).

If the team agrees there are concerns that affect the student's school performance, they must determine whether he or she needs occupational therapy services to achieve his or her goals. If services are needed, the team should indicate which of the student's annual goals and instructional objectives will be supported by occupational therapy. IEP goals should identify the educational areas in which the student has difficulty performing (e.g., completing written classroom assignments in a timely manner) rather than specific deficits (e.g., poor separation of two sides of hand). These goals are not occupational therapy goals; they are the student's goals as a part of his or her educational program that will be supported by occupational therapy as a related service.

The team should also discuss the amount, duration, and where occupational therapy services will be provided. Although IDEA does not require the team to identify how services are provided, it is good practice for the team to consider whether the student's needs can be managed through modification or remediation. It is important for the team and parents to know how occupational therapy will be provided. Services may include a combination of direct contact with the student and collaboration with school staff. Knowing what to expect is crucial to eliminating misunderstandings about service delivery and reducing potential future conflicts with parents.

Not Using Deficit-Based Evaluation

As defined in IDEA, occupational therapy is a related service that provides students with additional support to meet their IEP goals, as determined by the team. This is different than how services may be provided in a medical-based setting. Occupational therapists have traditionally been taught that, if a deficit is identified through the evaluation process, intervention should be provided to remediate the problem. Occupational therapy services in a school-based setting are not intended to address every identified deficit area.

In a deficit-based approach, occupational therapists typically determine the need for occupational therapy services, unilaterally, and recommend that services be provided through direct one-on-one intervention provided in isolation. Therapists using a deficit-based medical model mistakenly assume the occupational therapy intervention is equivalent to helping students achieve their

maximum level of independence in the school-based setting (Hanft & Place, 1996).

Providing Creative Services to Meet Changing Needs

As members of the team, occupational therapists should assume active roles when the needs of children are being discussed. Therapists are responsible for sharing the findings of the occupational therapy evaluation with regard to students' ability to function in the educational setting. As a part of that discussion, therapists can introduce strategies that can be used to address areas of concern, such as "Joey should be given an opportunity to put his coat on daily before the class goes out for recess." Discussion of strategies can assist the team in thinking about how to appropriately help the student.

For students added to the occupational therapy caseload, many parents will expect direct intervention because they believe their child is very needy and that intervention is the only way to meet his or her needs. When a specific service delivery model, such as direct service, is provided, it can be very difficult to reduce or change services for some students, as their parents may view these changes as "giving up" or not caring about their child. For students with significant needs, parents may expect continued direct intervention as they move through the educational system, particularly if they still have needs in fine motor and self-care due to their cognitive ability and overall developmental level. (The importance of understanding the child's cognitive abilities is discussed at length in Chapter 5.)

Occupational therapists need to understand the impact of a child's cognitive level but recognize that it should not be the reason for not recommending occupational therapy services. The team should consider its relevance, however, when deciding what services and supports are needed to allow the child to benefit from his or her educational program. It is critical that teams at each level within the educational system discuss service delivery "best practices" for very needy students, including students who have a significant cognitive impairment and those with autism.

It has been the authors' experience that, in the districts in which we provide occupational and physical therapy services, a collaborative role is identified as best practice, especially in addressing the needs of preschoolers. A combination of direct intervention and collaboration has allowed us to try specific intervention strategies, make suggestions, and identify strategies to be incorporated into student's daily school routines by classroom staff. This occurs in collaboration with staff; demonstrating specific techniques as necessary; and using existing equipment, materials, and activities already in the preschool. This approach helps facilitate the development and generalization of specific skills throughout the week.

Parents learn about the collaborative approach when their child is identified for services. This helps them understand the benefits of this approach in terms of affecting change. When parents understand that their child will actually receive more benefits from services provided in a collaborative model, they usually request individual direct services less frequently. It has also been easier as children transition from the preschool setting into the school-age program if collaboration is also used in that setting, as it is a method of intervention that the parents understand and realize the benefits for their child.

It is very important for occupational therapists to assume responsibility in discussing the need for adopting a philosophy for related service intervention that reflects best practice and meets the needs of the individual students. Other members of the team must

support this method of service delivery for it to work. For example, if a teacher believes that direct intervention is the only way to provide occupational therapy services and does not see the benefits of integrating therapist suggestions into the classroom routine, he or she will not support a collaborative approach when presented to the parents. Therapists need to be aware of the current research on the benefits of collaboration as a viable service delivery option so they can educate members of the team.

Another responsibility of occupational therapists is to continually evaluate the appropriateness of the services provided. This is an aspect of service delivery not often discussed or considered. The authors' experiences have lead to a desire to help districts contain costs, which has resulted in ongoing evaluation of the effectiveness of occupational therapy services. Instead of just providing services in the same way, we have been successful in exploring with administrators alternative, less costly ways to provide services that still meet student needs. It is critical that administrators support any proposed changes that will affect the provision of services and the role of classroom staff. Occupational therapists should not try to impose these changes if there is staff resistance to them.

Providing Occupational Therapy Input Into the IEP

Related services personnel, such as occupational therapists, play a vital role in helping the education team develop a student's IEP. This is true regardless of whether or not occupational therapy services are listed in the IEP. The IEP process, as described in IDEA, is intended to facilitate a smooth mechanism for developing an individualized, cohesive, comprehensive, and measurable education program for each student. This includes identifying each student's present level of performance and strengths and needs, developing measurable annual goals and instructional objectives, and determining what services and supports are needed to achieve those goals. Occupational therapy can also play an important role in helping plan for high school transition, including identification of the self-care/self-management, prevocational, vocational, and independent-living skills that will be needed. IDEA incorporates transition planning into the existing IEP process.

IDEA intends for the IEP to be mutually developed and agreed to at the team meeting. The reality, however, is that, for many reasons, most teams are not able to do this. The unfortunate consequence is that team members then write their own discipline-specific goals and objectives in isolation. Goals and objectives developed by occupational therapists in this situation become known as the "occupational therapy goals" rather than as the student's goals. It has been the authors' experience that, once this happens, teachers and other members of the team do not want to share responsibility for them, leaving occupational therapy as the sole implementer. At the very least, collaboration needs to occur between the teacher (usually the special education teacher) and the occupational therapist to jointly develop goals and objectives.

As indicated previously, the student's IEP should not include discipline-specific goals and objectives. The occupational therapist can provide information about a student's present level of performance specific to the goals and objectives that have been worked on by occupational therapy. The therapist can also indicate the student's needs from an occupational therapy perspective and recommend goals and objective areas based on the needs to be further discussed with the team (at minimum, the teacher). If the team agrees with the recommendations, the therapist can

assist in developing goals and objectives. This is the preferred process rather than having the therapist come up with the goals and then giving them to the teacher to be incorporated into the student's IEP.

Computer-Generated IEPs

Some school districts use computer-based programs, either those that are commercially available or that have been developed by the district, for writing IEPs (e.g., Gordon's [2001] Practical Solutions for Educators). The authors have found these programs very helpful because they provide an opportunity to input our information directly into the specific areas of the IEP (e.g., the PLOP, goals and objectives) once they have been discussed with the team. It also allows us to preview the information generated by other team members before the meeting. IEPs generated using a computer program appear to be more comprehensive, team-based documents rather than those having separate goal and objective pages, with each page in a different person's handwriting, which appears to fragment the student.

Writing the PLOP

The PLOP—a description of the student's strengths and needs and how his or her disability affects participation in school (e.g., academic, nonacademic, extramural) activities—is the starting point for the IEP. In addition, the PLOP provides baseline information for any proposed goals and objectives that are later identified in the IEP. It has been the authors' experience that occupational therapists do not always provide input into students' present level of performance. This information is critical for the team to develop a clear understanding of students' needs and to help identify appropriate proposed goals and objectives.

The PLOP must identify the child's unique needs and should be specific, objective, and measurable (Bateman & Herr, 2003). Occupational therapists can provide the following information for the PLOP:

- Evaluation results, such as legibility scores obtained on a handwriting assessment.
- For students already receiving special education and related services, information about a student's progress toward IEP goals and objectives. For example, the therapist might indicate that the student is able to independently copy the following prewriting shapes: circle, 70%; square, 53%; and triangle, 0%. These percentages can be used as a baseline to assist in determining criteria on the new IEP.
- Objective observations on a student's performance during therapy sessions. For instance, the statement "Alex is able to open and close the scissors independently to make consecutive cuts when cutting, but he does not stay on the line because he does not look at the paper while he is cutting" helps the team (including the parents) understand that Alex has the motor components needed for cutting, but his lack of visual attention affects the quality of his work.
- Information about instructional strategies or interventions that have and have not been successful in helping the student. For example, "After tactile and deep-pressure input, Zach is able to engage in tactile-based activities such as finger painting and playing with play dough and shaving cream. Without the input, he will resist participating in the activity."
- Information should provide logical cues for determining IEP goals. Information about a student's inability to "button his pants and tie his shoes when he changes for gym class" provides a logical cue a goal might be developed to address these areas (Gibb & Dyches, 2000).

Examples of PLOPs that include occupational therapy input are provided in Chapter 2.

Determining Needs

After the student's present level of performance has been determined, the next step for the IEP team is to discuss the student's educational needs and develop appropriate goals and objectives to address them.

As previously described, a student's present level of performance, including strengths and areas of concern and their affect on school success and participation, should be clearly understood by the team. The needs should require the provision of "specially designed instruction" (special education) and may need to be prioritized by the team. These priority areas are then reflected in the IEP goals and objectives. Remaining needs may be addressed informally within the daily curriculum or can be formally addressed as the prioritized needs are met.

Writing Measurable Goals and Objectives

After student needs have been identified and prioritized, the next step is to develop the annual goals and objectives to address those needs. According to Bateman and Herr (2003), IDEA requires goals and objectives be measurable but does not provide specific criteria to define measurability.

IEP goals and objectives should be written in such a way so that, if data were collected by different people, everyone would come to the same conclusion about a student's behavior or performance (Bateman & Herr, 2003). This is important for school-based occupational therapists to remember when assisting teachers in writing goals and objectives. Examples of specific IEP objectives are included throughout this book.

Annual Goals. Annual goals are what the team has determined to be reasonable for the student to accomplish during a school year. These goals should include measurable criteria. IDEA identifies four characteristics for annual goals (Gibb & Dyches, 2000):

1. They must be measurable.
2. They must tell what the student can reasonably accomplish in a year.
3. They must relate to helping the student succeed in the general curriculum or address other educational needs resulting from the disability.
4. They must be accompanied by benchmarks or short-term objectives.

It is important for the expected student behavior or performance to be clearly observable and not left to interpretation by data collectors. Vague words and concepts, such as "appropriate attention," "good behavior," and "improve writing skills," are not well defined and could be interpreted differently by different people who observe the child's behavior.

Short-Term Objectives and Benchmarks. Short-term objectives and benchmarks are the intermediate steps that need to be achieved to reach the annual goal. Benchmarks describe the amount of progress a student is expected to make within specific time periods during the year (e.g., every quarter, every semester; Bateman & Herr, 2003).

Gibb and Dyches (2000) have described three steps for writing short-term objectives:

1. Define the behavior to be measured, including the action the student is performing (e.g., writing, buttoning).
2. Explain the conditions under which the behavior will occur, including types of instructional materials used (e.g., when given a model of his name, when given a built-up handled spoon), levels of prompting needed (e.g., verbal cue, visual prompt), and where the student will be performing the behavior (e.g., in occupational therapy treatment sessions, in the classroom).
3. State the criterion for mastery or level set to determine if the student has learned the task (e.g., percentage of correct attempts, designated time frame).

Identifying Services Needed to Support Objectives

After the goals and objectives have been developed, the team identifies services and other supports needed to achieve the identified goals and objectives. The team should identify the following:

- Which service is to be provided (e.g., occupational therapy, school social work)
- Amount of time each service is to be provided (e.g., 30 minutes, 45 minutes)
- Frequency each service will occur (e.g., per week, every 2 months)
- Goals and objectives each service will address (e.g., occupational therapy services 30 minutes per week to support objectives 1a, 1b, and 1c; this particular format is not required by IDEA, but the authors have found it helpful to clarify for teachers and parents the specific objectives that occupational therapy will be supporting).

Team members should remember that, while occupational therapists may address specific IEP goals and objectives, these goals are also supported by other members of the team. Occupational therapy is a related service and as such helps support student progress; therapists should not be expected to be the only provider working on and collecting data on the objectives.

Considering Special Factors

IDEA also identifies special factors that must also be considered by the team. These include the need for assistive technology, use of Braille for students who are blind or have a visual impairment, language and communication needs for students who are deaf or hard of hearing, and need to address student behavior. Occupational therapy may play a role in each of these areas; however, the following discussion focuses on assistive technology.

IDEA distinguishes between assistive technology devices and services. An *assistive technology device* is defined as "any item, piece of equipment, or product system, whether acquired commercially, modified, or customized, that is used to increase, maintain, or improve the functional capabilities of a child with a disability" (§300.5). *Assistive technology services* are "any services that directly assists a child with a disability in the selection, acquisition, or use of an assistive technology device" (§300.6).

Devices can be "low tech" or "high tech." Low-tech devices include pencil grips, a slanted surface, or other adaptive equipment that allows the student to be more functional within the educational setting. High-tech devices include a computer or Alpha Smart, a word-processing device that is used for written output.

Occupational Therapy Services Under IDEA

When P.L. 94-142 was passed in 1975, approximately 5% of occupational therapists worked in school systems. That figure increased to 18% in 1991, and by 1993, approximately 15,000 (33%) AOTA members worked primarily with children and adolescents (Hanft & Place, 1996). According to AOTA (1999a), the school system was the primary employment setting for occupational therapists and the second-ranked setting for certified occupational therapy assistants (COTAs) in 1995.

The role of occupational therapy as an education-related service was defined by AOTA in 1981. This official position paper indicated that, as a related service, occupational therapy is provided to enhance students' ability to adapt and function in an educational program. In carrying out the mandates of the law, the primary goal of occupational therapy is to offer students a service that will improve their ability to adapt, thus enhancing their potential for learning. It indicated that occupational therapy services must directly affect students' abilities to learn and benefit from the educational program. To help school-based occupational therapists and occupational therapy assistants understand their role, AOTA developed guidelines that provide information on providing appropriate services in schools. These guidelines have been updated and revised over the years to reflect changes in the law and regulations. The most current guidelines were updated in 1997 and revised in 1999 to reflect the 1997 changes to IDEA and to provide a conceptual framework for best practices for occupational therapy services under IDEA. *Best practice* refers to approaches that go beyond those typically provided that result from research activities, model programs, or other types of innovative approaches (AOTA, 1997).

AOTA Guidelines

Five basic elements of occupational therapy practice, as it is governed by IDEA and in accordance with official AOTA documents, professional consensus, and a review of the relevant literature, were identified in the 1997/ 1999 guidelines.

1. Continuum of Services. One of the best practices under IDEA is the provision of a continuum of multifaceted services consistent with occupational therapy philosophy. Services should be adjusted to meet the changing developmental needs of the child and family. This continuum of care guarantees that children and their families will be supported during transition and will have access to multiple services and program options. AOTA believes it is the therapist's responsibility to recognize the dynamic nature of service needs by providing flexibility in promoting access to those services that respond to the changing needs of the child.

2. Clients of Services. Occupational therapy service delivery, including the type of service provided, is influenced by who is the recipient of service or who is the actual client. Factors that define the client are eligibility criteria, roles and responsibilities, service delivery options, and reimbursement policies. The client may change or the focus of service delivery may need to be modified throughout the continuum of service delivery.

To meet the developing and changing needs of the client, the process of service delivery must be interactive. Providing services that are family-centered as well as client-centered is important.

3. Context. It is essential for occupational therapists to understand the context in which they provide services. The student's interaction within the context in which services are provided (e.g., environmental, temporal aspects) must be considered. Environmental aspects include physical elements, social influences and expectations, and cultural aspects such as customs and beliefs. Temporal aspects are to be considered as well and include the child's age, developmental stage or phase, current place in the life cycle, and place in the continuum of disability. The child's performance is influenced by the value that the family, the child, the community, and school place on the child's context.

4. Collaboration and Partnerships. Developing effective partnerships by collaborating with team members is a central component for occupational therapy services under IDEA. Successful implementation of occupational therapy services depends on the occupational therapist's ability to communicate, cooperate, negotiate, coordinate, and integrate to promote effective teamwork. A collaborative service delivery model results in sharing the responsibility for student-specific outcomes. Collaboration enables team members to coordinate their efforts to maximize their potential impact.

5. Outcomes. Occupational therapists are concerned with both the process and product of their services. All occupational therapy services need to be directed toward and concerned with the effects or the outcomes of those services. The need to measure program-specific outcomes, as well as changes in student performance, are important to determine the overall effectiveness of occupational therapy services in early intervention and school system settings.

Part B

IDEA provides for a free appropriate public education in the least restrictive environment for children with disabilities ages 3 through 21 who require special education and related services. *Related services* offer "such developmental, corrective, and other supportive services as are required to assist the child with a disability to benefit from special education and includes . . . occupational therapy" (§300.16). *Special education* means "specially designed instruction" that is needed to meet the unique needs of the child with a disability (AOTA, 1997).

As defined in IDEA, occupational therapy services are provided by a qualified occupational therapist and include "improving, developing, or restoring functions impaired or lost through illness, injury, or deprivation; improving the ability to perform tasks for independent functioning if functions are impaired or lost; and preventing, through early intervention, initial or further impairment or loss of function" (§300.24(5)).

Part C

Under Part C, occupational therapy is considered a primary service and can be provided separately or along with any other early intervention services the child and family might need. Early intervention services are designed around an IFSP that "are decided to meet the developmental needs of the child . . . and the needs of the family related to enhancing the child's development" (§303.12(1)(2)). The need for occupational therapy services is selected in collaboration with the parents.

The IFSP, adopted by the family and the team, includes the expected outcomes for the child and family that should assist in guiding intervention. To receive occupational therapy services under Part C, the infant or toddler must meet eligibility criteria as established by the state of residency. The state is responsible for defining the amount of developmental delay, the specific conditions, and the type of risk that qualifies a child for early intervention services (§303.300).

Occupational therapy is defined in Part C as "services to address the functional needs of the child related to adaptive equipment, adaptive behavior, and play as well as sensory, motor, and postural development. These services are designed to improve the child's functional ability to perform tasks at home, school, and community settings" and include

- Identification, assessment, and intervention;
- Adaptation of the environment and selection, design, and fabrication of assistive or orthotic devices to facilitate development and promote the acquisition of functional skills; and
- Prevention or minimization of the impact of initial or future impairment delay in development or loss of functional ability (§303.12(8)(i)(ii)(iii)).

Early intervention providers, including occupational therapy, are responsible for

- Consulting with other service providers and representatives of appropriate community agencies to ensure the effective provision of services in that area;
- Training parents and others to provide those services; and
- Participating in a multidisciplinary team's assessment of a child and the child's family and in the development of integrated goals and outcomes for the IFSP.

Content of the IFSP

The IFSP emphasizes a family-centered approach to address the developmental needs of children and their families. The IFSP must include the following (§303.344):

- A statement of present levels of physical, cognitive, communication, social or emotional, and adaptive development based on acceptable objective criteria;
- A statement of the family's resources, priorities, and concerns related to enhancing the development of the child, with the concurrence of the family;
- A statement of the major outcomes expected to be achieved for the child and family and the criteria, procedures, and timeliness used to determine the degree to which progress toward achieving the outcomes is being made and whether modifications are necessary;
- A statement of the specific early intervention services necessary, including frequency intensity and the method of delivering services;
- A statement of the natural environments in which the early intervention services will be provided;
- The projected dates for initiation of services and the anticipated duration of those services;
- The name of the service coordinator from the profession most immediately relevant to the child's or family's needs who will be responsible for the implementation and coordination of the IFSP; and
- The steps to be taken to support the transition of the child to preschool services under Part B or other appropriate services that may be available.

Other Federal Laws That Affect Occupational Therapy Services

Even though a student may have a defined disability, he or she may not be eligible for services under IDEA and yet may need accommodations or modifications to be able to participate in benefits from educational programs. Section 504 of the Rehabilitation Act of 1973 and the Americans With Disabilities Act (ADA) of 1990 also provide rights to individuals with disabilities.

Section 504

The Rehabilitation Act of 1973 is a civil rights law to protect the rights of individuals with disabilities in programs that receive federal financial assistance from the U.S. Department of Education. A written educational accommodation plan is provided to any student who meets the definition of disabled and requires modifications to benefit from a free and appropriate public education (29 U.S.C. §706(8)).

General education is responsible for this law. Occupational therapy services may provide assistance with environmental adaptations, acquisition, or modification of equipment or devices and assistance in the development of the written educational accommodation plan.

ADA

The ADA is a civil rights law that provides a comprehensive national mandate to eliminate discrimination against individuals with disabilities. Title II of the ADA specifically covers services provided by state and local governments (e.g., education agencies). The district's Section 504 coordinator may administer this law. Occupational therapy services may address accessibility requirements, acquisition, adjustment, or modification of equipment or devices as needed.

Understanding the Roles of Occupational Therapy Services in School-Based Settings

Occupational therapy, as a related service provided in public schools, is mandated by and defined by federal and state laws. At the same time, IDEA does not identify the condi-

tions under which services are to be provided nor the criteria by which to decide when services are needed.

The question, How do students qualify for services? is common. It can be confusing for occupational therapists, parents, and education team members to know when students should receive services. Part of this confusion is due to the broad definition describing the numerous roles occupational therapy can assume in a school-based setting (e.g., improving, developing, restoring function).

Confusion about student eligibility for school-based occupational therapy is also related to a lack of understanding about IDEA eligibility. Under IDEA, students "qualify" for services if they

- Meet the definition of "child with a disability" in §300.7, and
- Because of that disability, require special education *and* related services to meet their unique needs.

Eligibility for school-based services is linked to the need for special education or specially designed instruction. In other words, a student must first be found to require specially designed instruction *before* the team can consider the need for other related services. If a student does not need special education, he or she cannot receive it under current law. In these instances, the school district can still choose to provide services at its discretion or under Section 504 if the student is eligible.

Related services can be provided to only those students who need them to benefit from special education. But what does it mean to "benefit from special education"? Does it mean that occupational therapy should support the academic component (i.e., writing, reading, arithmetic) of a student's education program? In this role the therapist would provide services to help the child write or align his or her numbers when doing math problems. Or, does it mean that occupational therapy services should help the student access and participate in all components of his or her education program, including his or her ability to function within the educational setting? In this role the therapist would have the latitude to support any area that is affecting the student's function in school. This could include managing his or her combination lock; being able to complete an art project that requires cutting, pasting, and coloring; or managing all the fasteners on his or her clothing needed to function within the school day.

The answer to both questions is "yes." The focus of school-based occupational therapy services depends on which IEP goals occupational therapy will be supporting. In addition to the requirement for special education, the need for occupational therapy is also based on the choice of annual goals and whether expertise is needed to help the student achieve those goals. In some instances, these goals will be academic in nature, while at other times the goals will focus on student function. At all times, occupational therapy should be focused on student participation and success in the school environment.

To further assist the IEP team in making appropriate decisions about the educational necessity of support services such as occupational therapy, Giangreco (1986) developed several criteria:

- Would the absence of this proposed service interfere with the student's access to or participation in his or her education program?
- Do the service recommendations of the team present undesirable or unnecessary overlap or contraindications?
- Can services provided in one context be adequately generalized to other settings without the direct involvement of the specialist?

Service Delivery Options for Occupational Therapy

IDEA does not stipulate how special education and related services are to be provided or listed in the IEP. Once the need for occupational therapy services has been identified, consideration should be given as to the most appropriate way to provide services (e.g., individual, group, or direct consultation or collaboration).

The 1987 AOTA school guidelines (AOTA, 1987) first identified three service delivery models that are still referred to today: direct, monitoring, and consultation. AOTA, however, no longer uses these terms. Instead, the continuum of service delivery is the preferred methodology as articulated in its 1997/1999 guidelines and the *Occupational Therapy Practice Framework* (AOTA, 2002). Therapists are encouraged to function as a member of students' educational teams so that collaboration between team members can occur, as this is an important component in the delivery of services within educational settings. Occupational therapy services may be delivered in different forms that vary according to the focus of services (AOTA, 1997).

No one service delivery method is better than another. When the team determines that occupational therapy services are needed, the occupational therapist and team must determine how to best serve those needs. Rather than relying solely on one way to provide services, the therapist should provide services using a variety of approaches depending on student needs and desired educational outcomes.

Direct Service Delivery. Direct service is the method of service that is most recognized. Direct service provided in a one-on-one situation is often requested by parents, as their perception is that only services provided by the occupational therapist can affect change.

Monitoring. Monitoring involves overseeing specific programs and intervention strategies that have been developed by the occupational therapist but are carried out by someone else.

Consultation. Consultation services include sharing information with other team members, including teachers and parents. In comparing service delivery models in school-based occupational therapy, Dunn (1990) found that consultative services were equally as effective as direct intervention for some students. Occupational therapists do not always know how to use a consultative approach. In school, therapists learn to provide direct intervention through fieldwork, practicum, and continuing education experiences, with little exposure or formal instruction on how to provide consultative services. Therapists quickly realize when they begin working in a school setting that they need to understand the consultation process (Hanft & Place, 1996).

Interventions using functional life skills that is provided in the student's natural environment and embedded within the classroom routine and structure have been shown to increase the efficacy of intervention, the achievement of IEP goals, and the student's motivation to participate (Dunn & Westman, 1995). This research provided the impetus to move from individual isolated direct therapy services to integrated collaborative therapy services. This change was accompanied by others, such as the movement of therapy services into the classroom and shift away from discipline-specific objectives to functional skills. Moving services out of the therapy area supports increased involvement of the therapists and team members in school activities and routines. This integrated approach provides both increased opportunities for team collaboration as well as for the student to practice the skill (AOTA, 1997).

Hanft and Place (1996) reviewed due process decisions indicating when consultation is an appropriate service model for individual students. These include

- Are school personnel qualified to implement the therapist's suggestions?
- Can the student's educational needs be met as well as or better than through direct service?

- Can therapy can be provided in the least restrictive manner in classrooms and regular school activities?

The authors caution that due process hearings affect an individual child and are not automatically applicable to all students. They do not guarantee that all other students should receive therapy using a consultative model.

Consultation is an important component of the following models (Hanft & Place 1996):
- *Integrated programming or therapy*—Working with team members to provide occupational therapy within the naturally occurring context throughout the school environment (Rainforth & York-Barr, 1997)
- *Monitoring or management*—Developing a student program implemented by team members in the educational setting with ongoing supervision from a therapist (Effgen & Klepper, 1994)
- *Consultation to other team members*—Recommending intervention strategies, equipment adaptation, or modifications of the classroom environment (Dunn, 1990).

Hanft and Place (1996) have identified four major benefits from using consultation to provide school-based occupational therapy:

1. *Makes effective use of available personnel*—Consultation expands the impact of direct service with the added benefit being that students receive the occupational therapist's recommendations throughout the school day. The consulting therapist can plan interventions to help the student enhance his or her skills.

2. *Supports inclusion and the IDEA mandate for providing services in the least restrictive environment*—Consulting therapists can suggest interventions that can occur in a variety of locations in the educational environment (e.g., classroom, lunchroom, gym).

3. *Builds or increases skills of other professionals*—By sharing knowledge through the consultation process, the consulting therapist can enhance the knowledge and skills of other team members that can then

be applied as appropriate to other students and settings.

4. *Enhances resources for problem solving*— Collaborative consultation is based on an exchange of information between two individuals who have different but equally important knowledge and experiences. By combining this talent, the consulting therapist can promote the development of creative programs to be used to achieve appropriate educational outcomes for each student.

The inclusion of students with disabilities into general education settings has required educational teams to recognize the need to adopt more collaborative and integrated approaches when providing services. The roles of teachers and therapists have shifted to evaluating student needs in the same environments as students without disabilities. This shift has resulted in active collaboration between teachers and therapists to help students achieve greater outcomes (Rainforth & York-Barr, 1997).

In support for full inclusion of individuals with disabilities, AOTA stated in a 1995 position paper that

> Occupational therapists assume a collaborative partnership with the person served and other team members to help ensure access to interventions and services in support of full inclusion. Interventions include use of activities designed to improve functional performance, utilizing adaptive equipment, and providing environmental modifications.

As previously indicated, as services can be provided in a variety of ways, it is the responsibility of occupational therapists to consider which of the approaches is the best match for the setting in which they are involved while meeting the philosophy of the team.

Providing Services on Behalf of the Student

In the school districts in which the authors provide services, there have been debates about what constitutes "services." At times, parents have requested individual or one-on-one service with a specific amount of time (e.g., individual direct services for 30 minutes once a week). Although the IEP process does not require this, the parents want it documented this way because they do not want the therapist counting the time spent on documentation, collaboration with the aide or teacher, or copying worksheets needed for handwriting intervention toward their child's therapy time.

According to AOTA (1999b), all activities or services that an occupational therapist or COTA may provide on behalf of the student should be considered occupational therapy services. The following activities can be considered as intervention:

- Working with the student directly
- Modifying the school environment (e.g., adjusting the student's desk height)
- Working with the teacher to identify ways for the student to perform a task
- Developing a dressing routine (e.g., shoe tying to be implemented by the aide on a daily basis)
- Contacting a physician about a student's recent surgery
- Reevaluating the student
- Meeting with the school psychologist to review evaluation data that will be included in the child's reevaluation
- Writing a note to the parent (e.g., to request that the child wears shoes with shoe laces to school to implement a shoe-tying program; AOTA, 1999b).

Each of these activities, which requires professional time and experience and knowledge, reflects the appropriate use and commitment of the resources that the team agreed needed to be provided on the student's behalf. It is important to document all the services and times that are provided for an individual student (in whatever format identified by the district or state).

This is another reason why specific models of occupational therapy service delivery (e.g., consultation, direct, monitoring) should no longer be indicated on the IEP. Occupational therapy service delivery is indicated by the ongoing needs of the student and should be flexible to meet those needs (AOTA, 1995a).

In terms of scheduling, providing a continuum of interventions can be challenging when the occupational therapist needs to be available at different times to meet the needs of the student. As an example, the therapist provides services to a student who has cerebral palsy by collaborating on a variety of areas with his aide. If the child is having difficulty accessing the computer in class, the therapist needs to be available at that time to assess the child is in his natural environment. However, if there are also feeding concerns, the therapist would need to be available during lunchtime to see the child in the cafeteria. Flexibility in scheduling is critical but not always possible, requiring problem solving by the team to identify other options and ways to address the needs.

Documenting IEP Outcomes

McClain (1991) stated that documentation results in goals that facilitate effective treatment; provide communication among team members, including the family; justifies reimbursement when applicable; and stands as a legal record. Poor documentation can have ethical, financial, and legal consequences. Specific federal legal requirements exist for documenting the provision of special education and related services under IDEA. (More information on documentation and occupational therapy's responsibility in the IEP process can be found in Chapter 2.)

Delineating and Describing the Roles of Occupational Therapists and Occupational Therapy Assistants

Using occupational therapy assistants in a school-based setting can be an effective way to provide services while allowing occupation-

al therapists to complete evaluations, meet with educational teams, and attend IEP or reevaluation meetings when needed without having to cancel intervention sessions.

Occupational therapists and occupational therapy assistants have important but distinct roles in the school-based setting. School personnel and parents do not always understand the differences between them. As such, parents may question the qualifications of the occupational therapy assistant to provide services to their child.

AOTA (1997) has identified roles for occupational therapists and occupational therapy assistants working in school settings (see Appendix 1.2):

- *Screening and evaluation*—Occupational therapists are primarily responsible for performing the evaluation, interpreting the results, and summarizing the information in a report. Assistants can help during various levels of this process.

- *Program planning*—Occupational therapists are primarily responsible for the development of the IEP and interpreting the child's performance and assisting the team in determining student needs in developing an intervention plan. Assistants can play an active part in providing assistance in this process by sharing information regarding the students for which he or she is responsible.

- *Intervention*—Occupational therapists are responsible for developing, directing, and overseeing intervention services. Assistants are active participants in this area as direct service providers. They are responsible for keeping therapists informed regarding the need to modify programs. They are able to attend meetings to share information and are responsible for maintaining daily documentation on students' performance during sessions. Assistants can provide training and supervision to non–occupational therapy personnel who would be responsible for providing these activities to students within their daily routine. Assistants are also capable of fabricating and modifying adaptive equipment.

- *Coordination*—Occupational therapists and assistants have equal roles in coordination, including determining when reviews are scheduled and demonstrating an awareness of legislation and best practice in school-based settings.

Supervising Occupational Therapy Assistants

Occupational therapists are legally responsible for all aspects of occupational therapy service delivery; occupational therapy assistants provide services under the supervision of occupational therapists. *Supervision* is defined as a process that fosters growth and development; ensures appropriate use of training; and encourages creativity and innovation through providing guidance, support, encouragement, and respect—all working toward a defined goal (AOTA, 1999a). Supervision occurs along a continuum that provides various levels and intensity of contact depending on the need within a particular setting.

It is critical for occupational therapists to be aware of specific supervision requirements defined in individual state practice regulations; these will take precedence over all other standards of practice. The level of supervision required by occupational therapy assistants depends on the therapist's experience, job responsibilities, and level of expertise. The frequency and amount of supervision can be mutually discussed and determined based on the service needs within the educational setting. Supervision should be provided to all occupational therapy assistants regardless of their experience and expertise. General supervision should be provided directly at least monthly, with ongoing supervision available (e.g., by phone) as needed (AOTA, 1997).

Once the occupational therapy assistant's level of competency has been determined, the type and frequency of supervision can be better defined. Input from the assistant is also important when determining a student's needs. Supervision can be provided using a combination of the following (AOTA, 1997):

- *Record review*—Reviewing daily documentation, including the occupational therapist's data, is essential in a school-based setting, because if a dispute arises about any aspect of programming, typically all documentation about the child is requested by administration. Record review also allows the therapist to make sure that the assistant is accurately documenting treatment data that will be used as part of the child's progress note.
- *Observation of intervention sessions*—The therapist can also observe the assistant working directly with students or when collaborating with staff, giving the therapist an indication of the assistant's ability to relate to the child at his or her appropriate level as well as the assistant's ability to effectively explain strategies or activities to be used with the student when talking to staff. The therapist can also use this opportunity to work directly with the child to demonstrate to the assistant specific strategies or techniques.
- *Meetings*—It is also important to meet with the assistant to review the students on his or her caseload, a critical step before the development of IEPs. This gives the assistant an opportunity to share information regarding the student's level of performance as well as to ask specific questions about intervention activities, strategies, documentation, or behavior intervention techniques. This meeting also can be used to discuss possible goal options for individual students' upcoming IEPs.

Summary and Conclusion

It is important for school-based occupational therapists to understand IDEA as the law that defines the rights of children with disabilities. The law guarantees a free appropriate public education and provides for the provision of related services, such as occupational therapy, if needed to help students benefit from special education. It is critical for therapists to understand their roles in the evaluation process and the importance of collaborating with the IEP team when determining the need for services. Therapists must also be aware of the variety in the ways that occupational therapy services can be provided in the school setting to provide the most effective services.

References

American Occupational Therapy Association. (1981). Position Paper: Occupational therapy as an education-related service. *American Journal of Occupational Therapy*, 35, 811.

American Occupational Therapy Association. (1987). *Guidelines for occupational therapy service in school systems*. Rockville, MD: Author.

American Occupational Therapy Association. (1995a). Concept Paper: Service delivery in occupational therapy. *American Journal of Occupational Therapy, 49*, 1029–1031.

American Occupational Therapy Association, Commission on Practice. (1995b). *Full Inclusion Position Paper: Occupational therapy: A profession in support of full inclusion*. Rockville, MD: Author.

American Occupational Therapy Association. (1997). *Occupational therapy services for children and youth under the Individuals With Disabilities Education Act*. Bethesda, MD: Author.

American Occupational Therapy Association. (1999a). Guide for supervision of occupational therapy personnel in the delivery of occupational therapy services. *American Journal of Occupational Therapy, 53*, 592–594.

American Occupational Therapy Association. (1999b). *Occupational therapy services for children and youth under the Individuals With Disabilities Education Act* (2nd ed.). Bethesda, MD: Author.

American Occupational Therapy Association. (2002). Occupational therapy practice framework: Domain and process. *American Journal of Occupational Therapy, 56*, 609–639.

Americans With Disabilities Act of 1990, P.L. 101-336, 42 U.S.C. §12134.

Bateman, B. D., & Herr, C. M. (2003). *Writing measurable IEP goals and objectives*. Verona, WI: Attainment.

Benner, S. (1992). *Assessing young children with special needs*. White Plains, NY: Longman.

Case-Smith, J. (Ed.). (1998). *Occupational therapy: Making a difference in school system practice*. Bethesda, MD: American Occupational Therapy Association.

Clark, D., & Coster, W. (1998). Evaluation/problem solving and program evaluation. In J. Case-Smith (Ed.), *Occupational therapy: Making a difference in school system practice* (pp. 2–46). Bethesda, MD: American Occupational Therapy Association.

Dunn, W. (1990). A comparison of service-provision models in school-based occupational therapy services: A pilot study. *Occupational Therapy Journal of Research, 10*, 300–319.

Dunn, W. (1993). Measurement of function: Actions for the future. *American Journal of Occupational Therapy, 47*, 357–359.

Dunn, W., & Westerman, K. (1995). Current knowledge that affects school-based practice and an agenda for action. *American Occupational Therapy Association School System Special Interest Section Newsletter, 2*, 1–2.

Education for All Handicapped Children Act of 1975, P.L. 94-142, 20 U.S.C. § 1401.

Education of the Handicapped Amendments of 1986, P.L. 94-457, 20 U.S.C.§1401.

Effgen, S., & Klepper, S. (1994). Survey of physical therapy practice in educational settings. *Pediatric Physical Therapy, 6*, 15–21.

Giangreco, M. (1986). Delivery of therapeutic services in special education programs for learners with severe handicaps. *Physical and Occupational Therapy in Pediatrics, 6*, 3–13.

Gibb, G. S., & Dyches, T. T. (2000). *Guide to writing quality individualized education programs:*

What's best for students with disabilities? Needham Heights, MA: Allyn & Bacon.

Gordon, R. (2001). Practical solutions for educators [Computer software]. Marysville, OH: Practical Solutions.

Hanft, B., & Place, P. (1996). *The consulting therapist.* San Antonio, TX: Therapy SkillBuilders.

Individuals With Disabilities Education Act, P.L. 101-476, 20 U.S.C. §1401 (1990).

Individuals With Disabilities Education Act, P.L. 102-119, 20 U.S.C. §1401 (1991).

Individuals With Disabilities Education Act Amendments of 1997, P.L. 105-17, 20 U.S.C. Chapter 33.

Individuals With Disabilities Education Act Final Regulations, 34 C.F.R., Parts 300 and 303, March 12, 1999.

Kupper, L., & Gutierrez, M. (Eds.). (2000). Questions and answers about IDEA. *NICHCY News Digest, 4,* 1–27.

McClain, L. H. (1991). Documentation. In W. Dunn (Ed.), *Pediatric occupational therapy: Facilitating effective service provision* (pp. 213–244). Thorofare, NJ: Slack.

McEwen, I. (2000). *Providing physical therapy services under Parts B and C of the Individuals With Disabilities Education Act (IDEA).* Alexandria, VA: American Physical Therapy Association.

Mills v. Board of Education of the District of Columbia. 348 F. Supp. 866 (D.D.C. 1972).

Pennsylvania Association for Retarded Children v. Commonwealth of Pennsylvania. 333 F. Supp. 1257 (E.D. Pennsylvania 1971).

Rainforth, B., & York-Barr, J. (1997). *Collaborative teams for students with severe disabilities: Integrating therapy and educational services* (2nd ed.). Baltimore: Paul H. Brookes.

Rehabilitation Act of 1973, Section 504, 29 U.S.C. §794.

Social Security Act of 1935, P.L. 74-271, Sections 701–710.

Waterman, B. (1994). Assessing children for the presence of a disability. *NICHCY News Digest, 4,* 1–27.

Appendix 1.1
OT/PT Referral Form

Date _____

Student _____   Birthdate _____

Parents _____   Address _____

District & School _____   _____

Grade Level _____   Phone _____

General Education Teacher _____   Special Education Teacher _____

Building-Level Contact _____   Is Student Currently in Special Education? ___ Yes ___ No

Referred by _____   Special Education Disability _____

Referral for
___ OT   ___ PT

Source of Referral
___ Team ___ General education teacher ___ Parent ___ Special education teacher ___ Psychologist ___ Other _____

Parent Permission Date Signed _____ (please attach)

Check the appropriate type of request.

1. Preschool Evaluation

   Is the request for OT/PT input part of ___ Initial MFE ___ Re-evaluation

   Planning (what areas does OT or PT need to evaluate?) _____

   _____

   What is area of suspected deficit? _____

   Approximate date for team meeting? _____

2. School Age

   ___ Initial MFE ___ Re-evaluation

   Planning (what areas does OT or PT need to evaluate?) _____

   _____

   Describe specific concerns (e.g., handwriting: poor spacing between words, can't write in the designated area) _____

   _____

3. Initial evaluation is completed but IEP not yet written

   Special Education Disability _____

   ___ Team is requesting additional information prior to writing the IEP. Information being requested _____

   _____

   Has team meeting taken place? ___ Yes ___ No

   Has IEP date been scheduled? ___ Yes date _____ ___ No

4. Student with ___ OT ___ PT on IEP needs further evaluation in the following area(s)_____

   _____

   _____

_____   _____
Signature of Pupil Services Administrator (or Designee)   Date

Appendix 1.2.
Fact Sheet: Understanding Occupational Therapy Services in a School Setting

The following fact sheet was developed and shared with parents and staff (special and regular education teachers) in an attempt to explain the role of occupational therapy services in the school setting.

What Is a Related Service?

As defined in the federal regulations, related services are transportation and such developmental, corrective, and other supportive services as are required to assist a child with a disability to benefit from special education (§300.24(a)). School districts are not required to provide related services to "maximize" a student's opportunities. They are only required to provide an "appropriate" education.

What Related Services Are Available to Students?

Occupational, physical, and speech therapy; psychological services; and counseling are a few of the related services as defined in Part B IDEA (§300.24 (a) Related Services). Who is eligible for related services? Related services are available to students being served in special education. While every child who is receiving special education is eligible for related services, the district is only responsible for providing related services that are necessary for the student to benefit from his or her special education program. *Special education* means specially designed instruction, at no cost to the parents, to meet the unique needs of a child with a disability (§300.26 Special Education). *Unique needs* means that each child's needs must be considered individually. Services should not automatically be provided based on the disability or special education classification.

How Do Students Qualify for Related Services (Occupational Therapy)?

Students do not qualify for occupational therapy services. Student's scores on an evaluation do not qualify the student for occupational therapy services, nor does the therapist completing the evaluation have the authority to determine the student's need for occupational therapy.

During the IEP process, the team identifies the student's strengths and needs based on his or her present levels of performance and then develops the goals/objectives to support those needs. The IEP team then determines the need for occupational therapy as a related service if it is considered necessary to assist the student to achieve his or her educational goals and objectives. The need for occupational therapy services should be determined when addressing the service area. The team should discuss what services are needed to support each objective so that the student can benefit from the educational program. The service and time is then listed in the service column. While parents, teachers, and therapists are equal participants in the IEP process, no one individual should dictate the type or amount of related services. The team should discuss all concerns and desires in an attempt to develop a plan that best addresses the student's strengths and needs.

Do Students Have Separate Occupational Therapy or Physical Therapy Goals/Objectives?

No, the role of occupational therapy as a related service supports the student's educational plan. IEP goals should be the student's goals; they are not occupational therapy goals. The occupational therapist can assist in developing the student's educational goals/objectives based on the identified needs but should not be the only person working on them or collecting data. The occupational therapist supports the objective, but the educational team is also responsible for implementation and data collection. The occupational therapist can act as a resource to assist the team with strategies/techniques.

Compiled by Lynne Pape, MEd, OTR/L

Writing Measurable Goals and Objectives for Effective Documentation and Data Collection

Occupational therapists who work in school-based settings evaluate students and work with educational teams to write measurable goals and objectives that relate to students' educational needs and performance. Occupational therapists and occupational therapy assistants also provide intervention to meet these goals and objectives and document students' progress toward mastery of those goals as established in their individualized education program (IEP).

This chapter discusses the importance of accountability in school-based occupational therapy services. Collaboration between occupational therapists and occupational therapy assistants in regard to students' progress and present level when developing goals and objectives is described, as well as the necessity for collaboration between occupational therapists and general education and special education teachers. The chapter also provides helpful information on how to write measurable annual goals and benchmarks and short-term objectives for the IEP. Finally, definitions are provided for data collection and documentation procedures in line with the *Guidelines for Documentation of Occupational Therapy* as outlined by the American Occupational Therapy Association (AOTA, 2003). Examples are included for specific intervention areas commonly supported by occupational therapists (e.g., handwriting, scissor skills, self-care tasks) in schools.

Individuals With Disabilities Education Act

The Individuals With Disabilities Education Act (IDEA, 1997) provides many rights to children who qualify for special education and their families (see Chapter 1 for an in-depth discussion of IDEA). These rights include the entitlement of students and their parents to evaluations by the school district to determine areas of qualification and individualized needs and the granting of a free and appropriate public education to children with special needs. A *free and appropriate education* is defined as "providing access to special education and related services that are provided at no cost to the parents and that are designed to meet the unique needs of the student" (IDEA, 1999, §300.13). The act also states that each student's needs must be individually and specifically addressed through an IEP that includes special education and related services (Bateman & Herr, 2003).

Special education is defined by the federal government as "specially designed instruction, at no cost to the parents, to meet the unique needs of the child with a disability" (§300.26). Bateman and Herr (2003) expanded on this definition and stated that the specifically designed instruction is comprised of

- *Adapted content:* This may include access to a modified curriculum, based on the school district's general education curriculum, or access to a separate curriculum to meet the student's needs.
- *Methodology:* This includes methods used to teach the skills. It may encompass access to assistive technology to achieve the skill, such as the use of Braille, a voice output computer program, or an augmentative communication device.
- *Delivery of instruction:* This defines what type of service is needed to assist students

in meeting the goals established in their IEP. It may include access to a small-group setting or one-on-one direct instruction. The need for related services to meet the stated goals and objectives also falls under the scope of this area.

Occupational therapy is considered a related service in a student's IEP. A *related service* is "transportation and such developmental, corrective, and other supportive services as are identified on the child's IEP that are needed to assist the child with a disability to benefit from special education" (§300.24). Such services may be occupational therapy, physical therapy, speech-language pathology services, counseling, social work services, psychological services, therapeutic recreation, orientation and mobility services, and school health services.

As service providers, occupational therapists are vital members of education teams, assisting with the development of a child's IEP goals and objectives. Following the IEP process as it was intended is important to the development of a cohesive, comprehensive, and measurable document. This includes determining a student's present level of performance, identifying areas of need, writing measurable goals and objectives, and determining what services are needed to achieve those goals.

The IEP Process

The IEP document is composed of numerous components that include

- The student's general background and identifying information;
- The future planning or vision statement section (parents and the educational team define their overall vision for the upcoming year and for the future);
- The present levels of performance;
- Measurable annual goals and short-term objectives or benchmarks;
- A statement of the student's progress;
- The services needed to support the stu-

dent's achievement of goals and benchmarks or short-term objectives; and
- The least restrictive environment in which the services will occur.

Other concerns that must be addressed in the IEP are the modifications that may be needed to support a student during testing situations or within the classroom on a daily basis (e.g., taking tests in a small group, having tests and assignments read to him or her, having access to technology for taking notes or completing classroom assignments and tests) and the planning for transition services for those students older than age 14. The IEP sections discussed in this chapter are the present level of performance, goals and objectives, services needed to support the IEP, and statement of student progress.

Present Level of Performance

The present level of performance, the starting point for the IEP, provides an overview of the student's current level of functioning. It also offers baseline information for the proposed goals and objectives outlined in the IEP. These goals and objectives usually are in effect for one calendar year from the meeting date. However, the team may decide to build in more frequent review dates throughout the school year to discuss a student's progress.

Gibb and Dyches (2000) mentioned that this section of the IEP should contain a statement about how the student's disability affects involvement and progress in the general curriculum (e.g., how a student's cognitive and developmental level affects his or her ability to learn phonics at the same rate as same-age peers in the general curriculum). Thus, special education instruction and modified methods of presenting the material are needed to meet his or her individualized needs. The present level of performance should also describe how the student's performance levels in the skill areas are affected by the disability and the logical cues for writing goals based on the information in this section. For example, if the information states that a student is unable to button his pants and tie his shoes, this provides a logical cue that these skills will be addressed in the goals and objectives section of the IEP.

Bateman and Herr (2003) noted that the present level of performance section of the IEP must identify the child's unique needs and should be specific, objective, and measurable and may incorporate information from recent testing, including standardized tests and statewide or districtwide assessments. This section also may provide objective data that outlines the student's progress toward goals and objectives written on the previous year's IEP and include objective observations by parents, teachers, or service providers about performance in general education and special education settings. Such observations could be descriptions of a student's behavior in objective terms. For example, "compared to his same-age peers who do not require breaks during instruction, student is observed to need on average 5 movement breaks within a 20-minute period as evidenced by him standing up or leaving the table to walk around the room" or "student demonstrates off-task behaviors during lessons, including looking around room, getting up out of his chair, and fidgeting with items from his desk."

In addition, the present level of performance material may provide information on instructional strategies or interventions that have been successful in helping the student to learn a skill. It also may identify if "special factors"—a behavior plan, assistive technology, modified instruction, or some combination of these—are needed for the student to achieve success. It should not include subjective information about the student's performance or behavior. Subjective information or opinions of the professionals do not assist the team in defining a baseline from which to develop new goals and objectives.

Present level of performance information needs to be objective, factual, and measurable to reflect the student's current level of functioning. Two examples are provided below, one that is measurable and one that is not.

Example 1: Present Level of Performance for Michael. Michael is right-handed and currently does not use a functional pencil grasp. He is able to write most alphabet letters. Michael has difficulty with orienting letters on the paper, which affects the overall legibility of his writing. He demonstrates difficulty cutting out shapes. His poor attention to the task affects his cutting. He continues to have difficulty managing clothing fasteners and managing his belongings in the classroom.

Example 2: Present Level of Performance for Michael. Michael is right-handed and uses a functional grip when holding a writing utensil. He is currently able to copy all 26 uppercase and lowercase alphabet letters in manuscript using proper letter formation. Without a model, Michael is able to form 15 out of 26 uppercase letters and 20 out of 26 lowercase letters using proper letter formation. Letters that he continues to have difficulty forming properly include A, D, G, K, M, N, Q, R, S, W, Z, a, b, d, k, q, and z. He continues to have difficulty writing letters using the appropriate size for the letter case to remain within the lines of second-grade paper. He is currently completing this task independently with 45% accuracy. His difficulty forming and aligning letters affects the overall legibility of his handwriting. Michael is able to position scissors correctly in his fingers in 100% of attempts. He is able to cut, remaining on a straight line with 100% accuracy, but continues to have difficulty cutting out shapes that require changes in direction (circle, square, triangle) to within 1/4 inch of the line with currently only 25% accuracy. Michael has mastered managing buttons and snaps on his clothing in 100% of attempts yet continues to have difficulty engaging the zipper on his coat (35% accuracy) and is unable to complete any of the steps in tying his shoes.

What is the difference between these examples? Measurability! In the first example, the description of Michael's present level of performance is general, subjective comments are made regarding his current skills, and it leaves room for questions such as

- What type of grasp is Michael using if his pencil grasp is not functional?
- When the author states that Michael can write most letters of the alphabet, does this refer to cursive or print letters? What letters does he continue to have difficulty writing? Does he use proper letter formation when writing the letters? Is he writing the letters independently or when given a visual model to reference?
- Why is Michael having difficulty cutting out shapes? Can he position the scissors correctly in his fingers? Is he able to open and close the scissors to cut the paper? Is he able to coordinate turning the paper when cutting out shapes that require changes in direction? Is his attention affected because he is leaving his desk during the occupational therapy session or fidgeting in his seat, or is he unable to remain on the lines because he does not visually attend to the cutting task?
- When the author states that Michael has difficulty managing his clothing fasteners, is the therapist referring to buttons, zippers, snaps, or shoe strings? More explanation, including what fasteners he is currently working on, and information on what is preventing him from completing these fasteners are needed.

In the second example, the team defined Michael's current performance in observable and measurable terms, including

- The type of grasp Michael was using was defined.
- Clarification of Michael's ability to write

when given a model and when writing independently was provided. The list of which letters he continues to have difficulty with offers good baseline information for developing the goals and objectives (i.e., targeting the letters of continued difficulty) for the upcoming school year. The team also discussed how his difficulty with writing affects his performance in the classroom.

- The team included specific percentages of current success Michael demonstrates for positioning scissors correctly in his fingers, for cutting a straight line, and for cutting shapes. This baseline information is important to reference when establishing criteria for a cutting goal on the new IEP.
- The team identified the fasteners that Michael had mastered, outlined the fasteners that he continues to have difficulty with, and provided baseline information on his current ability toward working on the fasteners of difficulty (e.g., coat zipping and shoe tying).

Determining Needs and Writing Measurable Goals and Objectives

After defining a student's present level of performance, the next step is to have the educational team, including parents, teachers, related service providers, and when applicable, the student, discuss the student's individualized needs. The team then determines what goals it would like to see the student work on and master during the upcoming school year.

Defining the Student's Needs. The educational team uses the student's areas of concern outlined in the present level of performance section of the IEP to identify his or her educational needs. These needs reflect those areas that require specially designed instruction. If numerous educational needs are defined for the student, the team should prioritize the most important and focus on these in the new IEP. The remaining needs possibly can be addressed as part of the daily curriculum, without the collection of detailed data, or may be addressed more specifically in an IEP format after the prioritized needs in the current IEP are mastered.

The needs should encompass the overall topic of what the goals and objectives are going to address. For example, if the student is unable to write his cursive signature, his need may be written as "Connor needs to learn to write his first and last name in cursive to have a functional signature." Another student may be unable to manage clothing fasteners. After defining which fasteners the team is going to work on over the next school year, the student's need may be written as "Becky needs to be able to manage buttoning and unbuttoning the riveted fastener on her jeans so that she can be independent in managing her fasteners in the school setting and in the community."

Writing Measurable Goals and Objectives. After identifying and prioritizing the student's needs, the next step is to develop the annual goals and short-term objectives, or benchmarks, to address these needs. Bateman and Herr (2003) stated that IDEA requires that goals and objectives be measurable, but the act does not outline specific criteria for what measurability means. This can lead to differing interpretations of "measurable." IDEA also does not give specific guidelines for writing goals and objectives in a measurable manner.

To compensate for this, the authors note that goals and objectives need a description of observable learner performance or behavior (e.g., writing, typing, counting) and a list of any conditions or equipment needed to master the goals and objectives, such as access to a typing tutor program or a calculator. Finally, they point out that goals and objectives need to include measurable criteria that specifies the level at which the student's performance or behavior is acceptable for mastery,

such as 80% of attempts using proper letter formation for each letter identified.

Bateman and Herr (2003) further stated that goals and objectives need to be written in such a way that, if data are being collected by different people, each will come to the same conclusion about the student's behavior or performance based on how it was defined in the goal. This is important for school-based occupational therapists to remember when assisting teachers in writing goals and objectives for students.

Components of Annual Goals. Annual goals are what the team has determined reasonable for the student to accomplish over one year. IDEA defines four characteristics of an annual goal (Gibb & Dyches, 2000):

1. It must be measurable.
2. It must tell what the student can reasonably accomplish in a year.
3. It must relate to helping the student be successful in the general curriculum and/or address other educational needs resulting from the disability.
4. It must be accompanied by benchmarks and short-term objectives.

McEwen (2000) further stated that annual goals should be functional, discipline-free, chronologically age-appropriate, and meaningful to the student and the student's family. To meet these requirements, they need to include established criteria that outlines the anticipated student progress in a year's time, according to the baseline data reported in the present level of performance. This criteria define what will be considered mastery of the goal (e.g., 80% of attempts, 75% for each step, 4 out of 5 opportunities independently). The goals need to indicate the subject (e.g., student's name) completing the goal and describe the action or behavior the student will do (e.g., write uppercase alphabet letters, complete the five steps in the shoe-tying task analysis, button and unbutton 1/2-inch buttons on pants). In addition, they must define the context in which the goal will occur (e.g., during occupational therapy treatment sessions, in the classroom setting, within the entire school environment, at school and home; Cuyahoga Special Education Service Center, 2003).

It is important that the student's anticipated behavior or performance is observable and is not left up to interpretation by the data collectors. Vague words and concepts, including such phrases as *appropriate attention, good behavior,* and *improve writing skills,* are not well defined. As such, the numerous people who provide intervention and observe the student's performance or behavior may interpret them differently.

Using levels of cueing as part of the criteria within a goal also can be confusing when it comes to collecting data on the student's performance. If the team feels that cueing needs to be incorporated for the student to achieve a goal, then the type and amount of cues need to be clearly defined. Terms like *maximum, moderate,* or *minimal assistance* in a goal or objective leave room for individual interpretations across the variety of people who take data on a specific goal.

There is no way to clearly define what "with moderate assistance given, student will be able to tie his shoes" means. Does this mean that, when provided with moderate verbal cueing (how many verbal cues equals moderate cueing), moderate physical prompting (how many physical prompts equals moderate cueing), or some combination of cues (physical, verbal, visual), the student will be able to tie his shoes? A more defined way to incorporate cueing may be, for example, "With no more than one verbal cue at each step, Mark will complete the five steps in the shoe-tying task analysis." This allows each person collecting data to know how many cues can be provided for the student to still meet the goal.

Writing goals and objectives without specific types of cueing or levels of assistance often lend to easier data collection. If the goal is for the student to complete the skill independently and the student required cueing for completion, then the criteria was not met and the student would not receive credit for mastering the skill. It is important to remember that providing the initial directive does not count as providing cueing. For instance, asking the student to tie his shoes is not a verbal cue. Defining each step verbally (e.g., first cross laces over, tuck under and pull through, then make the loop) would be considered verbal cueing.

Benchmarks or Short-Term Objectives. Benchmarks or short-term objectives are the intermediate steps needed to achieve the annual goal. Bateman and Herr (2003) explained how these can be related to either a ladder (benchmarks climbing up to the annual goal) or a pie (short-term objectives, or subtasks, that make up the pieces of the pie).

The authors wrote that benchmarks describe the amount of progress the child is expected to make within specific segments of the year (e.g., every quarter, every semester). An example of an annual goal may be "Tom will write his first and last name using proper letter formation so that it is readable to others." Benchmarks toward this goal may include "Tom will write the letters in his first name using proper letter formation so that it is readable to others by the end of the first semester" and "Tom will write the letters in his last name using proper letter formation so that it is readable to others by the end of the second semester."

Using this concept, the bottom of the ladder is the present level of performance, each rung is a benchmark, and the top is the annual goal. For instance, if tying shoes is the task being analyzed, a visual description will look like Figure 2.1.

Top rung of the ladder: Student will independently tie his shoes by the end of the fourth quarter (annual goal).
6. Pinch and pull tight (by end of fourth quarter).
5. Poke the lace through the hole (by end of the third quarter).
4. Cross laces over the loop (by the end of the second quarter).
3. Make a loop (by the end of the first quarter).
2. Cross laces over, tuck under, pull tight (by the end of the first quarter; first benchmark).
Bottom rung of the ladder: Student does not complete any steps to tie his shoes (present level of performance).

Figure 2.1. Benchmarks for Shoe-Tying Goal

When using the ladder concept to write benchmarks, Bateman and Herr (2003) indicated that the criteria for both the annual goal and the benchmarks need to incorporate the same unit of measurement.

Using the pie concept, the present level of performance is in the pie's center, each short-term objective is a piece, and the annual goal is the outer crust that encompasses all of the short-term objectives. The student has to achieve each piece of the pie (short-term objective) to achieve the overall annual goal. An example of the pie concept may be
- *Present Level of Performance:* Student is unable to correctly spell his first and last names independently and is unable to identify uppercase letters or use proper finger placement when typing on the keyboard.
- *Short-Term Objectives* (skills needed to complete the task):
  1a. Student will correctly spell his first and last names independently.

1b. Student will be able to identify uppercase letters as they are depicted on the keys on the keyboard.
1c. Student will use his left hand when locating and typing keys on the left side of the keyboard and use his right hand when locating and typing keys on the right side of the keyboard.
- *Annual Goal:* Student will type his first and last names independently using proper finger placement (left and right hands on the keyboard in home row position) when typing.

When using the pie concept, each short-term objective that makes up the annual goal may be assessed separately and in different units of measurement. This is because each objective may be measuring a different item that assists in getting to the annual goal.

Gibb and Dyches (2000) described writing short-term objectives as a three-step process. The therapist needs to
1. Define the behavior to be measured. This includes the action that the student is performing (e.g., writing, reading, buttoning).
2. Explain the conditions under which the behavior occurs. This may include the types of instructional materials used (e.g., math cubes, calculator, visual models), levels of prompting needed (e.g., verbal cues, visual prompts, physical prompts), and where the student performs the behavior (e.g., in occupational therapy treatment sessions, in the classroom setting, in performance across a variety of settings).
3. State the criterion for mastery. This is the level set to determine if the student has learned the task, including the percentage of correct attempts, number of correct attempts out of a specific number of opportunities, and the designated time frame.

The following are two examples of this three-step process:

- *Short-Term Objective:* When given a model, Matthew will copy the letters in his first and last names using proper letter formation with 80% accuracy for each letter.
  - *Behavior:* Matthew will copy.
  - *Conditions:* When given a model, the letters in his first and last names.
  - *Criteria:* Using proper letter formation, with 80% accuracy for each letter.
- *Short-Term Objective:* When presented with the opportunity during the school day (e.g., recess, getting ready to go home at the end of school day), Sarah will independently engage the zipper on a variety of coats in less than 2 minutes, 4 out of 5 attempts.
  - *Behavior:* Sarah will engage the zipper.
  - *Conditions:* Independently, on a variety of coats, throughout the school day.
  - *Criteria:* In less than 2 minutes, 4 out of 5 attempts.

When writing annual goals and benchmarks or short-term objectives, use measurable and observable terms such as *zips, cuts, writes, takes off,* and *puts on.* Nonmeasurable actions include *understands, knows, feels, thinks, demonstrates, tries,* and *believes.* Without measurable baseline information provided in the present level of performance, words like *improve* or *increase* should not be used. Anyone could look at the form and say "Increase or improve from what level?" See the data collection section for considerations when writing goals and objectives (including specific examples) and methods of collecting data toward the goals and objectives.

Identifying Services Needed to Support Objectives. After the goals and benchmarks have been written, the services needed to support them have to be identified. Services should be defined by the type of service to be provided (e.g., occupational therapy services); the duration of the service to be provided (e.g., 30 minutes, 45 minutes); the frequency of the service (e.g., per week, every 2 months); and the goals and objectives the service will be addressing (e.g., occupational therapy services 30 minutes per week to support objectives 1a, 1b, and 1c).

Occupational therapists may support individual goals and objectives in a student's IEP; however, the goals do make up the student's overall educational plan. Occupational therapists may support specific goals and objectives on the student's educational plan, but other team members also need to support the student in achieving these educational goals. As occupational therapy services are related services on the IEP, they should not be contained to an isolated service provider working on and collecting data on goals and objectives.

In the services section of the IEP, the special education or general education teacher working with the student (depending on the child's disability category and level of support) also is responsible for providing intervention toward the objectives outlined in the IEP and for collecting data on the objectives. The teacher usually has access to the student more frequently throughout the school week than the occupational therapist. The data the teacher collects can be compared to the therapist's data from occupational therapy intervention. Sometimes data can look very different. Usually, the student will have a higher percentage of success in a one-on-one or small-group intervention session in a quiet setting than when he or she has to apply these skills in the general education classroom. The occupational therapist should collaborate with the teacher who is reinforcing the objectives with the student to ensure that the method of measuring and collecting data is consistent among all service providers.

Identifying How the Student's Progress Will Be Measured. After the goals and short-term objectives are written, the educational team determines what methods will be used in collecting data, who will measure the data, how often the data will be collected, and when and how the progress will be reported to the student's parents. The method of collecting data includes reviewing the student's work samples, observing the student, consulting the student's teachers, charting the student's progress toward the goals and objectives, using a checklist to indicate performance, or taking a test to measure progress.

Occupational Therapy as a Consultative Service. Royeen (1992) noted that consultation with the student's teacher or other personnel is one of the most difficult areas to measure. If the occupational therapist is providing only consultation services toward an objective, the therapist should not be the primary source of data. How can data be collected if the therapist is not working directly with the student? In this case, the teacher or primary service provider working directly with the student is in charge of collecting the numerical data. The occupational therapist still can provide narrative information to the team and parents at reporting times in regard to suggestions and recommendations provided to the teacher about the objective and how the student is doing (based on teacher input) using the recommended techniques.

The authors of this book have developed a form (Figure 2.2) that can be used for consultations with teachers. The teacher can complete this form between consultations and document any questions or concerns about the student before the next consultation. At the next consultation meeting, these can be addressed, and the therapist can document on the form the recommendations provided. These recommended strategies or modifications can be attempted with the student. The therapist can follow up on the effectiveness of the strategies or modifications at the next consultation meeting with the teacher. This system also requires the teacher to become an active participant in the consultation process.

Occupational Therapists as Direct Service Providers. Occupational therapists working directly with a student on benchmarks or short-term objectives should collect specific data about the student's performance during intervention sessions. The student may be seen only an average of one to two times per week. The average reporting time lasts between 6 to 9 weeks. Therefore, it is critical to collect data on as many objectives as possible during intervention sessions. This provides more opportunities to factor into the overall count when calculating the student's progress.

Data from occupational therapy intervention sessions should be compared to the data collected by the teacher in the classroom to determine if the student is generalizing the skills learned to a classroom environment. If the student has handwriting goals, the therapist can create a work sample folder in a designated area in the classroom. The teacher can place several of the student's work samples into the folder each week so that the therapist can reference samples from the classroom if the student is seen by the therapist individually in a one-on-one setting outside of the classroom. If the student is seen within the classroom setting, the therapist not only has the work sample from the designated intervention time in the classroom but also has additional data from samples throughout the week when the therapist is not there.

A checklist also can be created for teachers to use for goals and objectives that do not produce work samples, like managing clothing fasteners (see Figure 2.3). If the student has a goal to manage the zipper on his coat, the occupational therapist can collect the data when working with the student in the

Student's Name_____   Teacher's Name _____

Therapist's Name _____   Therapist's Phone_____

Frequency of Consultation Per Student's IEP _____

Staff Present at Consultation Meetings _____

Date	Identified Concern(s)	Recommended Interventions or Modifications	Effectiveness of Recommendations

Figure 2.2. Classroom Consultation Sheet

Date	Task for Student to Complete	Completed Task Independently	Unable to Complete Task Independently	Type of Assistance Needed to Complete Task

Figure 2.3. Data Collection Checklist

classroom; the teacher or teacher's assistant can collect the data the remaining days throughout the week. The therapist can average the data from the entire quarter using the daily data sheet from the classroom.

What should the occupational therapist do if the teacher is not focusing on providing intervention toward the goals and objectives nor collecting data? This situation can be difficult for therapists to address. A teacher may approach the therapist and ask for data so that it can be placed on the teacher's progress note to the student's parents. This is a perfect opportunity for the therapist to address the issue with the teacher. The therapist should outline the importance of supporting the goals and objectives throughout the school week by providing intervention and collecting data on the student's performance across settings, explain how data can look very different across school environments (e.g., one-on-one vs. classroom setting), and describe how the therapist's data is based on intervention sessions that usually occur only one to two times per week.

The teacher often works with the student on a daily basis and therefore is presented with more frequent opportunities to collect data. The occupational therapist always should document in writing the number of consultations conducted with the teacher in regard to the importance of frequent data collection by all team members to support the goals and objectives of the student's IEP. This documentation also protects the therapist in the event that a parent accuses the team of lack of classroom data for goals and objectives that the therapist was supporting.

If the teacher continues to be unsupportive of the objectives listed in the IEP or fails to collect data after the occupational therapist has addressed the situation on multiple occasions, the occupational therapist may need to confer with the building administra-

tor or special education coordinator to address the continued concerns.

When and How Frequently Data Will Be Reported to Parents. Usually each school district has established timelines throughout the school year when student progress is reported to parents. This usually occurs at the end of each grading period or trimester. At this time, the occupational therapist, as a member of the educational team, is responsible for reporting progress that occurred over the past grading period on a standard form used by the district. If the district does not use standardized forms, the therapist may write a separate occupational therapy progress note that outlines the student's progress toward the goals and short-term objectives over the past grading period. Therapists also may collaborate with teachers and write a joint progress note from all team members who work with the student on the identified goals and objectives. For instance, if the special education teacher and occupational therapist have been supporting keyboarding objectives, these team members can collaborate at the end of the grading period and write a joint progress note.

The data gathered from each grading period can be compared over time to ensure that the student is making progress. If progress is not being made, the educational team should meet to determine why. Is it due to a high number of student absences, has the student come to school sick, does he or she demonstrate limited motivation toward working on or achieving the skill, or is the goal or objective too difficult for him or her to accomplish at this time? After concluding why the student has not made progress, the educational team needs to look at developing new or different strategies to address the goals and objectives, consider modifying the goal, or determine if the goal or objective should be discontinued and addressed at a later date.

Considerations When Writing Goals and Objectives

It is important to be aware of the student's overall developmental and cognitive levels when developing goals and objectives. Writing lofty goals and objectives with high criteria that the team knows the student will not achieve in a year's time is unrealistic. Instead, it is often easier to write short-term objectives that follow a progression. In this way, as the student achieves one part of the skill, he or she moves on to the next step gradually until the overall skill outlined in the annual goal is mastered. For example, a student beginning to draw the prewriting shapes needed for letter formation may not be able to master all nine (defined by the Test of Visual Motor Integration; Beery, 1997) in one school year. Instead of setting the student up for failure, the team can address the shapes in a developmental progression. As the student masters one objective that includes a few of the shapes, he or she can move on to the next objective. All of the shapes still can be included on the IEP so that the expectation is there. An example follows.

Annual Goal 1: When given a model, Brian will draw the prewriting shapes needed for letter formation (vertical line, horizontal line, circle, cross, square, right and left diagonal lines, X, and triangle) so that they are recognizable (80% for each shape).

Short-Term Objectives:

1. When given a model, Brian will copy a vertical line, a horizontal line, and a circle so that they are recognizable (80% for each shape).
2. On mastery of 1, when given a model, Brian will copy a cross, a right vertical line, and a square so that they are recognizable (80% for each shape).
3. On mastery of 2, when given a model, Brian will copy a left diagonal line, an X,

and a triangle so that they are recognizable (80% for each shape).

The same concept applies to self-care or other fine motor objectives. If a student is functioning cognitively at a three-year-old's level, it is unrealistic to write an objective that he will tie his shoes, as this is not a skill expected of a typical three-year-old. Instead, working on prerequisite components such as in-hand manipulation skills until the team feels that the student is ready may be more reasonable. This can be addressed during treatment sessions as preparation activities and does not necessarily require specific written goals and objectives to address the skills.

Self-care goals and objectives often can be broken into smaller increments or steps using a task analysis. The objectives can reflect the task analysis that the student should complete. Data can be collected and reported on each step of the task instead of for the task as a whole. An example follows.

Annual Goal 1: Kyle will complete the first three steps required in a shoe-tying task analysis (80% for each step).

Short-Term Objectives:

1. Kyle will cross laces over, tuck under, and pull through to make a knot (Step 1) (80% of attempts).
2. Kyle will make a loop (Step 2) (80% of attempts).
3. Kyle will place the lace over the loop (Step 3) (80% of attempts).

Once Kyle masters these steps, poking lace through (Step 4) and pinching and pull tight (Step 5) can be added to the IEP and worked on until Kyle masters the entire skill. The authors have observed that parents prefer objectives written this way, as it provides them with information on how their child is doing toward each step of the task. Kyle may be completing Step 1 with 50% accuracy, Step 2 with 25% accuracy, and Step 3 with 75% accuracy. This numerical data can be provided to the parent each quarter to indicate progress. It also allows the therapist to determine which step the student is having the greatest difficulty with so that intervention can be designed around the skills needed to complete it.

For example, many students have difficulty completing the fourth step, poking the lace through the hole before pinching and pulling tight. Intervention strategies and preparatory activities can be designed to work on this individual step that include having the student practice pushing coins through a resistive lid, placing pennies or marbles into resistive Theraputty, or using two different color laces to provide a greater contrast for the student to see the lace when poking it through the hole. These strategies can generalize to the "poking the lace through step" in the task analysis and promote further success with the student's ability to independently complete that step.

Remembering Not to Overload Goals and Objectives. Do not overload the goals and objectives with so many items, parameters, or other related tasks that it is impossible to collect data. Handwriting objectives often are written this way as in the following example:

> David will write using good handwriting mechanics, including proper letter formation, size, alignment, and spacing when completing writing tasks.

This objective covers many of the components of legible handwriting; it also provides more than 55 items for data collection. Writing "using proper letter formation" without defining for which specific letters implies that data will be taken on all 52 letters (uppercase and lowercase) of the alphabet individually. At the same time, data are collected on the size of the student's letters within the lines and the alignment of the letters within the lines of grade-level paper. The objective also states that the student will use good spacing. Does

this mean between letters, words, or both? This needs to be further clarified, so that the data collector is taking the data toward the student's actual problem correctly.

This cookie cutter objective appears to be addressing numerous components of handwriting within one objective. Does the student even have difficulty with all of these handwriting components identified in the present level of performance? If he doesn't, then these should not be included in the objective. Eliminating these components also will eradicate the need to collect data on them. On the other hand, if the student does have a problem with all of these components, then the team needs to prioritize the components that initially will be addressed and then focus on additional areas in the future.

In addition, self-care goals and objectives are written at times with numerous components. These may include globally mentioning that the student will manage clothing fasteners or writing that four different clothing fasteners will be worked on in one objective.

For example, "Kevin will manage buttons, snaps, zippers, and tying shoes with 75% accuracy." This requires that service providers address and collect data on four types of clothing fasteners and provide intervention toward that goal. It also requires that the student master all four fasteners before mastering the objective. What does "75% of managing a zipper" mean? Are the occupational therapist and the teaching staff measuring the individual steps in completing the task (i.e., task analysis) or just the end-product (i.e., zipped his coat)? If self-care and handwriting goals containing all of these components are written in the same IEP, then it will be very difficult to successfully address all of these areas within the limited amount of time that the therapist spends with the student each week. It is recommended that the team, including the parents, prioritize the fasteners that the student wears the most (usually zippers on coats and fasteners on pants) and address those first. After the student has mastered these fasteners, different ones can be addressed. An example follows.

Annual Goal 1: Logan will be able to button and unbutton the riveted button on his pants and engage the zipper on a variety of coats so that he is independent in managing his fasteners in the school environment 75% of attempts for each skill.

Short-Term Objectives:
1. Logan will button the riveted button on his pants (75% of attempts).
2. Logan will unbutton the riveted button on his pants (75% of attempts).
3. Logan will engage the zipper on a variety of coats (e.g., fall coat, winter coat, spring jacket, fleece jacket) (75% of attempts).

Relating Goals and Objectives to the Student's Grade-Level Curriculum

The educational team needs to determine when it is appropriate to write annual goals and benchmarks or short-term objectives that align with the student's grade level and curriculum. This is needed especially when writing handwriting goals for a student. Writing annual goals and benchmarks that focus on forming letters of the alphabet can present unique challenges. In kindergarten, a student usually receives initial exposure and instruction on letter formations. This will be reviewed again in first grade. Does the student need letter formation goals for all 52 letters in kindergarten, knowing that he will receive instruction again the following school year?

The team should think about waiting until after the student has received appropriate instruction in the general education classroom and has been provided with interventions in this setting for remediation of difficult letters before placing handwriting goals for all letter formations on the IEP document. If the student continues to demonstrate difficulty as the expectations of hand-writing increase, the occupational therapist may provide more intensive services. Waiting to initiate a referral provides the team with enough time to collect informational data on which letters the student continues to form with difficulty after interventions were tried. The therapist may be used as a resource during this time to suggest interventions and modifications to the teacher to try with the student in the general education classroom without having the therapist directly involved.

In the example of the kindergarten student, the occupational therapist and educational team need to keep in mind the expectations within the grade level when writing the objectives. This way, instead of addressing the entire alphabet, the team, including the occupational therapist, can support what is needed for that grade level. Kindergarten students are expected to be able to write their first names and last names by the end of kindergarten. Objectives may be written that focus on specific letters included in the student's first and last name, as this is a very important skill looking ahead to first grade. An example of how objectives could be written follows.

Annual Goal 1: When given a model, Valerie will write the letters in her first name and last name using proper letter formation (80% for each letter).

Short-Term Objectives:
1. When given a model, Valerie will write the letters in her first name (V, a, l, e, r, and i), using proper letter formation (80% for each letter).
2. On mastery of 1, she will write the letters in her last name (S, m, i, t, h), using proper letter formation (80% for each letter).

Writing "on mastery of 1" does not require the therapist or the teacher to work on all of these letters at the same time. Instead, it allows the occupational therapist or the teacher to introduce them gradually. It also does not require the therapist or the teacher to collect data on Objective 2 until Objective 1 is mastered.

For those students who receive instruction on letter formations across school years (e.g., kindergarten, first and second grade) and continue to demonstrate difficulty, the team can address within objectives the letters that the student continues to have difficulty forming instead of the entire alphabet. This can be done by looking at a variety of work samples from the student, the occupational therapy handwriting evaluation, and classroom writing samples. The therapist and teacher can identify which letters remain difficult for the student, and the teacher, with support from the therapist, can focus on those letters identified in the IEP. If there are many letters that continue to remain difficult for the student to form, the letters can be broken down into subgroups to teach them gradually. An example follows.

Annual Goal 1: Jeff will write the letters (A, K, M, N, R, S, Z, a, b, d, f, j, k, q, s, y) using proper letter formation (80% for each letter).

Short-Term Objectives:

1. Jeff will write letters A, K, M, N, R, S, and Z, using proper letter formation (80% for each letter).
2. Jeff will write letters a, b, d, f, j, k, q, s, and y, using proper letter formation (80% for each letter).

Using handwriting programs that sequentially introduce letter formation (Handwriting Without Tears, Olsen, 2001; Sensible Pencil, Becht, 2000; or Loops and Other Groups, Benbow, 1990) offers another way to write goals and objectives when using specific handwriting programs. Instead of stating that the student will write all lowercase letters in cursive, the team can break the letters down into groups as they are introduced in the curriculum defined by the handwriting program. An example follows.

Annual Goal 1: Bobby will write letters c, a, d, g, h, t, p, e, l, f, u, y, i, and j, using letter formation defined by the Handwriting Without Tears program.

Short-Term Objectives:

1. Bobby will write letters c, a, d, g, h, t, and p, using proper letter formation defined by the Handwriting Without Tears program (80% accuracy for each letter).
2. Upon mastery of 1, Bobby will write letters e, l, f, u, y, i, and j, using proper letter formation defined by the Handwriting Without Tears program (80% for each letter).

The Sensible Pencil handwriting program (Becht, 2000) uses this format. In that program, letters are divided into individual mastery tests. These tests group the letters based on how they are formed. The program has established criteria that outlines mastery. As the student achieves one mastery test, he moves on to the next test. The following is an example of how an annual goal and objectives are written using the Sensible Pencil handwriting program.

Annual Goal 1: Cameron will write letters as defined in Mastery Tests 3 and 4 in the Sensible Pencil handwriting program (Criteria—per criteria defined for mastery in the program).

Short-Term Objectives:

1. Cameron will write letters a, o, l, t, and i as defined in Mastery Test 3 in the Sensible Pencil handwriting program (Criteria—per mastery level defined by the program).
2. On mastery of 1, Cameron will write letters r, h, n, m, c, e, and s as defined in Mastery Test 4 in the Sensible Pencil handwriting program (Criteria—per mastery level as defined by the program).

It should be mentioned that personnel writing IEPs frequently are told by school administrators not to write specific titles of remediation programs used within the IEP goals and objectives. Instead, personnel are told to make the objectives more global (e.g., using a handwriting remediation program, Cameron will write letters a, o, l, t, and i using proper letter formation). The professional opinion of the authors of this book is that, if the district already has purchased a program (e.g., handwriting remediation books or a specific program) and the team knows that the program will be available throughout the school year, then objectives may include the name of the program. The special education teacher and occupational therapist should collaborate with the building administrator first to ensure approval. The teacher and therapist need to ensure that the student's parents are educated about the program that will be used so that they can provide reinforcement at home.

If the student moves to another building within the district or to a different district where the items may not be available, then the IEP may need to be revised. The objectives may need to be modified so that they are written in more global terms. When identifying the need to use a specific handwriting program that differs from the curriculum used by the school district, an IEP meeting should be held to discuss what program will be used and to reflect the change on the IEP if the change does not occur at the annual IEP meeting.

Finally, in regard to handwriting, goals and objectives can be written that address individual mechanics issues (e.g., size, alignment, spacing, erasing). These components should be separated into individual objectives to allow for easier data collection. An example follows.

Annual Goal 1: When writing a sentence, Brady will provide space between words so that all words are readable and will completely erase errors before writing over the same area so that his handwriting is readable by others (75% of spaces and erasures).

Short-Term Objectives:

1. When writing a sentence, Brady will provide space between words so that all words in the sentence are readable (75% of attempts).

2. When correcting work, Brady will completely erase each mistake before writing over the same area so that the correction is readable (75% of erasures).

Data Collection

According to Acquaviva (1996), documentation is the written record of evaluation and treatment provided. The American Occupational Therapy Association's (AOTA's) *Guidelines for Documentation of Occupational Therapy* (2003) state that documentation is necessary whenever professional services are provided to a client in the areas of evaluation, intervention, and outcomes:

- *Evaluation:* This section encompasses the documentation of the referral source and information and data gathered through the evaluation process. This includes a description of the student's occupational profile (current areas of concern, reason for seeking occupational therapy services, background information, and developmental history), assessments used and the results obtained, and analysis of the student's occupational performance. It also includes the identification of a student's strengths and those factors hindering the student from performing in certain areas of occupation, a description of recommendations or modifications based on assessment results, and the areas of occupation targeted for intervention if applicable. This same process is applicable for a reevaluation process during a student's multifactored evaluation.

- *Intervention:* This section includes documentation of the student's goals and objectives, intervention approaches, and the type of service provided to target the goals and objectives established for student based on the evaluation or reevaluation process. Documentation includes writing measurable goals and objectives for the student in collaboration with the team, defining intervention approaches (to create or promote, establish or restore, maintain, modify, or prevent) and services (e.g., consultation, direct services) used, and determining the outcomes measured, based on the student's progress toward the goals and objectives. Documentation should also occur for contacts made with private service providers, doctors, or vendors; collaboration between the occupational therapist and occupational therapy assistant who may be providing the intervention for the student; and any contact with the student's parents. When making contact with private service providers, the therapist needs to ensure that federal, state, and individual school district policies and procedures are being followed. Written permission needs to be obtained from the parents to speak to these private personnel. Progress reports should include a summary of services provided to the student, the student's performance toward goals and objectives, and recommendations for the need for continuation of service or plans for discharge.

- *Outcomes:* This section includes the discharge report (summary of occupational therapy services and outcomes). A discharge report should summarize the student's progress between the time of the initial evaluation and the discontinuation of services and make recommendations as needed toward the client's future needs.

Keep in mind that, if something is not written down, it will be difficult to prove that it occurred. If presented with a case in which the educational team's data needs to be reviewed (e.g., administrative review, mediation, due process) and given only a few days to assimilate data, the educational team needs to have on hand a concise and detailed account of the services that were provided to the student with data to back up the progress that the student has made as a result of the service. The school district's lawyers may want to review the student's data when presented with a high-profile situation.

The student's parents or legal representatives also have access to analyze all data and documentation (e.g., narrative notes, progress notes, documentation of phone conversations) collected on that student and that is in the child's record for his or her entire school career. The school district or the parents' representatives could call on the occupational therapist, as a member of the educational team, to explain data collection procedures used and to report on the student's progress. The possibility of being involved in this process substantiates the need for occupational therapists who work in a school setting to have a consistent data collection procedure that can be used for all students on their caseloads, not just with those students whose parents are knowledgeable and involved or who are requesting that numerical data be reported to them frequently.

Reasons for Collecting Data. Data collection provides accurate and current information about the student's progress toward goals and objectives and offers written proof that the goals and objectives are being addressed. It outlines the preparation activities and intervention strategies put into place to address the objectives and documents any other information related to providing a service to the student. For example, such services may include consulting with the student's teachers, providing materials or adaptive equipment, and consulting with private therapists or the student's parents.

Averaged data for each grading period can be provided and used to determine the student's progress toward goals and objectives during the school year. It also can be used as baseline data when writing the present level of performance the following year's

IEP. Examining data offers a way for the team to reflect on interventions that are working and an opportunity to look at those interventions that may need to be modified or changed due to lack of student progress.

Analyzing data allows the team to reflect on what services are needed to support the objectives. It provides a way for therapists to determine the effectiveness of their services and to determine when services are or are not needed to support the student's IEP goals and objectives. Finally, data provide an effective means of documenting the student's progress or lack of progress toward a certain skill. This is especially important when the educational team, including the occupational therapist, does not think that the student was developmentally ready to complete the task written as an objective in the IEP document. The team can use the data collected during intervention with the student, including numerical documentation and informational data that outline the preparation activities conducted, multiple intervention strategies attempted, and the student's performance, to go back to the parent to confirm that the student was not yet developmentally ready to complete the task.

Data Collection, Narrative Notes, and Progress Notes for IEP Objectives. On the following pages, data sheets are presented that provide examples and explanations on how to collect numerical data for intervention areas commonly supported by occupational therapists who work in schools. The short-term objectives are written on the data sheets, with data reported for sample intervention sessions. Data also are totaled at the end of the quarter to outline how to average the data to write a progress report. Sample progress reports are provided for the goals and objectives listed on the student's data sheet. A blank daily data and documentation note form is provided in Appendix 2.1.

Defining Cueing on Data Sheet

Always be aware of the types of cues used with students. Cues range from most restrictive (hand-over-hand assistance) to least restrictive (verbal prompt). The cues a student needs to complete a task should be coded on the daily documentation sheet either in the narrative section or in the reporting of numerical data. Remember that giving the initial direction (e.g., "Bobby, tie your shoes") does not constitute providing the student with a cue. The definitions of the types of cues used and the abbreviations used within documentation records are

- *Independent (I):* Student was able to complete the task without any assistance (either physical or verbal) from an adult.
- *Supervision (SUP):* Student was able to perform the task without any physical contact but needed to be supervised by an adult when completing the task to ensure his or her personal safety.
- *Verbal Cue (VC):* Student was given a verbal cue from an adult to complete the task (e.g., "Sarah, form the letter *a* by moving your pencil around and down").
- *Visual Prompt (VP):* Student was able to complete the task after the adult pointed out or gestured as to how to start or complete the task (e.g., Sarah is drawing a line down. The adult provides a visual prompt by pointing at the dot where she needs to start drawing and the dot where she needs to stop drawing).
- *Physical Prompt (PP):* Student needs physical assistance from an adult to complete the given task (e.g., during shoe tying, an adult initiates poking the lace through the hole, and then the student is able to grasp the lace to pull it tight).
- *Hand-Over-Hand Assistance (HOH):* In the most restrictive cue used with a student, the adult is physically completing the task

for the child, with little to no active participation by the student (e.g., helping a student cut a line by helping him or her open and close the scissors and holding the paper so that it can be cut).

The first daily data and documentation note provided in Figure 2.4 is for Ryan, a kindergartener. Ryan is developing his cutting skills and prewriting and writing skills. The numerical data, narrative note, and sample progress note are provided.

Information to Include in a Narrative Note

A narrative note describes information to support the numerical data on the front of the daily documentation sheet. The note should report the preparation activities conducted in the intervention session (e.g., putty activities, picking up and manipulating objects with fingers, using tongs to promote cutting skills), intervention strategies (e.g., using pencil gripper, forming shapes and letters on chalkboard or on clay tray), and any informational data on the student's performance or behavior for the tasks presented (e.g., observed to be able to turn the paper effectively when cutting around circle and square, visually attended to cutting task, demonstrated proper letter formation for three of the four letters in his name).

This section also may describe the types of cueing the student needed from the therapist to complete the task, such as "He needed two verbal cues to position the scissors correctly in his fingers." The narrative section of the daily documentation sheet can document when phone calls are made on behalf of the student (e.g., to student's parents or private therapists), when materials are made for the student to try, or if the therapist attended a meeting for the student. An blank narrative note is provided in Appendix 2.2.

Using a Preparation Activity Checklist

An activity checklist is another option to use in combination with a narrative note. The preparation activities can be listed along the left side of the document. The occupational therapist then records the date and checks the activities conducted during the intervention session. Data is not collected on the student's performance of the activity; rather, the checklist simply indicates which activities were conducted. This alleviates the need to describe the preparation activities within the narrative note. The narrative note can then cover the interventions used toward the specific goals and objectives and any other nonsubjective observations of the student during the intervention session.

Classroom staff also can use this activity checklist to document activities conducted with the student throughout the school week. For example, the occupational therapist develops a fine motor kit for the student that includes fine motor activities that target specific skills for the student to complete during the school day. The classroom teacher, special education teacher, or teacher assistant could check off the items conducted each day. This is a way for the team to document the activities conducted and reinforced consistently throughout the student's school week. An example of an activity checklist is provided in Appendix 2.3.

Ryan, whose preparation activity checklist is provided in Figure 2.5, has objectives to position scissors correctly in his fingers, cut out shapes that require changes in direction, copy prewriting shapes, and copy the letters in his first name. The numerical data reported on the sheet describes the number of times he completed the tasks independently, because that is how the objectives are written. The amount of assistance Ryan needs to complete the other attempts at the tasks can be mentioned in the narrative note section of the data collection form. Information regarding the preparation activities and intervention strategies also is mentioned in this section. The following is a description of how to structure an intervention session for these

Student Name __Ryan Martin__   Year __2003–2004__

Therapist Name __Kelly Ryba, OTR/L__   School __Snow Elementary__

                                                      Grade __Kindergarten__

Objectives and Criteria	Date							Total for 3rd quarter
	1-19-04	1-26-04	2-2-04	2-9-04	2-23-04	3-1-04	3-8-04	
3a. Ryan will position scissors in correct orientation in his fingers. (Criteria: 75% of attempts)	1/2	2/3	1/2	2/4	2/3	1/2	1/3	10/19 I = 52%
3b. Ryan will cut out a triangle, circle, and square within 1/4" of the lines. (Criteria: 80% of attempts)	△–1/1 □–1/2 ○–1/1	△–2/3 □–2/2 ○–0/1	△–0/2 □–1/3 ○–N/A	△–1/2 □–1/2 ○–1/1	△–1/1 □–2/3 ○–2/2	△–1/2 □–2/3 ○–2/4	△–1/3 □–1/3 ○–2/2	△–7/14 = 50% □–10/18 = 56% ○–8/11 = 73%
4a. When given a model, Ryan will copy a square, X, and triangle so that they are recognizable. (Criteria: 80% for each shape)	□–1/2 X–1/1 △–0/2	□–2/2 X–1/2 △–0/2	□–1/2 X–1/2 △–1/3	□–2/3 X–2/2 △–1/2	□–1/1 X–1/2 △–1/2	□–1/2 X–1/1 △–1/4	□–1/3 X–?/4 △–1/2	□–9/15 = 60% X–9/14 = 64% △–5/17= 29%
4b. Ryan will write the letters in his first name using proper letter formation. (Criteria: 80% for each letter)	R–1/3 y–2/3 a–1/3 n–3/3	R–1/2 y–1/2 a–2/2 n–2/2	R–1/1 y–0/1 a–0/1 n–1/1	R–2/2 y–1/2 a–2/2 n–1/2	R–N/A y–N/A a–N/A n–N/A	R–1/1 y–1/1 a–1/1 n–1/1	R–2/3 y–2/3 a–1/3 n–3/3	R–8/12 = 75% y–7/12 = 58% a–7/12 = 58% n–11/12 = 92%

Figure 2.4. Ryan's Daily Data and Documentation Note

(continued)

Daily Documentation Note

Date	Notes
1-26-04	Ryan participated in fine motor preparation activities, including working on in-hand manipulation skills by stabilizing coins in his palm and placing coins through slots in a container's lid prior to cutting and writing tasks. He was able to hold a total of three coins in his palm while bringing one coin to his fingertips. If given four coins to hold, he dropped them. Ryan positioned scissors correctly in his fingers 2/3 times independently but needed PP for remaining attempt to reposition correctly. Ryan had difficulty cutting around circles; his cuts remained rough and choppy. He reviewed writing letters in his first name and drawing shapes using the rainbow writing method on a mini-chalkboard. Ryan was able to form Xs and squares but continues to need PP and VC to form triangles. Ryan had difficulty forming the letters "R" and "Y" using proper letter formation. The two diagonal lines in the "Y" did not meet.
2-2-04	Ryan was observed placing his thumb in the large hole of the scissors and his fingers in the little hole. He required VC to reposition in half the attempts. Ryan was presented with two triangles and three squares to cut. He demonstrated difficulty turning the paper when cutting around the triangle and square—resulting in cutting off angles on the triangle and corners of the square. Ryan reviewed copying shapes on a vertical dry erase board and tracing shapes and letters made from Wikki Stix. He copied shapes on a worksheet and had difficulty using proper letter formation with the letters "y" and "a" in his first name. He uses a ball-and-stick method for "a" and the two strokes are not aligned properly, resulting in decreased legibility of the letter. His diagonal lines in the "y" appear horizontal.
2-9-04	Ryan participated in preparation activities, including using tweezers and a test-tube holder (for resistive open–close motion) to pick up objects and sort them by colors. He placed scissors in fingers two out of four times and needed a VC and PP to correctly orient the remaining two attempts. He continues to cut off corners when using scissors. The OT highlighted the corners with a contrasting color marker prior to him cutting it to assist with this problem. Ryan practiced prewriting shapes and letters in his first name using shaving cream on a table. He completed worksheets for name and shapes. His performance improved during this session compared to the last session for writing the letters "R" and "a." He drew more pronounced corners and angles on the triangle and square.
2-16-04	No school—President's Day
2-23-04	Ryan demonstrated ability to position scissors in fingers 2/3 times independently. Able to turn paper to accurately cut around variety of shapes. Practiced prewriting shapes using shaving cream and on chalkboard prior to paper-and-pencil task. Able to accurately draw square but continues to have difficulty consistently copying diagonal lines for X and triangle.

Key for Type of Assistance Given

I = Independent	VP = Visual Prompt	VC = Verbal Cue	SUP = Supervision
CG = Contact Guard	PP = Physical Prompt	HOH = Hand-Over-Hand	

Figure 2.4. Ryan's Daily Data and Documentation Note (continued)

Student Name Ryan Martin   School Year 2003–2004

Dates 3-15-04

Preparation Activity Conducted	Date					
	1-19-04	1-26-04	2-2-04	2-9-04	2-16-04	2-23-04
Tweezer scissors	✓				No school	
In-hand manipulation		✓				
Clay tray	✓					
Sand tray	✓					
Rainbow Writing		✓				
Chalkboard/ Dry Erase Board		✓	✓			✓
Shaving Cream				✓		✓
Wikki Stix			✓			
Tongs/Test Tube Holder/Tweezers				✓		

Figure 2.5. Ryan's Preparation Activity Checklist

objectives and how to collect data on Ryan's objectives.

Structuring Intervention to Promote Data Collection.

Positioning Scissors Correctly in Fingers. This requires the therapist or teacher observe the student picking up the scissors from the table and looking at how he positions them in his fingers. The therapist or teacher may set up the situation by placing the scissors in a variety of different directions on the table and then observing whether or not the student can pick up the scissors and perceptually orient them correctly to put them on. Intervention strategies may include providing a visual cue (e.g., a visual drawing of the scissors in correct orientation) on the table and allowing the student to align the scissors correctly on the table and then placing them in his hand. The therapist or teacher then totals the data by dividing

$$\frac{\text{the number of correct attempts}}{\text{Ryan has at picking up the scissors}}$$

by the total number of attempts that presented.

Cutting out Shapes That Require Changes in Direction. For this activity, the therapist or teacher may present preparation activities that focus on different aspects of cutting, including positioning the scissors, opening and closing the scissors, or following a line starting and stopping at designated points. Activities may include having the student use tongs or tweezers to pick up objects to play games. Intervention strategies may include providing a physical prompt or verbal cue to the student to position his forearms by his side, presenting adapted scissors, using thicker paper for added stability, using highlighting to further define where the student needs to cut, and slowly increasing the demands of the cutting tasks by having the student initially practice cutting a straight line and then moving to having the student cut out shapes that require changes in direction.

The therapist or teacher in this example focused on three shapes to chart data for a circle, a square, and a triangle. After the student completes the cutting tasks, the therapist or teacher reviews the work samples to see if the shapes cut out meet the criteria defined by the goal of being cut within 1/4 inch of the line. If they do meet the criteria, the student receives credit. If the student cut outside 1/4 inch of the line, he does not receive credit for completing the skill. The therapist or teacher calculates the data by dividing

$$\frac{\text{the total number of shapes cut}}{\text{within 1/4 inch of the line}}$$

by the total number of attempts at cutting out that shape.

Copying Prewriting Shapes. For this objective, the therapist or teacher may complete preparation activities that promote a three-finger (tripod) pencil grasp or increased hand strength. Intervention strategies may include having the student copy the shapes described in the objective using multisensory techniques like rainbow writing (having the student trace over letters numerous times using different colors of chalk, crayons, paint, or markers) on the chalkboard, drawing the shapes using the index finger on a paint bag, using a clay tray, air writing, or using a dry erase board. Other intervention strategies may include using dot-to-dot models to assist in the formation of the shapes, highlighting, various levels of cueing, and designated areas for starting and stopping when drawing the lines or shapes.

After these intervention strategies are conducted, the therapist or teacher collects a work sample for data collection purposes. A previously prepared worksheet that can be duplicated using the copy machine has the three shapes already drawn on it and may be presented to the student to copy (square, X, and triangle) after the intervention strategies are completed. Using this worksheet as the work sample, the therapist or teacher records the data based on whether the shape was recognizable. The therapist or teacher computes the data by dividing

$$\frac{\text{the number of times the individual shape was drawn so that it was recognizable}}{\text{by the total number of opportunities to draw the individual shape.}}$$

Writing First Name. For this objective, the therapist or teacher may use the same prerequisite and intervention strategies described previously for working on the prewriting shapes (e.g., paint bag, chalkboard) to practice individual letters. After providing the intervention, the therapist or teacher presents Ryan with a model of his first name and asks him to copy the letters. The therapist or teacher collects the data based on whether or not Ryan wrote the letters using proper letter formation, using the formula

$$\frac{\text{the number of letter } R\text{s that were written with proper letter formation}}{\text{by the total number of opportunities to write the letter } R.}$$

It is helpful for handwriting and cutting objectives, which produce work samples, to indicate directly on the work sample what type of assistance (e.g., verbal cue, visual prompt, physical prompt) and the amount of assistance (one, two, or three verbal cues) it took for the student to complete the task. This is especially important if the therapist or teacher has consecutive intervention sessions with students and does not have time to write down the data directly after each student's intervention session is over. Because the work sample has the types and amount of cueing needed written on the sample, the therapist or teacher has a record of the student's performance or behavior during the session to transfer to the data sheet during a break or at the end of the day.

Sometimes, if the student has a handwriting goal in his IEP, a teacher will ask the therapist to work on a classroom writing assignment during the student's scheduled therapy time. If using a pullout model for intervention, the therapist always needs to make a copy of the work sample before the student returns to class. Without a work sample, data cannot be collected and the therapist will not have the work sample to show as proof. Even if providing intervention within the student's general education classroom when the class is working on a handwriting task, a copy of the handwriting work sample conducted within this class time that the therapist supported still should be photocopied so that a written document is available within the therapist's file.

Writing Progress Notes

According to AOTA's *Documentation Guidelines* (2003), a progress report summarizes the intervention process and documents the client's (student's) progress toward goals and achievement. This report should include new data that has been collected, modifications that have occurred to the treatment, and the statement of need for continuation of the plan and services or discontinuation of services. When reporting a student's progress to a parent, it is always important to indicate the totaled percentage for the designated goals and objectives that the student has achieved over the given grading period. To total the data, the therapist divides

$$\frac{\text{the total number of correct attempts}}{\text{by the total number of opportunities provided to the student over the grading period.}}$$

In addition to reporting the numerical data, providing narrative informational data to a parent helps further define the numerical data as to whether progress has or has not been made. Informational data that can be reported include what preparation activities and intervention strategies are being done during intervention sessions to work on the skills, what carryover activities are being done in the classroom setting, factual observations of the student's behavior while completing the activities, what is holding the student back from achieving the goals and objectives (e.g., student continues to have difficulty correctly forming the letter *a,* which affects the overall legibility of his name), and if substantial progress has been made from the previous quarter.

Teachers and therapists often use global terms, including "making adequate progress, not making progress, and mastered," to indicate the student's progress on a quarterly progress note without having the numerical data to back up the statement. How can those statements be used if there are no numerical data being collected based on the criteria? These types of codes should not be used if the therapist does not have the data to back it up. A sample progress note is provided in Figure 2.6 to reflect Ryan's progress during the third quarter of school.

The next example addresses a student named Samuel who has self-care goals on his IEP. Samuel currently is working on managing a riveted fastener on his jeans that he wears to school and also is working on the steps to tie his shoes. A sample data sheet and narrative note (Figure 2.7), and progress note (Figure 2.8) for Samuel are provided.

The therapist needs to begin a new narrative note page to continue the note on a second page for sessions on 3-1-04 and 3-8-04.

In the sample, Samuel has objectives to button and unbutton his jeans and to complete the steps in tying his shoes. The numerical data reported on the data sheet describe the number of times he completed the tasks independently, because that is how the objectives were written. The amount of assistance Samuel needed to complete other attempts at the tasks is mentioned in the narrative note section of the data collection form. The following is a description of how to structure a treatment session for the objectives listed and how to collect data on Samuel's objectives.

Structuring Intervention to Promote Data Collection.

Buttoning and Unbuttoning a Riveted Fastener on Jeans. For this objective, the therapist or teacher may provide preparation activities that focus on in-hand manipulation skills, pincer grasp, and finger strengthening. These may be the skill deficit areas that the therapist determined as preventing the student from being able to finish the task after completion of the Self-Care Functional Checklist (see Chapter 4). Intervention strategies may include having the student practice fastening the jeans when they are placed in correct orientation in front of him on the table. This eliminates Samuel having to look down when completing the task and also allows him to practice the skill without the resistance of having the jeans around his waist. Other intervention strategies may be the enlargement of the button hole to decrease the amount of resistance when buttoning or unbuttoning or only partially completing the task, using a backward chaining method of instruction. That means starting to push the button through the hole for Samuel and requiring him only to finish pushing the button through the hole. Data then is collected based on dividing

$$\frac{\text{the number of times the student buttoned the riveted fastener}}{\text{by the total number of attempts he was given to complete the task}}$$

and

$$\frac{\text{the number of times the student unbuttoned the riveted fastener}}{\text{by the total number of attempts he was given to complete the task.}}$$

Shoe Tying. Preparation activities completed before the task may include providing support to the student in learning how to tie a knot, completing bilateral tasks (e.g.,

Name of Student Ryan Martin   School Year 2003–2004

Date of Note 3-15-04   Grade Kindergarten

School Snow Elementary

Goal	Objective	Comments
3	a	Ryan is able to position scissors correctly in his fingers in 52% of attempts. He required either a verbal cue or physical prompt from an adult to assist with positioning the scissors correctly in his fingers in the other attempts. He tends to place his thumb in the large hole and his index and middle fingers in the small hole, needing cues to correct.
3	b	Ryan has been working on cutting out a circle, triangle, and square. The following data are reported for cutting these three shapes within _" of the line: circle: 73%, square: 56%, triangle: 50%. Ryan does at times deviate more than _" over the line and will require multiple verbal cues to find the black line in order to reposition his scissors on the line of the shape.
4	a	Ryan has been practicing copying the prewriting shapes using a variety of multisensory techniques, including painting and writing on a chalkboard, dry erase board and sand tray and also in shaving cream. The following data are reported for his ability to copy a square, X, and triangle so that they are recognizable: square: 60%, triangle: 29%, X: 64%.
4	b	Ryan has been using the same intervention techniques described in 4a to practice copying the letters in his first name. The following data are reported for his ability to copy the letters using proper letter formation: R: 75%, y: 58%, a: 58%, n: 92%. He continues to have difficulty aligning the diagonal lines to form the "y." We will continue to work on his name next quarter.

Additional Comments

Ryan is a very hard worker and is a pleasure to work with during occupational therapy. He continues to make good progress from the second quarter (please reference second-quarter progress note) in writing the prewriting shapes and letters in his name. We will continue to work on the above-mentioned goals and objectives until he meets the criteria established in his IEP.

Signature of Therapist_____   Page _____ of _____

Figure 2.6. Ryan's Student Progress Note

Student Name Samuel Banks   Year 2003–2004

Therapist Name Kelly Ryba, OTR/L   School Mayfair Elementary

                                                      Grade 4

Objectives and Criteria	Date							Total for 3rd quarter
	1-19-04	1-26-04	2-2-04	2-9-04	2-23-04	3-1-04	3-8-04	
1a. Samuel will independently button the riveted fastener on his jeans. (Criteria: 80% of attempts)	0/2	1/3	2/4	1/2	2/3	2/2	3/3	11/19 = 58%
1b. Samuel will independently unbutton the riveted fastener on his jeans. (Criteria: 80% of attempts)	0/2	0/3	0/4	1/2	1/3	1/2	1/3	4/19 = 21%
2a. Samuel will independently complete the 5 steps in the shoe-tying task analysis (Criteria: 80% for each step): 1. Cross over, pull through 2. Make the loop 3. Put the lace over the loop 4. Poke the lace through 5. Pinch and pull tight.	1. 5/5 2. 5/5 3. 3/5 4. 0/5 5. 4/5	1. 3/3 2. 3/3 3. 2/3 4. 0/5 5. 5/5	1. 2/2 2. 2/2 3. 1/2 4. 0/2 5. 2/2	1. 4/4 2. 4/4 3. 4/4 4. 1/4 5. 2/4	1. 1/1 2. 1/1 3. 1/1 4. 0/3 5. 3/3	1. 2/2 2. 2/2 3. 2/2 4. 1/2 5. 2/2	1. 3/3 2. 2/3 3. 3/3 4. 1/3 5. 3/3	1. 20/20 = 100% 2. 20/20 = 100% 3. 16/20 = 80% 4. 3/24 = 13% 5. 21/24 = 88%

Figure 2.7. Samuel's Daily Data and Documentation Note

(continued)

Student Name **Samuel Banks**   Year **2003–2004**

Date	Notes
1-19-04	Prep activities done prior to practicing buttoning include moving objects from palm to fingertips and shifting objects among fingertips (e.g., coins, pegs, marbles). Samuel is able to stabilize three objects in his palm when bringing object to fingertips. Prep activity also included practicing buttoning on pair of jeans positioned in correct orientation on the table. He buttoned and unbuttoned twice I on the table. When wearing jeans, Samuel was unable to complete either skill. He has difficulty aligning the sides to button and pulls at the fabric when attempting to unbutton. He completed the first two steps in shoe tying I, needed VC to wrap lace around loop twice, and was unable to poke lace through; he let go of the loop, resulting in the lace falling apart.
1-26-04	Prep activities completed prior to self-care tasks include pushing coins through resistive lid and shifting coins within fingertips to put into a piggy bank (in-hand manipulation). After reviewing buttoning on jeans positioned on table, Samuel was able to complete this I. When wearing the jeans, he was able to button on his first attempt I, but required VC for finger placement on jeans for second attempt. He continues to be unable to unbutton; he just pulls at the fabric. He requires PP from OT to complete the task. He is independent with the first two steps in shoe tying. He needed 1 VC to complete one attempt at wrapping lace around loop. He was unable to poke lace through on any attempts I and continues to need both VC and PP to complete. He completed last step I.
2-2-04	Prep activities done prior to buttoning included finding coins in therapy putty (finger-strengthening exercise). Samuel then had to stabilize five coins in his palm and shift them in his fingertips to put into container. He was able to stabilize four objects but dropped coins while holding five in his palm. Samuel was able to button two out of four times I. He needed VC to visually attend to task twice. He was unable to unbutton riveted fastener even after visual demo and VC were provided. He continues to need PP to complete. Samuel continues to need assistance with Step 4 in shoe-tying task analysis. The OT tried using contrasting-color laces today with Samuel for better visual cue. Even with contrasting-color laces, he continued to need VC and PP to complete Step 4.
2-9-04	Prep activities completed prior to buttoning included pinching clothespins to put on board held horizontally in front of the student (pinching and wrist extension). Prep activity also included practicing buttoning jeans with enlarged buttonhole. When wearing these pants Samuel was able to button and unbutton one out of two times I. He required VC from OT for the remaining attempt. He completed first three steps of shoe tying each attempt I and was able to poke lace through one out of four times I. The remaining attempts required VC and PP. Samuel continues to use contrasting-color shoelaces for better visual of where the lace needs to be poked through.
2-16-04	No school—President's Day
2-23-04	Prep activities done prior to self-care practice include working on in-hand manipulation skills by stabilizing objects in the palm while manipulating objects in hands. Practiced buttoning on model on table, then on self. He buttoned two out of two times I while wearing jeans without enlarged buttonhole. Samuel was able to unbutton one out of two times I. He had good visual attention to task and completed steps 1, 2, 3, and 5 I in shoe tying. He continues to need VC for poking the lace through the hole.

Key for Type of Assistance Given

I = Independent	VP = Visual Prompt	VC = Verbal Cue	SUP = Supervision
CG = Contact Guard	PP = Physical Prompt	HOH = Hand-Over-Hand	

Figure 2.7. Samuel's Daily Data and Documentation Note (continued)

Name of Student **Samuel Banks**   School Year **2003–2004**

Date of Note **3-15-04**   Grade **4**

School **Mayfair Elementary**

Goal	Objective	Comments
1	a	Samuel is currently buttoning the riveted fastener on his jeans 58% of attempts over the third quarter compared to 29% during the second quarter. The remaining attempts, Samuel continues to need verbal cues for proper finger placement when attempting to button.
1	b	Samuel continues to demonstrate difficulty with unbuttoning the riveted fastener on his jeans. He currently completes this task independently in 21% of his attempts. Samuel continues to need both verbal cues and physical prompts from the therapist to unbutton his jeans. He pulls at the fastener when trying to unbutton and does not use proper finger placement of pinching both sides and pulling up and over to release the button from the hole.
2	a	Samuel continues to make great progress with tying his shoes. He has mastered (80% or greater criteria) Steps 1, 2, 3, and 5. He continues to have difficulty with the fourth step of "poking the lace through," requiring physical prompts from the therapist. Continued practice has been provided with this step, as well as engaging in preparation activities focused on placing an object through a hole. Contrasting-color shoelaces also have been used. The following data is reported for Samuel's ability to independently complete each step in the shoe-tying task analysis: Step 1 (Cross over and pull through): 100% Step 2 (Make the loop): 100% Step 3 (Wrap lace around loop): 80% Step 4 (Poke lace through): 13% Step 5 (Pinch lace and pull tight): 88%

Additional Comments

Samuel continues to be very dedicated to gaining independence in his self-help skills. He works very hard during his occupational therapy intervention sessions. He has made very good progress this quarter with buttoning the fastener on his jeans and with mastering all but one step in the shoe-tying task analysis. We will continue to address those goals that he has not mastered. Way to go Samuel—keep up the great work!

Signature of Therapist_____ Page _____ of _____

Figure 2.8. Samuel's Student Progress Note

stringing beads, lacing, cutting) if the student has difficulty using two hands together, and practicing pinching objects (e.g., clothespins, tweezers, coins, bingo chips) through a hole on a container lid. Intervention strategies may include working on steps in isolation, if certain steps are more difficult than others; completing a backward chaining model, which involves starting with last step and working backward to the first step; or using adapted methods that include an adapted shoe-tying technique, contrasting-color laces, and thicker laces. In Samuel's example, he is given more opportunities to practice Steps 4 and 5, because these are the steps that he continues to have difficulty completing independently. It makes sense to focus the intervention on tasks the student is unable to complete versus focusing the same amount of attention on steps he already is able to do independently. To tally the data the therapist or teacher would divide

$$\frac{\text{the total number of attempts the student completed each step independently}}{\text{by the total number of attempts the student was given to complete each step.}}$$

Data should be collected for each step of the task to show progress with each individual step on progress notes. A sample of a quarterly progress note for Samuel is provided in Figure 2.8.

Writing a Discharge Summary

Once the student's goals and objectives are mastered and the team (including the student's parents) decides that occupational therapy services are no longer needed to support the student's educational needs as defined by his or her goals and objectives in the IEP, the therapist needs to write a discharge summary note. The *Documentation Guidelines for Occupational Therapy* (AOTA, 2003)

state that the discharge report should summarize the changes in the student's ability to engage in occupations between the initial evaluation and discontinuation of services and make recommendations as applicable. The discharge note may include how long occupational therapy services were provided, the type of service provided (e.g., direct, consultation), a summary of the student's progress toward goals and objectives, and any recommendations that pertain to the student's future needs. These recommendations may describe if a follow-up by the occupational therapist is needed or may also suggest modifications or equipment that may be needed for the student to engage in his or her occupations (e.g., activities at home, school, or in the community).

The therapist should ensure that the discharge report is distributed appropriately. Copies need to go to the student's parents and teachers, into the occupational therapist's file for the student, and into the student's permanent record that is usually kept at the school building or with the board of education. This way there is a permanent record within the student's file that identifies when and why services were discontinued in the event that the student changes buildings or moves out of the district.

Summary and Conclusion

Occupational therapists working in a school-based setting are required to evaluate students, assist in writing goals and objectives for each student's IEP, design intervention strategies to support each student in mastering the goals and benchmarks or short-term objectives, collect data to show student progress over the course of the school year, and report to each student's parents through progress notes at the end of each grading period. Therapists must become knowledgeable of the evaluation and IEP processes.

Occupational therapists are accountable for their services through data collection and documentation. These require the therapist and the educational team to take the time when writing a student's present level of performance and goals and objectives to ensure that they are observable and measurable. It is impossible to collect accurate data if the annual goals and benchmarks are not measurable. The occupational therapist needs to collect numerical data on those students receiving direct intervention. The special education teacher or classroom teacher who also is working on the goals and objectives should collect data that reflects each student's performance and progress toward the goals and benchmarks, or short-term objectives, within the classroom setting. This numerical data assists the team in determining what interventions are working, the amount of progress that has been made, and if the goals or objectives need to be revised or discontinued. The occupational therapist is responsible for documenting all consultation meetings held with staff members on a student's behalf, if materials were made for the student, and the effectiveness of the recommendations provided by the therapist based on the teacher's report.

This chapter outlined the overall components of a student's IEP and the considerations to take into account when writing measurable present levels of performance and goals and objectives. It also provided examples of how to record numerical data and transfer it to a data sheet and of totaling the data to report within a quarterly progress note. Samples of measurable short-term objectives for specific intervention areas (e.g., self-care, handwriting) can be found in other chapters.

References

Acquaviva, J. D. (1996). Documentation of occupational therapy services. In *The occupational therapy manager* (Rev. ed., pp. 424–436). Bethesda, MD: American Occupational Therapy Association.

American Occupational Therapy Association. (2003). Guidelines for documentation of occupational therapy. *American Journal of Occupational Therapy, 57,* 646–649.

Bateman, B. D., & Herr, C. M. (2003). *Writing measurable IEP goals and objectives.* Verona, WI: Attainment.

Becht, L. C. (2000). *Sensible pencil.* Birmingham, AL: EBSCO Curriculum Materials.

Beery, K. E. (1997). *The Beery–Buktenica Developmental Test of Visual Motor Integration* (4th ed., rev.). Parsippany, NJ: Modern Curriculum Press.

Benbow, M. (1990). *Loops and other groups: A kinesthetic writing system.* San Antonio, TX: Therapy SkillBuilders.

Cuyahoga Special Education Service Center. (2003, October). *IEP Guide.* Paper presented at an occupational therapy and physical therapy networking meeting, Parma, OH.

Gibb, G. S., & Dyches, T. T. (2000). *Guide to writing quality individualized education programs: What's best for students with disabilities?* Needham Heights, MA: Allyn & Bacon.

Individuals With Disabilities Education Act Reauthorization of 1997, Pub. L. 105–17, 20 U.S.C. § 1400 *et seq.*

Individuals With Disabilities Education Act Assistance for Education of All Children, 34 CFR § 300 (1999).

McEwen, I. (2000). *Providing physical therapy services under Parts B and C of the Individuals With Disabilities Education Act.* Alexandria, VA: American Physical Therapy Association.

Olsen, J. Z. (2001). *Handwriting without tears* (8th ed.). Potomac, MD: Author.

Royeen, C. B. (1992). Measuring and documenting all services. In C. B. Royeen (Ed.), *School-based practice for related services* (pp. 8–22). Rockville, MD: American Occupational Therapy Association.

Appendix 2.1.
Daily Data and Documentation Note

Student Name _____   Year _____

Therapist Name _____   School _____

Grade _____

Objectives and Criteria	Date							

Key for Type of Assistance Given

I = Independent	VP = Visual Prompt	VC = Verbal Cue	SUP = Supervision
CG = Contact Guard	PP = Physical Prompt	HOH = Hand-Over-Hand	

(continued)

Student Name_____   Year _____

Date	Notes

Appendix 2.2.
Student Progress Note

Name of Student _____   School Year _____

Date of Note _____   Grade _____

School _____   Building _____

Goal	Objective	Comments

Additional Comments

Signature _____   Page _____ of _____

Appendix 2.3.
Preparation Activity Checklist

Student Name_____   School Year _____

Dates _____

Preparation Activity Conducted	Date								

Understanding Children With Dyspraxia: Identification, Evaluation, and Intervention

The *Occupational Therapy Practice Framework: Domain and Process* (American Occupational Therapy Association [AOTA], 2002) stated that

> Occupational therapists and occupational therapy assistants help individuals link their ability to perform daily life activities with meaningful patterns of engagement in occupations that allow participation in desired roles and life situations at home, school, workplace, and community. (p. 611)

The *Framework* continues on to say that these "individuals engage in occupations because they are committed to performance as a result of self-choice, motivation, and meaning" (p. 611). Attending and participating in activities at school are two of the most important occupations for children, adolescents, and young adults. School, as an occupation, has multifaceted expectations for students. Some of these expectations are managing academics, including language arts, math, science, and social studies; managing nonacademic activities, including recess, lunch, and time spent on the bus; establishing and maintaining social relationships with peers and adults; and participating in extracurricular activities such as athletics, clubs, or committees.

Occupational therapists who work in a school-based setting evaluate students. With the help of occupational therapy assistants, they provide intervention to those students (both in preschool and in school-age programs) who demonstrate deficits in their motor planning abilities. These students may present a wide variety of deficits in their per-formance skills, including motor skills, processing skills, and communication/interaction skills, that affect the quality of the skill and the overall ability to complete the expectations of the school day. These students may appear clumsy and have difficulty with

- Organizational skills in the classroom and managing personal belongings (e.g., coat, book bag, folders, and books);
- Following classroom routines and completing tasks that involve single or multistep directions;
- Visual–perceptual and visual–motor skills;
- Fine motor skills that affect the ability to complete classroom tasks, including handwriting, scissor skills, pasting, drawing, and using classroom manipulatives (e.g., math cubes, protractors, rulers);
- Self-care skills that affect the student's ability to manage clothing fasteners (e.g., zippers, buttons, snaps, shoe tying), use utensils appropriately, open small containers and packages at lunch, and manage a combination lock to access a locker;
- Gross motor skills that affect the ability to participate in games and activities in physical education class and to manage playground equipment; and
- Establishing and maintaining social relationships with same-age peers.

This chapter describes the characteristics of a student with dyspraxia to help occupational therapists better understand students with motor planning problems in schools. Evaluation techniques, intervention strategies, and suggested modifications that can be used within the classroom setting also are discussed.

69

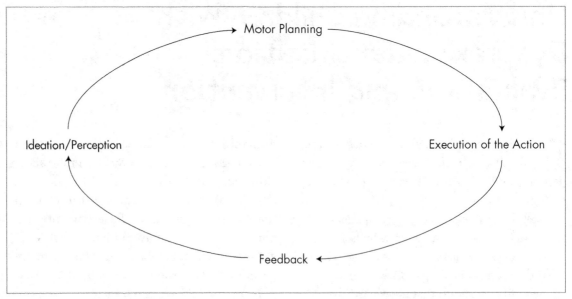

Figure 3.1. Aspects of Praxis

Graphic adapted from *Dyspraxia 5-11: A Practical Guide*, by C. Macintyre, 2001, p. 11. © 2001 by David Fulton. Adapted with permission of Fulton Publishers, www.fultonpublishers.co.uk.

Aspects of Praxis

To understand dyspraxia, aspects of praxis (Figure 3.1) first must be defined. Dr. A. Jean Ayres (1989) defined *praxis* as a "uniquely human aptitude that underlies conceptualization, planning, and execution of skilled adaptive interaction with the physical world" (as cited in Blanche & Parham 2001, p. 184). There are four aspects to praxis: ideation, motor planning, execution, and feedback.

Ideation

Ayres (1985) defined *ideation* as the cognitive process used to create an idea or concept to allow for purposeful interaction with the environment (cited in May-Benson, 2001). Liepmann (1966) described it as a process in which a person develops an idea (or a gestalt image) that consists of a purpose (or goal), an action, and ways of performing the action to meet the goal (cited in May-Benson, 2001). Both definitions describe ideation as a cognitive process that consists of developing an

idea and plan in order to complete an action and interact with the environment.

Dysfunction in ideation may or may not coincide with impaired cognitive ability and sensory integration dysfunction. In a student with significant cognitive deficits, it may be the student's inability to perceive and apply meaning to the sensory input and to the overall experience that interferes with the ability to plan motor functions. When this is the case, the student's inability to apply meaning to the experience (cognitively) affects the ability to generate a plan. May-Benson (2001) explained that the ideation process begins with an intentional process in response to both internal and external stimuli. She stated that an idea results from a cognitive awareness of the need for a goal-directed action.

For example, a child goes bowling with her family and sees a bowling ball, a bowling lane, and pins at the end of the lane. These should provide the external stimulus for the action. The internal stimulus is the child's desire to bowl with her family. The child should be able to use her previous knowledge to realize that the ball is rolled down the lane to knock down as many pins down as possible. This idea is then the basis for the process of motor planning. A student with deficits in ideation does not understand the function of the bowling ball or know what to do with it and so is unable to generate a plan. It does not occur to her that it can be picked up, that she can put her fingers in the holes, and that it can be rolled down the alley to knock down the pins.

Children with ideation deficits appear to not understand how to interact with their environment or play purposefully with toys or use objects for their intended uses. These children may wander around the room; may watch other children engage in an activity and try to imitate the movement; or may complete repetitive, nonpurposeful movements with toys or other objects (e.g., pushing cars back and forth on the floor with no intent to race one car with another, go around a race track, or drive up or down a hill).

Motor Planning

The second step in praxis is the ability to interpret the sensory information to plan for the motor response. May-Benson (2001) noted that a student with difficulties in *motor planning* is able to identify ideas and goals for play but is unable to organize a plan to achieve the goals. To motor plan, the student needs to know what he wants to do and what resources he needs to carry out the plan (Portwood, 1999). Students who have difficulty with the planning part of the process know what they want to do but do not know what resources they need to organize themselves to complete the motor part of the task.

Applying the example just presented in the ideation section to a deficit in motor planning, the student understands that she needs to pick up the ball and put her fingers in the

holes and also knows that the ball needs to be rolled down the lane to hit the pins. This student, however, does not know how to approach the lane, does not know how to hold and release the ball to roll it down the lane to hit the pins, and is unable to coordinate the stepping pattern needed to walk up to the lane and release the ball in a coordinated fashion that allows the ball to roll down the middle of the lane to hit the pins.

Execution and Feedback

Execution is the completion of the movement or the carrying out of the task. In *feedback,* the body provides sensory information to the brain and body after the movement has occurred. This helps the body make any needed adjustments for the next time the movement occurs.

If a breakdown occurs at any level in the process, the entire cycle is affected. If the body does not perceive sensory information effectively, then planning for the movement is very confusing and difficult, and thus the motor response is accurate but laborious and awkward. Feedback to the brain regarding the movement also is affected.

Definition of Dyspraxia

Cermak (1991) pointed out that health care professionals often use the terms *dyspraxia* and *motor planning* interchangeably. Numerous definitions of dyspraxia are described within the literature. The Dyspraxia Foundation defined it as "an impairment or immaturity in the organization of movement, which leads to associated problems with language, perception, and thought" (Macintyre, 2001, p. 1). Portwood (1999) stated that it is a difficulty in planning and carrying out skilled, novel motor acts in the correct sequence with the problem arising more in planning of the action than in the actual execution of the motor response.

The *Diagnostic and Statistical Manual of Mental Disorders* (American Psychiatric Association, 1994) defined criterion for diagnosis of dyspraxia (or what it refers to as a "developmental coordination disorder") as a marked impairment in motor coordination development that significantly interferes with the child's academic achievement and activities of daily living. Further, it stated that the coordination difficulties are not due to a general medical condition (e.g., cerebral palsy) and that, if the child has a cognitive or developmental delay, the motor difficulties must be in excess of those usually associated with the developmental delay to be classified as a discrepancy between ability and performance, or dyspraxia.

Ayres conducted extensive research on the relationship among sensory integration of tactile, proprioceptive, and vestibular input and motor planning. Through her research, she defined dyspraxia as

> a brain dysfunction that hinders the organization of tactile, and at times, proprioceptive (providing information from the joints and muscles) and vestibular (providing the body with information about how the body acts in relation to space) sensations, and interferes with the child's ability to motor plan. (Ayres, 1979, p. 101).

A child with dyspraxia often has very poor *tactile discrimination,* or the ability to localize touch stimuli and assign meaning to the sensation. This affects the perception of tactile information, body scheme, and overall motor planning abilities. Because the body does not take in and register the tactile sensory input effectively, dyspraxia also affects the feedback given to the body regarding the experience.

Ayres (1979) described certain types of movements (e.g., crawling or walking) that are innate and defined them as "centrally programmed movements." A child does not have to plan for centrally programmed movements; they are just a part of the typically developing nervous system. She goes on to state that, when initially learning a novel motor skill, a child has to motor plan for the movement. After the skill is learned and becomes familiar (e.g., writing the alphabet, riding a bike), the child no longer has to motor plan to complete the skill, as it comes naturally, and he or she is able to generalize the skill to related situations.

Ayres (1979) described motor planning as "one of the highest and most complex forms of function in children" that involves attention and complex integration of sensory information. She referred to it as "the bridge between the sensory motor and intellectual aspects of brain function" (p. 94). Cermak (1991) stated that a child with motor planning problems displays difficulty learning novel tasks within an environment. The child requires repeated practice to be able to complete a particular task, and when the task is learned, this performance does not generalize to similar tasks. The student must continue to learn each new task (even if it is similar to another, previously learned task) as if it is entirely new.

Neurological Background

The central nervous system consists of many structures, including the spinal cord, brain stem, cerebellum, and the cerebral hemispheres. Neurons (nerve cells) carry information to and from the brain so that the body responds to specific impulses. Sensory neurons carry a multitude of information from our body (e.g., tactile, proprioceptive, visual, auditory input) to the brain to be processed. After the brain processes the information, the motor neurons carry this information from the brain through the spinal cord to specific areas to produce a motor response. This process helps the body learn about the environment and how to interact with it.

Ayres (1979) explained that more than 80% of the nervous system is involved in processing sensory input. She stated that this complex process must work effectively if the brain is to be well organized. When the brain is well organized, this process results in effective learning and coordinated movement. As a child develops within the first few years of life, neurons begin to establish connections and interconnections. This allows more complex processing and more refined motor responses to occur (e.g., the infant goes from banging the spoon on the highchair tray to spilling the food when scooping and bringing the spoon to the mouth to being able to feed himself independently without spilling).

Connections are reinforced even as others are weaned. This allows certain movements to be reinforced, so that the child can build on these experiences and apply them to similar experiences. Thus, the movement becomes more automatic and requires less energy the next time the child needs to complete it. Portwood (1999) theorized that, in the child with dyspraxia, fewer specialized connections are reinforced, which results in the brain's cortex remaining in a state of immaturity. Because connections are not specialized, information taken in and processed remains confusing (e.g., information taken in to be processed by one limb instead is processed by all four limbs), which results in the child's motor response not being accurate or efficient and contributes to the presence of associated responses when completing motor movements (e.g., sticking tongue out or opening and closing mouth when cutting).

Role of Sensory Integration in Motor Planning

Ayres (1979) conducted extensive research in sensory integration and established an association between deficits in motor planning and the tactile, proprioceptive, and vestibular systems. She observed that, as children develop and expand their experiences, neural memories are created within the brain. These neural memories consist of all of the things experienced within an environment, including the language used, faces of people, and motor acts completed. Such experiences go into making what she defined as a person's "body percept." This body percept also is referred to as "body image" or "body scheme." The body percept consists of all of the information people need to know about their bodies. It acts on objects within the environment to perform familiar and unfamiliar body movements. Children with dyspraxia often have poor body percepts that are the result of poor tactile discrimination and poor processing of proprioceptive sensory input.

Tactile discrimination is a specific type of tactile input that is usually localized to the mouth and hands. This specific tactile input is processed at the cortex level and enables the child to respond accurately to the input. In a child with dyspraxia, the tactile information entering the system to be processed remains vague and cannot be processed in a precise way. This affects the child's ability to identify objects by touch alone (e.g., identifying the difference between a penny and a quarter when the coins are in the child's pocket) and also affects the child's ability to use tools effectively. The child may have to continue to rely on his or her sense of vision to complete tasks, including having to look at his or her feet when tying shoes or having to look down at his or her coat to engage the zipper. Poor tactile discrimination affects the child's overall body percept.

Proprioceptive input not only provides the brain with information from the joints and muscles, it also contributes to body percept by letting people know where and how their body parts are moving in space so that movements can be coordinated (Ayres, 1979). A student with dyspraxia often has difficulty processing proprioceptive input. The information he or she is receiving from his or her proprioceptors is jumbled, and the result is not being able to perform movements efficiently.

The student may overshoot or undershoot his or her efforts when completing tasks. The student may clutch his or her pencil tightly, break the lead from too much exerted force, smash a paper cup while exerting too much effort when holding it to take a drink, or easily break toys by being too rough in his or her movements. Poor processing of proprioceptive input also affects the student's ability to navigate his or her body within space. The student may bump into objects or others, trip and fall, and have difficulty managing changes in body position or moving in a coordinated way (e.g., moving from standing to sitting in a chair or on the floor, running, skipping, climbing steps to go down a slide). He or she often must rely on his or her sense of vision to help coordinate movements.

The vestibular system also plays an important role in the development of body percept. Ayres (1979) wrote that vestibular input is instrumental in the formation of the "maps" that assist in navigating body movements. The vestibular system assists in the generation of the adequate muscle tone needed to complete muscle movements. A student with dyspraxia often prefers more sedentary play as a result of having a poor body percept, which has contributed to poor balance, difficulty navigating throughout environments, and awkwardness or clumsiness with movement. The student seldom chooses to engage in movement activities. He or she may have gravitational insecurity that results in the student wanting to be grounded by having his or her feet touching the floor (e.g., not wanting to swing, go down a slide, or be picked up or thrown up in the air). A "fight-or-flight" response to the vestibular input may cause the student to overreact to such movements.

Perceptual–Motor Development as It Relates to Motor Planning

As an infant develops his or her body percept through the integration of tactile, proprioceptive, and vestibular input, he or she begins to assign meaning to his or her experiences. Perception is the cognitive understanding of the information that the senses take in to interact and understand the external world (Kranowitz, 1998). It is important to understand the distinct functions of each side of the brain and how the two sides work together to integrate information.

As shown in Table 3.1, Portwood (1999) explained that the left hemisphere processes information sequentially, processes verbal information more efficiently than the right hemisphere, and specializes in recognizing parts that make up a whole. The right side processes information simultaneously and specializes in combining parts of images to create a whole picture. The left side is more efficient in processing verbal information; the right side is better at processing visual and spatial information. The two sides must work together to form a complete picture (Portwood, 1999).

Many perceptual–motor skills are needed to help the body obtain a body percept. An infant begins to develop postural stability and mobility to be upright so that he or she can

Table 3.1. How the Left and Right Hemispheres of the Brain Process Information

Left Hemisphere	Right Hemisphere
• Processes information sequentially	• Processes information simultaneously
• More efficient at processing verbal information	• More efficient at processing visual and spatial information
• Recognizes parts that make up a whole	• Combines parts that make up a whole

Adapted from *Developmental Dyspraxia: Identification and Intervention*, by M. Portwood, 1999, p. 15. © 1999 by David Fulton. Adapted with permission of Fulton Publishers, www.fultonpublishers.co.uk.

interact and learn from objects in his or her environment. The child's ability to visually attend to objects within the environment increases. Hand preference, known as *lateralization,* is established. Through lateralization (using one side of the body), the brain establishes a dominant side for directing efficient movement on the opposite side of the body. This affects the child's ability to use his or her two hands together (bilateral integration), to interact with objects, and to cross the midline of the body to reach for and retrieve objects. Around age 8, a child begins to direct the concept of laterality outside of himself or herself. A child develops directionality, or the understanding of an external object's position in space in relationship to himself or herself (Schneck, 2001). This helps the child understand the concepts of left and right and being able to apply this not only to himself or herself but also to another person (e.g., imitating a mirror image when playing Simon Says).

Many visual–perceptual components build the foundation for higher-level language and academic skills. A child with poor visual–spatial skills often has difficulty understanding spatial concepts (in, under, on top of, over, down). This affects his or her ability to follow directions that include these terms (as is needed when playing gross motor games), to follow directions from a teacher to place objects in designated locations in the classroom, or to apply directional terms when learning to write shapes and letters.

Difficulty with visual memory (remembering visual information in both short-term and long-term memory) and visual discrimination can affect a student's ability to remember and identify letters when reading and writing. This can affect his or her reading and writing abilities, including remembering information long enough when copying from the chalkboard or from a paper positioned on his or her desk. Poor figure ground abilities can cause the student to struggle with organization skills (e.g., locating a folder within a crowded and disorganized desk), affect his or her ability to complete worksheets that are full of visual information, and may affect his or her ability to copy information from a chalkboard or a book (Case-Smith, 1996).

Causes and Incidence of Dyspraxia

Numerous theories exist on the actual causes of dyspraxia, including poor prenatal care and nutrition, birth trauma, genetics, and a failure of cells within the brain to develop and mature. How many students are affected by dyspraxia? According to Kirby (1996), almost 8%–10% of children are affected by some degree of dyspraxia. Two percent of these students are severely affected. Putting that statistic into perspective, if an average class in the United States has at least 20 students, 2 or more students could be affected. The need for teacher education on this disorder is evident. Kirby went on to note that boys are affected by the disorder four times more than are girls. However, he reported that when girls do have dyspraxia, they usually are more severely affected.

Characteristics of a Child With Dyspraxia

Portwood (1999) examined the birth histories of children with dyspraxia and found that the children demonstrated similar characteristics even as infants and toddlers. These characteristics are presented in Exhibit 3.1. Children generally are not identified as having dyspraxia until they reach school age or older, if they ever are officially diagnosed. During the school-age years, teachers, with the help of special education personnel (including occupational therapists, physical therapists, speech therapists, psychologists, and special education teachers) may identify that a student is demonstrating difficulty in completing activities in the classroom. Remember,

---

Exhibit 3.1. Early Signs of Dyspraxia: From Birth to Age 3 Years

- May be irritable, easily distressed, and difficult to comfort
- Often requires frequent adult attention due to anxiety
- May experience sleeping problems
- May experience delays in early motor milestones, including sitting, crawling, and walking
- May experience delays in expressive language development
- Has poor concentration, fleeting attention to task
- Has sensory sensitivities, including sensitivity to sounds and tactile, oral, and visual input
- May have feeding problems, including colic, milk allergies, and difficulty with independent feeding using utensils or cup
- Avoids constructional play (e.g., blocks, puzzles, pegboards).

Adapted from *Developmental Dyspraxia: Identification and Intervention*, by M. Portwood, 1999, p. 27. © 1999 by David Fulton. Adapted with permission of Fulton Publishers, www.fultonpublishers.co.uk.

however, that children affected by dyspraxia do not always have consistent profiles, so the number and severity of the characteristics may vary.

Infants with dyspraxia may or may not acquire developmental milestones at the same rate as other infants. They may be late to sit up independently and may never achieve a reciprocal crawl. Crawling requires the child to coordinate opposite extremities (right leg and left arm, left leg and right arm) in a reciprocal manner. Frequently these children scoot on their bottoms or bunny hop for early mobility. Sometimes they move directly from sitting to pulling themselves up to a stand to walking without ever crawling.

There has been research to support that infants with dyspraxia have a higher frequency of colic behavior and often have milk allergies (Portwood, 1999). This can lead to the child experiencing difficulty sleeping and result in irritable behavior. The child also has delayed language development, especially stringing words together into beginning phrases and sentences. These children may not play with toys appropriately and avoid constructional play (e.g., building blocks, puzzles, pegboards). When reviewing these char-

acteristics for a child from birth to age 3 years, it is important to keep in mind that all children naturally develop at different rates. Examining the characteristics to determine if the child's overall profile includes a variety of the items listed may assist in the early identification process and could possibly aid in providing the child with early intervention and preschool services to meet his or her individual needs.

Characteristics of a Preschool Child

Many new demands and routines are introduced to children when they enter preschool. Children must follow a daily schedule (e.g., circle time, free play period, learning center periods, snack time, story time, preparing to go home) and be able to participate in the structured activities planned by the teacher. This presents many challenges to students with dyspraxia or other motor planning conditions. The following characteristics are common among children with motor planning deficits during the preschool years (Exhibit 3.2):

- Preschool children with motor planning difficulties often struggle with following the multistep directions that accompany

---

Exhibit 3.2. Characteristics of a Preschool Child With Dyspraxia

- Is clumsy, bumps into others or objects, has difficulty managing playground equipment, is awkward when completing gross motor tasks
- Has difficulty with fine motor tasks, such as using classroom tools (e.g., writing utensils, scissors, spoons), using a consistent hand, completing bilateral tasks, crossing midline, completing art projects, and developing prewriting shapes and letter formations of own name
- Has difficulty with self-care tasks, including managing clothing fasteners, personal belongings, and eating neatly
- Avoids creative and constructional play within the classroom
- Has difficulty following multistep directions
- Has delayed language abilities, (e.g., continues to use one-word responses or short word phrases), poor auditory memory
- Has behavioral issues
- Has sensory issues, including tactile defensiveness, poor tactile discrimination, and gravitational insecurity.

Adapted from *Developmental Dyspraxia: Identification and Intervention*, by M. Portwood, 1999, p. 31. © 1999 by David Fulton. Adapted with permission of Fulton Publishers, www.fultonpublishers.co.uk.

the everyday class routine. They may understand the directions being given by an adult but may remember and complete only the first or last step in the task due to short auditory memory. For example, a student enters the school building and gets ready to start the school day. He or she must take off his or her coat and book bag, remove any needed items from the bag, place his or her take-home folder in the appropriate container, and begin to engage in the first activity of the day (e.g., free play, circle, centers).

- The number of steps required in this familiar routine already can be challenging. If the student has difficulty completing routine tasks, then it is even more difficult to complete the novel tasks introduced in the classroom each day. These new tasks may include imitating motor movements to accompany a song at circle time or completing a multistep color, cut, and paste project at the art center. The student with motor planning difficulties is able to generate an idea for a goal-directed action and knows what needs to be done to complete the action but cannot organize and sequence the steps to formulate a plan and then perform the individual steps to complete the action independently. This can lead to the child becoming easily frustrated in the classroom setting and at home.

- In the classroom, the student may gravitate to similar toys each day. He or she avoids constructional toys that involve fitting objects into designated locations (e.g., puzzles, building blocks, pegboards). Again, the student may generate the idea that he or she wants to do a puzzle and may know exactly how the puzzle pieces fit together but is unable to sequence the steps to organize a plan to complete the puzzle. The student also may avoid unstructured imaginative play (e.g., dressing up, playing house) due to poor interaction with peers, concrete thinking patterns that often limit his or her imaginative play skills, and difficulty with the self-help task of independently putting on and taking off the dress-up clothing.

Characteristics of a School-Age Child

Many changes occur when students graduate from preschool and enter elementary school. They transition to a longer school day, participate in new classes (e.g., music, physical education, computer, art), eat lunch with their peers in the lunchroom, and adjust to an academic workload that increases dramatically throughout the school-age years. During the first few years in elementary school, students will learn handwriting skills (including printing and cursive), be expected to increase their independence in completing classroom routines, and be expected to manage their personal belongings independently. The following are characteristics of a school-age student who demonstrates difficulty with motor planning (Exhibit 3.3):

- A school-age student with motor planning problems may have difficulty following a school routine that includes frequent transitions between subject areas that may involve switching classrooms. This requires the student to finish working in a timely fashion to move on to the next activity or class. He or she may appear disorganized and have difficulty bringing the correct materials to class. He or she may take longer to gather his or her materials and may lose papers or needed materials due to disorganization. The teacher may need to provide additional time for him or her at the end of a class period to organize his or her belongings and go to the locker early so that he or she can be on time to the next class.

- Handwriting instruction usually begins in kindergarten or first grade. The student with motor planning problems often demonstrates an inefficient pencil grasp and poor forearm stability when learning to write. If the student also has deficits in his or her visual–perceptual skills and understanding of spatial terms, then he or she may have trouble learning the prewriting shapes and incorporating and applying

---

Exhibit 3.3. Characteristics of a School-Age Child With Dyspraxia

- Has difficulty following school routine (including managing frequent transitions both within and between classes, organizing materials for classes, and completing tasks within designated time frame)
- Has continued difficulty following multistep tasks and multitasking
- Has continued deficits in self-care tasks required during school day (e.g., managing clothing fasteners, changing for physical education class, managing belongings, opening combination lock)
- Experiences fine motor delays (e.g., while using classroom manipulatives, scissors, rulers, protractors, compass)
- Has handwriting deficits, such as poor pencil grasp, difficulty being able to form letters of the alphabet, difficulty transitioning from manuscript to cursive, and problems with other handwriting mechanics (spacing, alignment, size of letters)
- Has difficulty with gross motor skills needed to participate in activities in physical education class or sports activities
- Has poor social skills and difficulty relating to same-age peer group (tends to gravitate toward younger children)
- Has continued behavioral concerns, including somatic complaints and resistance to coming to school due to frustration.

Adapted from *Developmental Dyspraxia: Identification and Intervention*, by M. Portwood, 1999, p. 37. © 1999 by David Fulton. Adapted with permission of Fulton Publishers, www.fultonpublishers.co.uk.

these strokes to form letters. The student often struggles to understand lined paper and to align letters within the space appropriate for the size of the letters. In addition, understanding margins and leaving adequate space between letters and words in a sentence may be an issue.

- Using classroom tools across subject areas can be problematic. The student may have difficulty working with a protractor or compass during math class and using a ruler to measure an object or draw a straight line in science. He or she also may struggle when playing an instrument (e.g., recorder) during music class. In the same way, novel gross motor tasks within physical education remain challenging. The student may be unable to follow the basic warm-up exercises and will have difficulty following the directions and remembering the rules when playing interactive games (e.g., basketball, badminton, bowling, dodgeball).

- The student with dyspraxia often cannot relate to other students of the same age or engage in reciprocal conversation about common interests and activities. Subsequently, he or she may have problems establishing good friendships with same-age peers and may be made fun of or taken advantage of by others. This can affect the student's self-concept and overall self-esteem. The student usually becomes a follower within his or her peer group. He or she may seek out children who are younger because his or her interests often are similar to those of younger children. Interacting with younger children also provides the student with motor planning problems the ability to control situations (e.g., to not engage in situations that are difficult). The child with motor planning problems may be playing with toys geared toward younger children. In addition, younger children may not make fun of a child with motor planning problems as much as older children.

As students move through elementary school and into middle and high school, the demands on students steadily increase. It is often difficult for students with motor planning problems to keep up. A student who is bright and can recognize those tasks that are challenging for him or her to complete may modify his or her own behavior to compensate for his or her deficits. Continued frustration with tasks can lead to the student exhibiting behavioral issues in the classroom. The student may complain that he or she does not feel well (e.g., headache, stomachache) so that he or she can go home. This type of anxiety can lead to the student displaying "school phobia," or not wanting to come to school each day. All of the characteristics of a student with motor planning conditions need to be considered when the educational team evaluates and designs programming for him or her.

Cognitive Profile of a Student With Dyspraxia

Gubbay (1978) stated "a child with dyspraxia has normal intelligence" (cited in Cermak, 1991). Cermak stated that the issue of using intelligence as a diagnostic criterion remains controversial. Does this mean that a student with mental retardation cannot have dyspraxia? Cermak noted that if a student's motor planning abilities are consistent with his or her cognitive and motor development, the student is not considered to have dyspraxia. A student with mental retardation would be considered to have dyspraxia only if his or her motor planning abilities are significantly below his or her performance in other areas and if the motor deficits are specifically a result of poor motor planning and not a deficit in motor skills.

To better understand the overall profile of student with dyspraxia, it is important to consider cognitive ability. A common cognitive assessment given by school psychologists to determine a student's IQ (intelligence quotient) is the Wechsler Intelligence Scale for Children (WISC; Wechsler, 1991). The WISC examines the student's ability to complete both verbal and nonverbal tasks. It reports a verbal IQ, a performance IQ, and a full-scale IQ for the student. Portwood (1999) found that similar patterns emerged in the cognitive profiles of students with dyspraxia who were administered the WISC. These students usually were found to be of average intelligence. They almost always displayed a higher verbal IQ compared with their performance IQ.

The research evidence also found that these students had difficulty completing 4 of the WISC's 11 subtests. Two of the subtests (arithmetic and digit span) were within the verbal component of the test, and two others (coding and block design) were within the performance area. In the arithmetic subtest, the student has to orally respond to mental arithmetic problems. The digit span subtest requires the student to remember a series of numbers (of increasing length) and be able to verbally repeat the numbers back to the examiner both forward and backward. Both of these verbal subtests require sustained attention by the student and the ability to remember information given orally by the examiner. In the coding subtest, the student must copy a series of symbols within a designated area that correspond to numbers. This test is timed and relies heavily on visual memory and eye–hand coordination. The block design subtest requires students to replicate a series of block designs using cubes from a two-dimensional model.

When an occupational therapist evaluates a student within a school-based setting, it is important to review the student's cognitive assessment to look for the similarities to the profile described previously. Although not every student with motor planning deficits presents this type of cognitive profile (higher verbal than performance IQ), reviewing a student's test results on the WISC, and observ-

ing this pattern may help provide insight into the student's performance on other assessment tools.

Completing an Occupational Profile

Using Developmental and Comprehensive Questionnaires

When initiating the evaluation process, the occupational therapist needs to complete an occupational profile of the student. This is done by obtaining information from the student (if possible) and from the student's teacher and parents. An *occupational profile* is defined in the *Occupational Therapy Practice Framework* (AOTA, 2002) as "information that describes the client's occupational history and experiences, patterns of daily living, interests, values, and needs" (p. 616). Completing a profile helps the therapist understand the student's current issues and problems and aids in the identification of the targeted outcome.

Obtaining information from parents about the student's birth history, acquisition of motor skills, current language skills, independence in activities of daily living, play skills, and overall emotional development helps the therapist identify if the student exhibits characteristics of dyspraxia. Information from the teacher provides insight into how the student is functioning within the educational setting, including academic skills, language and social skills, ability to complete fine motor and visual–motor tasks, ability to be independent with activities of daily living required during the school day, and gross motor skills.

Information should be gathered from all personnel involved with the student (e.g., general education teacher, special education teacher, speech-language pathologist, physical therapist, physical education teacher) to get a complete picture of how the student is managing within the school environment.

The authors of this book have developed questionnaires for this purpose, and these are included at the end of the chapter (see Appendix 3.1 and Appendix 3.2) to assist in this process. They are designed for use in an interview format between the evaluating occupational therapist and the student or the parents and educational staff. The therapist can use the results to identify specific areas that warrant further assessment.

Evaluating Occupational Performance

The *Occupational Therapy Practice Framework* (AOTA, 2002) defined *occupational performance* as "the ability to carry out activities of daily life, including activities in the areas of occupation: activities of daily living…, education, work, play, leisure, and social participation" (p. 617). When evaluating occupational performance, the student's performance skills and patterns are identified and assessed, and the context in which the performance occurs is taken into account. When evaluating a student with motor planning deficits, both formal and informal types of assessments may be used to assess a variety of skills related to the student's performance in a school setting.

Completing a Motor Screening

It is important to obtain baseline information on the student's ability to perform age-appropriate gross motor skills. Consulting the school's physical education teacher is helpful in determining if the student is able to complete the skills needed to participate in the warm-up exercises and other gross motor activities in class compared with same-age peers. Such information also is helpful in understanding the student's ability to follow directions and rules to participate in novel and routine gross motor games in physical education class. In addition, a gross motor screening to observe a student's ability to complete selected tasks is recommended.

Portwood (1999) has developed a simple motor skills screening that can be administered in less than 15 minutes. This screening examines the student's ability to complete a variety of gross motor tasks, including hopping on one foot, walking on heels and toes, walking on the insides and the outsides of the feet, and jumping. The therapist observes the student to determine if the student exhibits any associated movements (e.g., tongue movement, awkward hand movements, posturing of the body) when completing the tasks. The therapist also can observe the student to see if there are any movement patterns (e.g., one side is posturing or displaying more associated movements than the other side). This is not a tool with strict guidelines of pass or fail, and if a student performs poorly on the screening it does not mean that he or she has dyspraxia. However, the screening does provide additional information to the therapist about the student's motor performance during the evaluation process.

Using Standardized Assessments and Observations

Numerous assessments can be completed to gain further information about how a student is functioning. If issues are present in the student's ability to complete activities of daily living (e.g., dressing, managing belongings, feeding, hygiene), it may be beneficial to observe him or her engaging in these activities to determine what is preventing him or her from successfully mastering them. The Self-Care Functional Checklist (see Chapter 4) also can be used to structure observation of the student for activities conducted at school and can be used to interview the student's parents. Baseline information needs to be obtained on the student's visual–motor, visual–perceptual, and handwriting abilities if the student's parents or teachers identify concerns in these areas.

Evaluation of Visual–Motor, Visual–Perceptual, and Handwriting Skills. The Beery Developmental Test of Visual–Motor Integration (Beery, 1997) is a commonly used and well-recognized assessment that measures a student's visual–motor skills. It requires the student to copy a variety of shapes and geometric designs to help determine if the student has visual–motor deficits. Through research conducted by the authors of the test, nine basic prewriting strokes needed for letter formation have been identified: a vertical line, a horizontal line, a circle, a cross, right and left diagonal lines, a square, an X, and a triangle. The test provides developmental age equivalents for acquisition of the skills necessary to copy the individual shapes and designs. There is a short format for students ages 3 to 7 years and a long format for students ages 3 to adult.

The test also has standardized supplemental tests that measure a student's visual perception and motor coordination. They may be administered after the Beery test if it is suspected that the student has deficits in these two areas. Frequently, it is helpful to reference performance on this assessment when developing goals and short-term objectives for a student who remains unable to form prewriting strokes. These strokes may be targeted as part of an annual goal and short-term objectives on an individualized education plan (IEP).

Tests of Visual Perception. It often becomes evident after completing the motor skills questionnaires with the student's teachers and parents that visual–perceptual difficulties exist. The teacher or parents may reveal that the student has difficulty copying from the chalkboard, writing letters that remain within the lines, using scissors, completing puzzles, and navigating around people and objects. Numerous standardized tests can provide information on a student's visual–perceptual abilities.

Test of Visual–Perceptual Skills. The Test of Visual–Perceptual Skills (Nonmotor–Revised; Gardner, 1996) is a norm-referenced assessment that examines seven aspects of visual perception, including visual discrimination, visual memory, visual–spatial relationships, visual–form constancy, visual-sequential memory, visual figure ground, and visual closure. This assessment does not require motor involvement from the student to complete. The student simply points to the response on the test booklet. The test is to be used with students ranging in age from 4 years to 12 years and 11 months. The Test of Visual Perceptual Skills (Nonmotor–Upper Level) can be used with students who range in age from 13 to 19 years.

Developmental Test of Visual Perception. The second edition of the Developmental Test of Visual Perception (Hamill, Pearson, & Voress, 1993) is used with students ages 4 to 10 years. This norm-referenced assessment examines eight aspects of visual perception: eye–hand coordination, copying, spatial relations, position in space, figure ground, visual closure, visual–motor speed, and form constancy. Another version of the test, the Developmental Test of Visual Perception–Adolescent and Adult, can be used with individuals between the ages of 11 years and 74 years, 11 months.

Information obtained from any of these tests of visual perception is important when planning remediation. A student's scores within the different subtests often can guide a therapist's intervention strategies and the suggested modifications parents and teaching staff need to implement with the student to make him or her more successful in school and home environments.

Assessing Handwriting. A combination of observation and standardized assessment may be used when evaluating a student's handwriting skills (depending on the student's age). It is important to keep in mind what the student has been exposed to at different grade levels so that the assessment accurately reports his or her skills in an age-appropriate manner. For a preschool student, an occupational therapist may observe the student copying or independently drawing the prewriting shapes needed for letter formation. If the student is working on kindergarten readiness skills, the therapist also may observe the student writing his or her name and review work samples from the preschool classroom. The therapist may consider such factors as, Is the student forming letters and shapes properly, is he or she able to write their shapes and letters within a designated area (e.g., a box or line), and is he or she using left-to-right progression when writing the letters in his or her name?

When evaluating a school-age student, the occupational therapist needs to consider what handwriting curriculum the district uses (if there is a specific adopted program) or determine if a student has been exposed to numerous methods of forming letters. In a majority of school districts, students are exposed to manuscript letter formations in kindergarten and first grade. Cursive handwriting instruction may begin in second or third grade. It is inappropriate to evaluate a student on writing letters if the student has not received formalized instruction on the letter formations. The Evaluation Tool of Children's Handwriting (Amundson, 1995) requires that the student has been exposed to all of the letters (either in print or cursive) and has been using them within the classroom for at least six weeks before a handwriting assessment can be administered. The student's work samples from the classroom should be reviewed to examine the student's ability to use proper letter formation; to properly size letters; to use proper spacing between letters and words; and to use margins and write letters within the lines of lined paper, notebook paper, or on worksheets.

A student with motor planning problems often has difficulty transitioning from print to cursive writing. After becoming proficient forming letters in print, cursive instruction is introduced. Cursive handwriting requires the student to be able to recognize the letters and match them to their print equivalents, read in cursive, and remember letter formations and connect letters to write words. The occupational therapist should speak with the student's general education and special education teacher to determine what the expectations for handwriting are in the classroom.

Sometimes, even after students are exposed to cursive, students are not required to use this form of handwriting to complete classroom assignments. The teacher often will allow students to write using whichever form of handwriting they feel most comfortable using and will produce the most legible work. Other teachers place a greater emphasis on cursive handwriting and require students to complete some, if not all, assignments in cursive. Obtaining the classroom expectations from the student's teachers assists the therapist and the team in planning for intervention or modifications. A formal standardized assessment also may be needed to gain further information on the student's handwriting abilities.

Evaluation Tool of Children's Handwriting. This handwriting assessment, created by Amundson (1995), evaluates both print and cursive handwriting skills. The occupational therapist examines a student's pencil grasp to determine if it is functional for writing and studies his or her in-hand manipulation skills as they relate to pencil control. The assessment looks at common writing tasks that a student is expected to complete within a given school day. It requires the student to write the uppercase and lowercase alphabet from memory, complete a near-point and a far-point copying task, write letters and numbers as dictated by the examiner, and compose a sentence and write it on the paper. Specific scoring parameters are established to determine appropriate use of letter case, letter formation, size of letters, spacing, and alignment within the lines of the paper. The assessment also looks at the student's writing speed when completing the tasks.

Assessing Sensory Processing Skills

The student's sensory processing abilities also must be assessed. After completing the Identifying Characteristics Associated With Motor Planning Deficits Questionnaire (Appendixes 3.1 and 3.2) with the student's teacher and parents and observing the student, it may become evident that the student is displaying sensory processing issues at home, at school, or both. Completing a structured sensory assessment or informal questionnaire (see Chapter 8 for information about structured sensory assessment tools) with both the student's parents and teachers helps the therapist determine what specific sensory issues are affecting the student's ability to benefit from his or her educational programming.

Observing the student in a variety of school settings (e.g., playground, classroom, lunchroom, physical education) provides insight into how he or she is managing throughout the school day across school environments. Interviewing the student's parents offers insight into what sensory issues the student is experiencing at home (that may or may not be observed within the school setting) with regard to the toleration and participation of grooming tasks; transitions among places, people, and activities; overall activity level; sleeping habits; and whether emotional outbursts are occurring. Items to consider are

- Is the student able to independently complete multistep tasks as they apply to completing activities of daily living (e.g., getting up in the morning, taking a shower, brushing teeth, applying deodorant, comb-

ing hair, getting dressed, eating breakfast, catching the bus)?
- What type of assistance does the student require to complete these tasks?
- Does the student need visual cues (e.g., a checklist), or can he or she rely on verbal reminders and directions to complete the tasks (e.g., "Cameron, go upstairs, get your shoes and your book bag, and then put these items on")?

There are many assessment tools and options that can be used when evaluating a student with motor planning problems. A combination of observation and direct assessment using standardized tools may be needed to understand a student's overall profile. To further define what individualized areas need to be assessed, begin by having the student's parents and teachers complete the Identifying Characteristics Associated With Motor Planning Deficits Questionnaire (teacher and parent versions) found at the end of this chapter (see Appendixes 3.1 and 3.2). The results of these questionnaires provide information about the student's independence and success during his or her school day (these include behavior and attention, fine and gross motor skills, self-care skills, visual–perceptual abilities, and sensory issues). Based on the information obtained from the questionnaires, the occupational therapist can decide how to structure a classroom observation and determine which standardized assessment tools need to be administered. Potential areas to assess are
- Completion of informal questionnaires with the student's parents and teachers;
- A review of the student's cognitive profile (done through testing done by the school or a private psychologist);
- Completion of a motor screening;
- Evaluation of the student's visual–perceptual and visual–motor skills;
- Evaluation of the student's prewriting and handwriting skills;

- Observation of the student's independence activities of daily living; and
- Examination of sensory processing skills, especially tactile, proprioceptive, and vestibular processing.

Considerations for Interventions and Modifications

The final step is planning and implementing interventions to target performance skill deficits and putting modifications into place in both the classroom setting and in the home to increase the student's success. Keep in mind that a student with motor planning problems often has difficulty across performance domains, including with gross and fine motor skills, language development, social skills, activities of daily living, and academic tasks. These deficits can affect the student's ability to complete expected tasks at school and at home. An occupational therapist needs to work collaboratively with the educational team and the student's parents to be consistent in the terminology and methodologies used in the intervention process. Students with dyspraxia need consistency, and the therapist can stress this concept. The therapist can provide intervention strategies and suggest recommended classroom modifications to be incorporated into the student's IEP to help the student be successful within the classroom.

Assisting With Attention and Organization Skills

The teacher must ensure that the student is seated in the front of the classroom facing the chalkboard so that he or she does not have to turn to see the chalkboard. This will limit the number of distractions in front of the student when he or she is looking at or copying information from the chalkboard. The student also may benefit from being positioned near the teacher's desk. The teacher will be better able to see the student to determine when he or she may need additional assistance or clarification. The teacher should not position the student in an area that is noisy or has frequent distractions (e.g., by a doorway or the pencil sharpener). If the student is distracted easily, he or she may benefit from having a separate quiet area within the classroom where he or she can sit when completing class work. This may include providing the student with a study carrel to block visual distractions.

Make certain that the student is seated in a functional position. Pay attention to desk height and the support provided for his or her feet. If the student slides forward in his or her seat, which results in a posterior pelvic tilt position, a piece of nonskid material (dycem or shelf liner) or a Movin' Sit cushion (Gymnic Line: The Way to Move, Ledraplastic S.p.a., Via Brigata Re nr. 1, 33010 Osoppo (UD), Italy) can be attached to the chair to prevent this position in the chair.

The student may continue to struggle with organizing his or her materials and accessing the appropriate materials in a timely fashion to transition between classes. One or more of the following may be helpful:

- *Color coding:* Matching the color of the textbook cover with the corresponding folder can help the student locate items by subject area.
- *Use of resealable plastic bags:* Having the student fit his or her folder and book in a large, resealable plastic bag (one bag can be used for each subject area, and the bags can be labeled for easy recognition) can help the student retrieve the correct materials when transitioning to the next subject.
- *Use of binders, accordion folders, and portfolios:* Using a binder, accordion folder, or portfolio that contains individual folder compartments for each subject can help older students who are changing classrooms for different subjects. The folders or

compartments can be labeled or color-coded so that the student knows where to put papers for each subject.

- *Weekly cleaning of desk and locker:* Cleaning out the student's desk and locker weekly, to help him or her be organized for the next week, can help the student with motor planning problems. Being organized can reduce the amount of time it takes the student to locate materials needed for class. A peer or the teacher can assist the student, and incentives (e.g., extra recess, free time in the classroom) can be used for the student if his or her locker remains organized and clean throughout the week.

Allowing for Additional Time

Students may require additional time to complete tasks, whether it is a handwriting task or retrieving needed materials from their cubby or locker. Teachers can allow additional time (within reason) to complete classroom tasks.

Providing Additional Cueing

Because of poor auditory memory and a greater reliance on visual skills, the student with motor planning problems benefits from having directions repeated and also from visual cues. These cues include labeling common areas or objects in classroom, teaching the student to self-talk, using a picture schedule to define the student's day, using visual checklists with daily routines listed on them or step-by-step directions for how to complete an assignment, and establishing a classroom routine.

Repeating Directions. The student with motor planning problems may need directions repeated for routine or novel activities. The student often may appear at the teacher's desk directly after the directions were given to clarify the expectations of the assignment. The teacher needs to understand that the student is not being defiant and should repeat the directions simply and clearly to allow the student to better understand them.

Labeling Objects and Common Items. Labeling common objects or areas (e.g., the student's desk, locker, or cubby; the restroom; the homework basket) provides the student with a visual cue to reference and may allow him or her to not have to ask the teacher where particular items need to be placed or where a specific area is located.

Teaching the Student to Self-Talk. The student also will benefit from being taught to "self-talk," a method that may prove helpful when he or she is presented with a novel or a familiar task in the classroom or at home. The teacher or parent provides the directions and then encourages the student to repeat them in the correct order out loud before completing the task. After applying this intervention technique repeatedly, the goal is to have the student use this rehearsal strategy automatically to follow directions and complete tasks.

Using Visual Checklists. A dry-erase board, laminated index cards, or a journal can be used at the student's desk or locker to list the steps of the task or activity. The student reads the steps and then checks them off once they are completed. This can be applied to a variety of classroom tasks, including a morning routine—for example, (1) Take off your coat and book bag. (2) Take the materials out of your book bag. (3) Hang up your coat and book bag. (4) Sit at your desk. (5) Begin the morning work—or a multistep activity—for example, (1) Color in the worksheet. (2) Cut out the shapes on the worksheet. (3) Glue the items onto a separate piece of paper. (4) Turn the project in to the teacher.

Establishing a Classroom Routine. Students with motor planning problems like to have predictable environments in which they can learn the routine and be successful.

Providing structure and consistency in the classroom environment helps alleviate the student's anxiety because he or she can learn and follow the classroom routine.

Using Handwriting Interventions and Modifications

Encouraging Hand Preference. The student may still have difficulty establishing hand dominance. If he or she continues to switch hands to complete tasks at the end of the preschool years and into kindergarten, the teaching staff and parents need to determine which hand the student appears to use more frequently. They can monitor which hand the student uses to initially pick up objects and hold feeding utensils. He or she should be encouraged to use whatever hand results in the most success. This may include consistently positioning materials on the apparent dominant side and verbally cueing the student to reposition the materials to the dominant hand if he or she is observed to switch.

Using Pencil Grips. The student with motor planning problems can use a nonfunctional grip when holding a writing utensil. Because of poor tactile feedback, he or she may continue to use all of his or her fingers around the shaft of a pencil to gain stability. A variety of pencil grippers can be tried to determine if any of them help the student have more success. Breaking crayons in half and using shortened pencils (e.g., the small pencils used to fill out golf scorecards or lottery cards) may help the student use a three-finger grasp, as these do not have a long shaft that the student can wrap his or her fingers around. The student can use a Handiwriter™ (HandiThings, P.O. Box 41, New Melle, MO 63365; 636-398-4081), a device that promotes a three-finger grasp (tripod grasp) by positioning the pencil into the child's web space and allowing him or her to

hold on to an object with the ring and fifth fingers.

All of these strategies can be tried to determine if they help the student change his or her grasp to a more functional position on the writing utensil. If the student's grasp is not changing, instruct him or her to use the "monk's grasp," a modified yet functional way to hold the writing utensil that may provide further stability (see Figure 3.2). The student stabilizes the pencil between his or her index and middle fingers with both fingers placed on top of the utensil in opposition to the thumb. The difference between a tripod and monk's grasp is that, instead of the utensil resting between the thumb and index fingers, it is positioned between the index and middle fingers.

Stabilizing the Student's Forearm. "Flying forearms" are common among students with motor planning problems. This condition often accompanies a poor pencil grasp and the use of whole-arm movements when writing. A student may benefit from being allowed to complete assignments in different positions in the classroom (e.g., prone on the floor to allow for weight bearing through the shoulders and stability at the forearm). He or she also may benefit from using a slant board that provides a vertical surface on which to rest the forearm when writing. Weighted wrist cuffs can provide additional proprioceptive input to the student to keep the forearm stabilized.

Instructing on Letter Formations. Students with motor planning problems often have difficulty with visualization skills, including remembering how to form letters of the alphabet. The student may benefit from daily reinforcement in practicing letter formations for 10 to 15 minutes (either at school or home) to write the letters using proper letter formation.

Multisensory Instruction. A variety of multisensory techniques can help the student

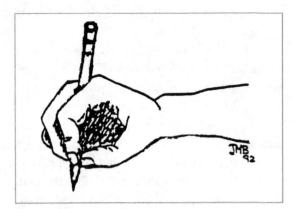

Figure 3.2. Adapted Tripod Grip or "Monk's Grasp."

From *Loops and Other Groups: A Kinesthetic Writing System,* by M. Benbow, 1990, San Antonio, TX: Therapy Skillbuilders. Copyright 1990 by Harcourt. Reprinted with permission.

visualize letter formations and implant the formations into his or her motor memory. Techniques include writing letters in the air, in shaving cream, or hair gel; using a paint bag; writing in a sand tray; using rainbow writing (having the student trace over letters numerous times using different colors of chalk, crayons, paint, or markers); and using the chalkboard or dry-erase board in combination with paper-and-pencil tasks.

Simple and Consistent Terminology. Directional concepts (up, down, around, left, right, across, over) involved in teaching letter formations may be difficult for students with motor planning conditions to understand. Keep any terminology used simple and consistent among all people working with the student on writing (e.g., parents, teachers, child care providers). Occupational therapists can collaborate with the teacher and speech therapist regarding the directional terms used so that all team members can reinforce them.

Visual Model. A visual model may need to be used by students with motor planning problems as a reference for letter formation. Individual letter strips are available in both print and cursive and can be placed on the student's desk for easy reference.

Handwriting Programs. For students who continue to have difficulty learning the formation of letters using the curriculum put in place by the school district, an alternative handwriting program may need to be explored. A program like the Sensible Pencil (Becht, 2000) provides limited terminology and a consistent format and worksheets for learning prewriting shapes, lowercase and uppercase letters, and numbers. The program groups letters that use similar strokes and combines these letters into individual mastery tests. The student must master the letters within the mastery tests before moving on to the next set of letters. This not only benefits the student by providing daily reinforcement of given letters and providing smaller steps to mastery, it also benefits the special education staff (including the occupational therapist) by not requiring the team have the student master all 52 letters of the alphabet in an objective in the student's IEP.

Transitioning to Cursive Handwriting. Sometimes it seems that, as soon as a student gains success with print writing, cursive instruction begins. This often is a difficult transition because a new language accompanied by new motor movements are being introduced. To write individual letters, students must be able to recognize the cursive letters to their print equivalents, be able to read the cursive letters when they are combined to form words and sentences, and be able to understand the terminology used to describe the formations to be able to write the individual letters. Occupational therapists and teachers stress that letters need be formed from top to bottom when printing, but a majority of cursive handwriting programs teach cursive letters starting from bottom to top so that the letters can be connected. This can be a confusing concept. For students taught a "ball-and-stick" method to forming manuscript letters, writing letters with continuous stroke (as is required in cursive) becomes difficult. The student may struggle with writing letters like a, b, d, p, and q using one stroke instead of two. They also may have difficulty connecting and bridging letters together.

The educational team needs to decide if a student should be required to learn and write in cursive. The team can expose the student to cursive by working on the letters in his or her name to determine if he or she understands the formations. After observing the level of mastery, the team can decide whether to continue to teach the student all letters of the alphabet or to allow the student to continue printing.

Alternative programs, including *Loops and Other Groups* (Benbow, 1990) and *Handwriting Without Tears* (Olsen, 2000), can be attempted to see if the student is more successful with a different curriculum. If it is determined that he or she is becoming frustrated by cursive and continues to struggle with forming the letters, then the team can choose the option of focusing on the student's cursive signature only and helping him or her learn to read cursive handwriting.

Sizing, Spacing, and Alignment. Students may continue to struggle with writing letters in the correct size for the letter case, providing spaces between letters and words, and aligning letters on the baseline of paper. Many paper modifications and strategies exist to help the student organize his or her writing on paper.

Type of Paper Used. Often in the lower grades, varying sizes of lined paper are used. Students are now expected to write in a daily journal as early as kindergarten and first grade. These journals usually are only a spiral-bound notebook of wide-ruled notebook paper. This type of paper can be confusing for young students, especially those with motor planning problems, because there are no clear lines to differentiate the sizes between upper-

and lowercase letters. Older students may continue to struggle with writing on notebook paper. Taping or gluing a sheet of lined paper into a student's notebook may help him or her organize letters within the lines, because he or she is not expected to write on notebook paper. If the student is having difficulty aligning math problems, have him or her try using graph paper, or allow him or her to turn the notebook paper vertically to provide columns.

Highlighting. A great visual cue, highlighting the baseline on lined paper helps students who have difficulty aligning letters in the lines. Skipping lines on notebook paper is suggested for a student who writes large, which allows for additional room between lines for easier readability. For students who continue to write large, highlighting every other line on notebook paper defines the space to write within.

Box Technique. Students who continue to struggle with understanding the size and position of letters (difference between uppercase and lowercase letters or tail vs. tall lowercase letters) on lined paper or notebook paper can be given boxes to write letters in. This helps students define the size and the position of the letters in the lines. Boxes can be drawn for individual letters, or one box can be drawn for each word. This technique works only when the teacher or occupational therapist can predict what the student is writing (e.g., spelling words or copied information from the chalkboard). When the student is composing work, another technique such as highlighting may need to be used.

Margins of Paper. When the student demonstrates difficulty in the use of margins on paper, providing a visual or tactile cue (e.g., highlighting margins, placing stickers or green and red dots at the margins) can create a better understanding of when the student needs to move to the next line to continue writing.

Providing Reduced Written Assignments, Oral Responses, and Additional Time

For the student who has continued difficulty copying information from the chalkboard or who writes at a very slow pace, the educational team needs to determine if he or she should have modified written assignments. The student also could be presented with options to decrease the amount of written work, including receiving copies of class notes, providing oral responses on tests that require extended answers, or having a scribe available for lengthier written assignments in the class. The student still has to generate the correct answers or the thoughts but can orally present the material for a scribe to put into written form.

Teaching Keyboarding Skills

For students who continue to struggle with writing (both with formation and writing speed), teaching keyboarding skills during the elementary years is a proactive way to provide another means of legible written output. Many typing tutor programs are available that move students progressively through lessons to learn proper keyboarding techniques. Some students may demonstrate difficulty coordinating all of their fingers to perform the traditional "home row" technique of typing.

Students still can be more efficient and successful if instructed on keyboard placement and encouraged to use both index fingers to press keys on the corresponding sides of the keyboard. Once the student meets the criteria within the lessons of the typing tutor program, he or she can begin to type selected assignments in the classroom. The student can use an Alphasmart (Alphasmart Inc., 973 University Avenue, Los Gatos, CA 95032), a laptop computer, or a traditional computer, depending on the assignment and setting. With repeated practice throughout the week and the opportunity to use the keyboard, the student's accuracy and speed with typing can increase.

Assisting With Self-Help Skills

Managing Clothing Fasteners. When managing fasteners on clothing (e.g., buttons, zippers, snaps, riveted buttons, shoe tying), students may benefit from interventions that target these skills at school and at home. A student is presented with natural times throughout the day to practice clothing fasteners, including after using the restroom or when changing for physical education class. At these times the teacher or assistant can monitor his or her success and can provide assistance if needed.

The student also may benefit from occupational therapy services to work on this skill. The therapist can look at what is preventing the student from mastering these skills (e.g., poor bilateral skills, inability to complete in-hand manipulation tasks, poor visual attention) and provide intervention or adapt methods to manage the fasteners. The therapist can educate the student's teachers and parents on the method being taught or modifications needed so that all adults involved in the learning process are consistent.

Prioritizing fasteners to master usually proves more successful for the student. The occupational therapist can collaborate with the student's parents to determine which fasteners need to be addressed first (e.g., a zipper on a coat worn three seasons out of the year). Once the student masters this fastener, another can be introduced (e.g., buttons on pants). Parents need to be informed about the benefits of limiting the variety of fasteners that the student uses each day. By doing this and focusing on mastering one fastener at a time, the student can feel successful for the individual accomplishments made instead of feeling overwhelmed. If the child is older and has received intervention on managing fasteners but continues to be unable to perform the task, the educational team (including the student's parents) needs to determine if modifications to his or her clothing are needed (e.g., Velcro® or slide shoes, elastic pants, pullover shirts and jackets).

Opening Containers. Occupational therapists can educate parents on appropriate types of containers to send the student's belongings in so that he or she can manage them independently. This includes the student's lunch box, food and drink packages and containers, and art box or pencil case. Using containers that are easy to open but secure are good options for food items. The student also may be able to keep a pair of scissors in his or her lunch bag (permission must be obtained from the school) to open difficult packages. Another option is to have the parent cut a small hole in the package to allow the student to open it independently.

Managing Lunch Money and Tray. The occupational therapist also needs to look at the coin purse or wallet the student uses for lunch money. Sometimes it is difficult for a student to manage the fasteners on small wallets and access the money in a timely fashion. The student may not exhibit the in-hand manipulation skills needed to get the money out of the coin purse. Walking through the lunch line and balancing the lunch tray as food items are added to it and then carrying it to the table without spilling anything also may be difficult for a student to manage. The teacher can position the student closer to the end of the lunch line so that he or she does not hold it up. Some schools use styrofoam lunch trays, which are not stable. If this is the case, the student may need to use a plastic tray to carry to the table to avoid spilling. In addition, he or she may need instruction on how to hold the tray to provide increased stability and support.

Managing the Locker or Cubby. A student with motor planning problems benefits from having his or her locker or cubby positioned at the end of the row. This provides more room and prevents him or her from bumping into other students or their belongings. Some students have lockers that require them to manage a combination lock. Remembering the code and performing the precise movements needed to access the code can be difficult, and the student may benefit from having the code written down to recall if he or she forgets (e.g., in an assignment pad or in his or her desk). Highlighting the individual notches on the student's combination lock helps him or her know where to start and stop when performing the code. If the student still is unable to manage the combination lock, a key lock or number lock can be tried. When using a key lock, the student needs to have a consistent place to keep the key to avoid losing it. The number lock only requires that the student align a series of three numbers instead of having to manage all of the steps required with a combination lock. Both of these locks allow for less motor movement to open the locker.

Assisting With Gross Motor Skills

Students with motor planning problems often struggle with playground equipment and following exercises and playing games in physical education class. They often are the last chosen to be on teams when playing a sports activity. Studies have shown (e.g., Portwood, 1999) that working with students with motor planning problems on daily exercise programs can help them over time become more coordinated and able to follow tasks in physical education class.

These activities increase the student's overall body awareness, bilateral coordination, timing and rhythm, eye–hand coordination, imitation skills, and ability to follow directional terms. They can be conducted when the student is in preschool and during the school-age years and may include climbing through a tunnel, walking on a balance beam, riding a tricycle or bike, balancing on wobble boards, managing an obstacle course, throwing a ball to a designated target, and hitting a ball with a bat.

These activities can be incorporated into the student's occupational therapy treatment session, sensory plans (if needed), physical education class or adapted physical education class, and a home program. Please see Portwood (1999) for a program description.

Preteaching Gross Motor Skills. Another intervention strategy is to have the student meet with the physical education teacher before having physical education class. This enables the teacher to preteach the games or gross motor skills focused on that week in class. The teacher also can provide the student's parents with information on what activities will be conducted so that they can practice with the student at home. This strategy has proven successful for many students with motor planning difficulties, as it provides them with an opportunity to learn and practice the skill before having to complete it with peers. It is a good way to support the student in his or her self-esteem and self-image.

Programming for the Student's Sensory Needs. After completing a sensory assessment and determining that a student requires a sensory plan during the school day, appropriate activity suggestions should be given to classroom staff to incorporate daily into the student's schedule. The student often has a high activity level and a limited attention span. He or she also can become easily overwhelmed and may "shut down" when tasks become too difficult. Providing calming or alerting strategies during the day can help the student be better organized when attending to classroom tasks. It also can provide a "break" between work tasks when he or she shows signs of frustration.

Ensure that the activities in the sensory plan are at the student's level so that they can be successfully completed. This provides students with a sense of accomplishment and something to look forward to when completing activities. Please refer to Chapter 8 for sensory strategies that can be implemented in a school setting.

The teaching staff, with the support of the occupational therapist, can determine which activities to suggest that the student completes at certain times during the school day. The team can collect informational data to determine if the activities help the student better attend to tasks.

Summary and Conclusion

This chapter has given background information and a description of dyspraxia. The characteristics of a student with dyspraxia and the areas to consider during the evaluation process have been reviewed. Treatment interventions and suggested modifications have been discussed. The educational team needs to treat each child with motor planning deficits individually. Each student presents unique and individualized needs that must be supported and programmed for throughout his or her educational career. Providing appropriate interventions and modifications as needed helps alleviate the student's anxiety and helps promote success in all areas related to his or her school day.

References

American Occupational Therapy Association. (2002). Occupational therapy practice framework: Domain and process. *American Journal of Occupational Therapy, 56,* 609–639.

American Psychiatric Association. (1994). *Diagnostic and statistical manual of mental disorders* (4th ed.). Washington, DC: Author.

Amundson, S. J. (1995). *Evaluation tool of children's handwriting.* Homer, AK: OT Kids.

Ayres, A. J. (1979). *Sensory integration and the child.* Los Angeles, CA: Western Psychological Services.

Ayres, A. J. (1985). *Developmental dyspraxia and adult onset apraxia*. Torrance, CA: Sensory Integration International.

Becht, L. C. (2000). *Sensible pencil*. Birmingham, AL: EBSCO Curriculum Materials.

Beery, K. E. (1997). *The Beery–Buktenica Developmental Test of Visual Motor Integration* (4th ed., rev.). Parsippany, NJ: Modern Curriculum Press.

Benbow, M. (1990). *Loops and other groups: A kinesthetic writing system*. San Antonio, TX: Therapy SkillBuilders.

Blanche, E. I., & Parham, E. D. (2001). Praxis and organization of behavior in time and space. In S. S. Roley, E. I. Blanche, & R. C. Schaaf (Eds.), *Sensory integration with diverse populations* (pp. 89–108). San Antonio, TX: Therapy Skill-Builders.

Case-Smith, J. (1996). *Occupational therapy for children* (3rd ed.). St. Louis, MO: Mosby.

Cermak, S. A. (1991). Somatodyspraxia. In A. G. Fisher, E. A. Murray, & A. C. Bundy (Eds.), *Sensory integration theory and practice* (pp. 137–165). Philadelphia: F. A. Davis.

Gardner, M. F. (1996). *Test of Visual–Perceptual Skills* (nonmotor, rev.). Hydesville: California Psychological and Educational Publications.

Gubbay, S. S. (1978). The management of development dyspraxia. *Developmental Medicine and Child Neurology, 20,* 451–454.

Hammill, D., Pearson, N., & Woress, J. (1993). *Developmental Test of Visual Perception* (2nd ed.). Austin, TX: Pro-Ed.

Kirby, A. (1996). *Dyspraxia: The hidden handicap*. London: Souvenir Press.

Kranowitz, C. S. (1998). *The out-of-sync child: Recognizing and coping with sensory integration dysfunction*. New York: Skylight Press.

Macintyre, C. (2001). *Dyspraxia 5-11: A practical guide*. London: David Fulton.

May-Benson, T. (2001). A theoretical model of ideation in praxis. In S. S. Roley, E. I. Blanche, & R. C. Schaff (Eds.), *Sensory integration with diverse populations* (pp. 89–108). San Antonio, TX: Therapy SkillBuilders.

Olsen, J. Z. (2001). *Handwriting without tears* (8th ed.). Potomac, MD: Author.

Portwood, M. (1999). *Developmental dyspraxia identification and intervention: A manual for parents and professionals*. London: David Fulton.

Schneck, C. M. (2001). Visual perception. In J. Case-Smith (Ed.), *Occupational therapy for children* (4th ed., pp. 382–411). St. Louis, MO: Mosby.

Wechsler, D. (1991). *Wechsler Intelligence Scale for Children* (3rd ed.). San Antonio, TX: Psychological Corporation.

Appendix 3.1.
Identifying Characteristics Associated With Motor Planning Deficits
Parent Questionnaire

Student's Name _____   Student's Date of Birth _____

Name of Person Completing This Form _____   Student's Grade _____

Relationship to Student _____   Date of Completion _____

I.   Developmental History

1.   Were there any complications during the labor or delivery of your child? _____
_____
_____
_____

2.   At what stage of the pregnancy was your baby delivered (e.g., 34 weeks)? _____

3.   What was your child's birthweight? _____

4.   Were there any concerns immediately after the birth of your child (e.g., low Apgar scores)? _____
_____
_____
_____

5.   Were there any feeding or weight gain issues when your child was a baby (e.g., allergies, poor sucking ability, poor weight gain, colic, lactose intolerance)? _____
_____
_____
_____

6.   Was your child a good or a poor sleeper (i.e., did or did not sleep through the night)? _____
_____

7.   Was your child difficult to comfort when upset? _____
_____

8.   Describe your child's activity level as a baby. _____
_____
_____

9.   At what age did your child achieve the following motor milestones?

    • Sitting independently _____

    • Crawling _____

    • Walking _____

(continued)

10. At what age did your child develop language?

  • One word _____

  • Simple phrases _____

11. At what age was your child toilet trained? (If delayed, please explain.)_____

_____

_____

Other Areas to Consider:

II. **Overall Behavior**

Answer Yes or No; if Yes, please describe. Does your child:

1. Become easily frustrated? _____

    _____

2. Have outbursts of uncontrolled behavior? _____

    _____

3. Do better with a structured routine?_____

    _____

4. Have difficulty with organization skills? _____

    _____

5. Have difficulty following directions or following rules? _____

    _____

6. Need to change activities frequently or do something that someone else is doing?_____

    _____

7. Need immediate gratification? _____

    _____

8. Have difficulty taking turns with others? _____

    _____

9. Have difficulty forming relationships, making friends, or being accepted by peers? _____

    _____

10. Complain of physical problems (e.g., headache, stomachache)? _____

    _____

11. Have immature social interests?_____

    _____

12. Try to control situations? _____

    _____

13. Display a heightened sensitivity to sensory input (e.g., to touch, smell, sounds)? _____

    _____

III. Fine Motor and Self-Care Skills

1. At what age did your child establish hand dominance? What is your child's dominant hand? _____

_____

2. Does your child participate in constructional or building activities (e.g., puzzles, building blocks)? _____

_____

3. Does your child have difficulty manipulating small objects? _____

_____

4. Does your child have difficulty grasping and managing a writing utensil? _____

_____

5. Does your child have difficulty completing tasks that require both hands working together (e.g., stringing beads, lacing and managing fasteners)? _____

_____

6. Does your child have difficulty using scissors to cut paper? _____

_____

7. Does your child create immature drawings compared to other children of the same age? _____

_____

8. Is your child a messy eater?_____

_____

9. Does your child have difficulty using eating utensils appropriately (e.g., stabs food with fork, scoops with a spoon, cuts food using a fork and knife together)? _____

_____

10. Does your child have constipation issues? _____

_____

11. Does your child have difficulty dressing independently? Does your child assist with dressing when not dressing independently?_____

_____

12. Does your child have difficulty accurately orienting clothing to put it on the correct way?_____

_____

13. Does your child have difficulty tying shoes? _____

_____

IV. Gross Motor Skills

1. At what age did your child begin walking? Did your child walk late? _____

_____

(continued)

2. Can your child jump up, clearing both feet off of the ground? _____

_____

3. Does your child fall easily? Does he or she seem fearful of movement? _____

_____

4. Does your child appear uncoordinated or clumsy? _____

_____

5. Does your child have difficulty maneuvering on the playground or gross motor equipment? _____

_____

6. Does your child have difficulty balancing on one foot? _____

_____

7. Is your child able to ride a bike? Does he or she have difficulty pedaling the bike? _____

_____

8. Does your child dislike climbing (e.g., on furniture, playground equipment)? _____

_____

9. Does your child have difficulty with reciprocal movements (e.g., alternating arm and leg movements, climbing steps)? _____

_____

10. Does your child bump into objects or other people when walking? _____

_____

V. Visual–Perceptual Skills

Answer Yes or No; if Yes, please describe. Does your child:

1. Have difficulty visually tracking a moving object (e.g., a ball being thrown to him or her)? _____

_____

2. Have difficulty with identifying background from foreground (e.g., bumps into objects, unable to find the "hidden pictures" in books, unable to find something in a crowded drawer)? _____

_____

3. Have difficulty with visual–spatial skills (e.g., completing puzzles, placing letters on the writing lines, spacing between words in a sentence during handwriting activities)? _____

_____

4. Prefer to print (even after being exposed to cursive instruction in the classroom)? _____

_____

5. Mix letter cases when writing (e.g., combine using uppercase and lowercase letters within words)?

_____

_____

(continued)

6. Have poor spacing between letters and words when writing? _____

_____

7. Have difficulty writing legibly?_____

_____

8. Write at a slow pace?_____

_____

VI. Language and Auditory Memory

1. Does your child have poor articulation when talking?_____

_____

2. Does your child have poor short-term auditory memory, or ability to follow a single or multistep direction after it is given? _____

_____

3. Does your child require additional time to process information (i.e., takes a while to understand and respond to what is being asked)?_____

_____

4. Does your child visually watch others for cues (i.e., to see what they are doing for him or her to complete the same task)?_____

_____

Questionnaire compiled by Lynne Pape, MEd, OTR/L, with information referenced from Developmental Dyspraxia, Identification and Intervention *by Madeleine Portwood, 1999.*

Appendix 3.2.
Identifying Characteristics Associated With Motor Planning Deficits
Teacher Questionnaire

Name of Student _____ Teacher_____

Date of Birth_____ Age_____

Grade_____ Date _____

I. Classroom Behavior

Yes　No　　Does the child have difficulty:

__ __　　1. Attending or concentrating

__ __　　2. Following directions (2–3-step task)

__ __　　3. Adapting to a more structured classroom routine

__ __　　4. Staying focused

__ __　　5. Practicing organizational skills

__ __　　6. Sequencing tasks

__ __　　7. Completing tasks within an allotted time

__ __　　8. Initiating work when a direction has been given

Comments:

_____

_____

_____

_____

II. Social–Emotional Behavior

Yes　No　　Does the child:

__ __　　9. Get easily frustrated or distressed

__ __　　10. Complain of physical problems (e.g., headache, stomachache)

__ __　　11. Display outbursts of uncontrollable behavior

__ __　　12. Need immediate gratification

__ __　　13. Display a high level of activity

Yes　No　　Social–Emotional Behavior (continued):

__ __　　14. Have difficulty forming relationships with classmates

__ __　　15. Act immature

__ __　　16. Have a poor self-concept and low self-esteem

__ __　　17. Try to manipulate and control situations

Comments:

_____

_____

_____

_____

III. Gross Motor Skills

Yes　No　　Does the child:

__ __　　18. Appear clumsy or awkward with movement, falls easily

__ __　　19. Have evident difficulties in physical education class

__ __　　20. Have difficulty using equipment along with motor skills (e.g., dribbling a ball, jumping rope, hitting a baseball)

__ __　　21. Have difficulty playing on the playground equipment

Comments:

_____

_____

_____

_____

(continued)

IV. Fine Motor Skills

Yes   No   Does the child:

___ ___   22. Avoid activities that require building/construction (e.g., blocks, LEGOs™)

___ ___   23. Have difficulty managing tools and manipulating scissors, pencils, utensils, math cubes

___ ___   24. Have difficulty writing legibly

___ ___   25. Prefer to print (even after being formally instructed in cursive)

___ ___   26. Mix cases when printing

___ ___   27. Have problems using the mouse on the computer

Comments:

_____

_____

_____

_____

V. Visual–Perceptual/Visual–Motor Skills

Yes   No   Does the child have difficulty with:

___ ___   28. Placing letters and numbers on the lines or within a designated area

___ ___   29. Providing adequate space between letters and words

___ ___   30. Drawing tasks

___ ___   31. Completing worksheets with a lot of visual information

___ ___   32. Completing puzzles

___ ___   33. Walking around people or objects

Comments:

_____

_____

_____

_____

VI. Self-Care Skills

Yes   No   Does the child have difficulty:

___ ___   34. Managing fasteners

___ ___   35. Orienting clothing/coat to put it on

___ ___   36. Eating neatly

___ ___   37. Managing a combination lock (if applicable)

Comments:

_____

_____

_____

_____

VII. Language/Auditory Memory

Yes   No   Does the child:

___ ___   38. Have articulation problems

___ ___   39. Have difficulty understanding spatial terms (i.e., on, behind, in front of)

___ ___   40. Have poor auditory memory (following 2–3-step directions)

___ ___   41. Have difficulty with more abstract concepts and language

___ ___   42. Please describe the student's areas of academic difficulty (e.g., math, language arts)_____

_____

_____

_____

_____

Checklist compiled by Lynne Pape, MEd, OTR/L, with information referenced from Developmental Dyspraxia, Identification and Intervention *by Madeleine Portwood, 1999.*

Activities of Daily Living: Evaluation and Intervention

4

The *Occupational Therapy Practice Framework* (American Occupational Therapy Association [AOTA], 2002) includes activities of daily living (ADLs) as one of its primary performance areas. Achieving independence in self-care and instrumental activities of daily living (IADLs) is fundamental for a student's independence at home and at school. Self-care skills in a school setting include feeding, dressing, and hygiene. IADLs include tasks that students are expected to perform in school, such as managing personal belongings, participating during lunch and snack time, and managing items in the school environment (e.g., getting items out of the desk).

From the time students enter the school building in the morning until they leave at the end of the day, they are expected to participate in the educational program and manage a variety of other tasks critical to their success and independence. These may include opening school or gym locks and lockers, taking off coats and boots and putting them in a designated area, and removing items from book bags and folders. Students also are expected to perform a variety of additional tasks, such as

- At lunch or snack time, managing lunch boxes, money or tickets, and lunch trays; opening food and drink packages and containers; and using utensils;
- Managing clothing and fasteners when using the restroom or changing for physical education class;
- Washing hands before snack time, during art class, or after using the restroom; and
- Sharpening pencils or getting a drink.

A student who is unable to complete these tasks independently may have to rely on another student or an adult for assistance. This can adversely affect the student's self-esteem, ability to develop peer relationships, and overall level of independence. A dependency, or "learned helplessness," on adult support may be created that can interfere with the peer relationships that are a natural part of school.

Numerous factors affect students' abilities to achieve independence in self-care-related tasks, including students' level of motivation, their cognitive level in relation to their ability to complete self-care tasks, and their overall developmental level in relation to the expectations of the tasks. Other factors are overall physical status (e.g., whether the student has a physical disability that might affect his or her ability to achieve independence) and the family's expectations and desire to have their child become self-sufficient.

The role of school-based occupational therapists is to help identify areas of concern in the performance of self-care and IADL skills. This role extends to helping students function within the context of their daily routine. This chapter describes the overall skills needed to acquire self-care and IADLs. The developmental ages for the acquisition of specific self-care tasks and the prerequisite skills needed for them are presented to help readers understand the foundation needed for the development of these skills.

School-based occupational therapists need to evaluate self-care tasks, and this chapter includes descriptions of both formal and informal assessments. Service delivery options, such as the role of the therapist, also are discussed. Intervention approaches, strategies, and modifications are provided. Measurable objectives that relate to various self-care tasks are listed; these can be used when developing a student's individual education program (IEP). In addition, the Self-Care Functional Checklist (SCFC) developed by the authors is included in Appendix 4.1.

Development and Acquisition of Skills Needed for Self-Care Tasks

The performance of many self-care tasks is dependent on the development of hand skills. Even when children possess the fine motor performance components needed for the completion of self-care tasks, they still need several years to reach an automatic level of skill execution in terms of speed and precision. A fisted grasp is adequate for removing a hat and socks. However, pulling up pants requires more skills than pulling them down. This is why young children are able to undress themselves (except for managing fasteners) before they can dress themselves.

Acquisition of self-care skills and participation in daily living skills also depends on other related factors, including the student's perceptual and cognitive skills and the ability to motor plan and to complete tasks that require multiple steps. Henderson (1995) has indicated that aspects of self-care skill acquisition include grip abilities, bilateral hand use, proper hand positioning, and the execution of motor sequences.

Infants and toddlers have developed the whole-hand and pincer grasps before they begin to acquire self-care skills. They use the whole-hand grasp to hold spoons and get food to their mouths. As fine motor skills become more refined, such as development of the ability to supinate the forearm and hand, so does the efficiency and precision of the self-care acquisition. The grasp on the spoon changes from a palmar grasp to a finger grasp that allows more precise hand and wrist movements (supination) and increases the efficiency of spoon use.

Self-care skills require the bilateral use the hands—both hands working together in a complementary fashion. For selected activities, the hands need to work together (e.g., to pull a shirt over the head). At other times, the hands need to work separately, each performing a different task at the same time (e.g., forming a bow when tying shoes).

According to Henderson (1995), two factors have been identified in regard to the position of the hands that may influence the child's ability to perform a self-care task. The first is performing tasks, such as buttoning, without being able to see the hands. The second is performing a task with the hands in awkward positions, such as buttoning a button on the side of the body.

In addition to the motor components required, many self-care tasks have multiple steps that need to be learned for task completion. Depending on the task, different fine motor components can be required for each step (e.g., the steps needed to tie shoes). The ease in which a skill is mastered depends on the number of motor steps required and the ability of the child to be able to plan, understand, and replicate each step.

The ability to organize and create a motor plan for sequencing the steps is critical in the execution of self-care skills. Motor planning also is needed to perform the task automatically. When learning the sequence of the steps initially, the child must actively think of each step as it is being performed, while visually attending to the task for additional feedback. After many repetitions and much practice, the child does not have to think through each step or use vision to provide feedback. The task becomes efficient and automatic. Self-care tasks that require tool use add another dimension to the activity demands for the execution of motor sequences. Tool use demands the understanding of the tool's purpose, the ability to sequence the steps needed, and the motor ability required to use the tool.

Mastery of several skills is necessary to the dressing process, and good body awareness, or body scheme, is critical. Kinesthetically, a child needs to know where his or her body parts are in relation to space and to be able to recognize what part he or she is moving without depending on vision. He or she must be able to translate the spatial terminology into motor output, such as "put the lace over the loop." The child has to be able to distinguish the front from back, right from left, and inside from outside of any item to orient the clothing correctly and be able to cross midline to assist in dressing and undressing the opposite side. Visual discrimination is needed to help identify clothing parts (e.g., front of the garment). To recognize a specific piece of clothing when it is not correctly oriented, such as when it is upside down or folded, visual form constancy is required. Visual figure ground also is needed, to be able to find and differentiate clothing items (e.g., finding a navy pair of socks vs. a black pair in a drawer).

Children with cognitive deficits may have difficulty with all of the factors needed for dressing. They may need support to remember directions, especially if there are many steps, and thus they may not be able to attend to the activity long enough to complete it. In these instances, a picture schedule can be helpful. Sometimes, children may have difficulty understanding the perceptual components (e.g., spatial and perceptual terminology, such as "right from left") needed to learn specific skills. Visual cues, for example, buttons sewn on the inside of coat so the child knows where to grab it, may prove beneficial in these cases. In addition, children's fine motor skills may be delayed, and they may not be able to perform bilateral tasks efficiently or have the finger dexterity needed to manage fasteners.

A compilation of typical developmental ages for the acquisition of self-care skills is provided in Table 4.1.

Feeding

Gross motor components are needed for feeding: To develop self-feeding skills, a child needs to have head control and trunk stability. This allows the arms to move out and away from the body to grasp and carry the finger food, cup, or utensil up to the mouth. The fine motor components needed for finger feeding are whole-hand grasp to manage a cracker and ability to take it to the mouth, and pincer (thumb and tip of the index finger) and lateral grasp (thumb held on the side of the index finger) to manage smaller pieces of food.

Fine motor components also are needed for utensil use. Initially, a palmar grasp is used with forearm pronation and shoulder abduction. This pattern results in a spoon being inserted in the side of the mouth because of lack of wrist movement and supination. With increased lateral wrist movement, the child discovers that the spoon can be dipped into the food. At approximately ages 15 to 18 months, the child learns to insert the point of the spoon into the food. A 2-year-old is able to hold the spoon in his or her fingers with a supinated grasp, and a 3-year-old can insert the spoon into the front of mouth (Morris & Klein, 1987).

Cup drinking requires that the child be able to visually direct his or her hand to grasp the cup with four fingers and the thumb as a stabilizer and determine the amount of pressure or force needed to be able to pick up the cup. The child must be able to take the cup to the mouth, tilt it by rotating the forearm and the wrist, and return it to the table without spilling.

Dressing

Visual and tactile feedback; perceptual factors; active movement; coordination and balance;

Table 4.1. Developmental Ages for Acquisition of Self-Care Skills

Feeding

7 months	Finger feeds dry cereal
9 months	Feeds self cracker; whole-hand grasp
10 months	Feeds self finger foods; pincer grasp
	Drinks from cup, returns it to table
2–2 1/2 years	Scoops food, uses spoon well with minimal spilling
2–2 1/2 years	Spears and shovels food with fork, little spilling
4 years	Holds spoon with fingers
5–5 1/2 years	Uses knife to cuts soft foods and spread

Undressing

1 1/2–2 years	Removes socks or unties shoes
2–2 1/2 years	Removes pants with elastic waists and pulls over tops
	Removes unfastened coat
3 years	Undresses self

Dressing

3–3 1/2 years	Puts on coat, shoes (although possibly on wrong feet), socks, pullover garments; pulls up pants
4 years	Distinguishes front/back and clothes that are inside out; orients clothing and puts clothing on; can turn clothing right side out
7 years	Discriminates inside and outside of clothing

Unfastening

1 year	Unsnaps front snaps
2–2 1/2 years	Unzips and zips unseparating zipper
3 years	Unbuttons front buttons
3 1/2 years	Unzips front-opening zipper

Fastening

3 1/2 years	Buttons small buttons
3 1/2–4 years	Snaps most snaps—front
4 1/2 years	Zips front, separating zipper
5 1/2–6 years	Zips, unzips, hooks, unhooks separating zipper
6–6 1/2 years	Ties bows on shoes

Hygiene

2–2 1/2 years	Wipes nose on request
3 1/2–4 years	Completes hand-washing routine without supervision
4 1/2–5 years	Applies toothpaste and brushes teeth thoroughly
5 1/2–6 years	Manages all aspects of toileting
6–6 1/2 years	Blows and wipes nose by self

Adapted from *Hand Function and the Child: Foundations for Remediation*, by A. Henderson & C. Pehoski (Eds.), "Self-care and hand skills," pp. 164–183, © 1995. Adapted with permission from Elsevier.

arm and hand control; and reach, grasp, and release abilities are the prerequisite sensory and motor performance skill components needed to dress successfully (Klein 1983). These skills need to be considered as part of the overall assessment process to assess the child's needs. The child needs to be able to attend to the task visually and use visual and tactile feedback to adjust or modify his or her approach. He or she also needs to be able to identify objects by touch alone without vision (stereognosis). This enables the child to locate and manipulate buttons or zippers that are out of sight. An understanding of various spatial terms and concepts, including top, bottom, in, out, front, and back, also is necessary to efficiently participate in the dressing process. The child needs to have an internal awareness of his or her body and where his or her body parts are in space, realize that the body has two sides, and know how all parts relate to each other.

To dress themselves properly, children must have the range of motion and strength to actively move their extremities against gravity to complete the dressing process. They need to maintain their balance while changing positions and postures, shift their weight to free up specific body parts, stabilize the joints needed for support, and isolate the individual body parts needed to perform the dressing task in a fluid and coordinated fashion. Dressing also is more efficient if the child has a preferred hand and can perform bilateral hand skills, including the hands working together performing the same task and the hands working cooperatively, with each hand performing a different task. Finally, the child needs to be able to reach forward, above his or her head, and behind the back. He or she also needs to be able to use his or her hands in a variety of positions to grasp and release at times without visual feedback.

Undressing. Undressing skills are developed before dressing skills because they require less refinement of hand skills. Only a gross grasp, pulling and pushing, is needed to remove clothing (Klein, 1983). Pulling off hats and socks and pushing down pants can be managed with a gross grasp and require less bilateral coordination and strength than putting on the same clothes. The clothing is already on the child, so he or she does not have to deal with any perceptual components. In terms of fasteners, it is easier to untie, unsnap, unzip, unbuckle, and unbutton most fasteners than it is to close them. Of course, success is affected by the type of clothing worn. Loose tops with larger openings for the head and loose pants with elastic

waists may make undressing easier and less frustrating for the young child. Complete independence in undressing depends on the child's ability to undo fasteners, a skill that does not develop until after age 3 years (Henderson, 1995).

Dressing. Dressing skills require more refined fine motor and perceptual–motor skills than undressing. Perceptually, children need to be able to understand the front and back of clothing and the concepts of left and right and inside and outside. Until children are age 7 years, they are not able to discriminate the inside and outside of clothing in terms of being able to correctly orient and put it on (Brigance, 1991). Difficulty with some tasks is related more to perceptual–motor skills, such as finding the heel of a sock or locating the front of a top, than to the motor components needed to complete the task.

In addition, dressing requires the ability to motor plan. Gaddes (1980) has indicated that some children with disabilities have difficulty dressing because of a lack of the tactile and kinesthetic awareness critical to putting on one's own clothes. They do not lack the strength, but rather, they lack the ability to plan a sequence of actions when the goal is understood (the ideomotor image).

Managing Fasteners. Bilateral finger manipulation skills are needed to manage all fasteners. To be successful, children need to be able to complete the motor components and perform the task in the correct sequence. For example, both hands need to work together to align snaps and maintain this alignment as the child attempts to close them. Touch and vision are critical to providing feedback about the alignment. Considerable finger strength also is needed to close the snaps.

Buttoning requires a precision pincer grip, in which both hands work together to push the button through the opened hole and pull it out to fasten it. Success is affected by the location of the button. It is easier for children to button buttons on a strip on the table than on themselves. They are able to use their vision for feedback more easily when the button strip is in front of them and away from the body. In addition, buttoning requires perceptual skills. Children must be able to align the button with the correct hole, and this is dependent on vision. Front buttons are easier to manage, especially if they can be seen. Only after the skill has been perfected can back buttons be accomplished using touch and kinesthesia alone (Henderson, 1995).

Like buttoning, zipping requires a precision grip and the ability of both hands to work together in addition to pinch strength. Vision also is a critical component, as it is needed to provide feedback about location and alignment when trying to thread the zipper. Tactile feedback helps children know when they have engaged (locked) the shank into the base of the zipper, which is necessary before the zipper can be pulled up.

Shoe tying is itself a complex task that requires motor planning, perceptual–motor skills, isolated finger use, and bilateral finger manipulation. Vision is needed to help children identify how big to make the loop, which lace to poke through, and where to grab the lace to pull it tight. Tying shoes and engaging a zipper are the most difficult of fastening tasks to manage and are the last to be perfected. Generally, children master these skills between ages 5 $\frac{1}{2}$ and 6 $\frac{1}{2}$ years, and it is not uncommon for kindergarten students to still require help.

Hygiene and Grooming Skills. Hygiene and grooming skills require a series of steps to complete because a tool or object is incorporated into the task (e.g., toothbrush, comb). Some of the motor components (e.g., rubbing hands together when washing hands) are present within the first 18 months to 2 years of life. Complete mastery and independence, however, do not occur until middle childhood. Children have the motor ability to complete the grooming and hygiene skills before they

accept the responsibility for performing them (Henderson, 1995).

Hygiene and grooming skills encompass the hand skill development factors described previously. A variety of grips are required to manage the objects involved with grooming and hygiene tasks, including in-hand manipulation (e.g., rotating the toothbrush to change the orientation of the bristles). Bilateral hand skills also are an integral part of such tasks as washing hands or applying toothpaste to the toothbrush. The position of the hands when completing tasks sometimes requires using the hands without the benefit of seeing what is being done (e.g., when washing or combing hair). Motor planning is needed to complete the multiple sequences of actions. Continued practice allows the development of the automaticity needed for efficiency.

IADLs

In addition to the ADLs already identified, there are additional life skill tasks (IADLs) that students must be able to manage throughout the school day. Difficulty performing these skills can affect their independence. The SCFC provided in this chapter includes a list of IADLs in addition to the dressing, feeding, and hygiene skills just discussed.

The Evaluation Process

The evaluation process measures a student's occupational needs in specific ADLs and IADLs. This is done to determine if any problems exist in occupational performance.

Choosing Assessment Methods

Occupational therapists can use a variety of methods to examine a student's occupational needs. A therapist may rely on data from a standardized or formal assessment, checklist, or questionnaire and then supplement this information with informal testing and observations of specific performance skills in the context of the school setting. To help understand the contexts in which task performance occurs and to identify the concerns and expectations of the team in relation to the child's ability to function in school, additional information should be obtained through collaboration with the parent, classroom teacher, or classroom aide.

Formal Assessments. Numerous assessments are available commercially that can be used to evaluate a student's ability to complete self-care tasks. These assessments include the self-care subtest of the Brigance Diagnostic Inventory of Early Development, the Battelle Developmental Inventory, the Pediatric Evaluation of Disability Inventory (PEDI), and the School Function Assessment (SFA).

Brigance Diagnostic Inventory of Early Development. The self-care subtest of the Brigance Diagnostic Inventory of Early Development (Brigance, 1991) examines a student's performance in a variety of self-care tasks: feeding and eating, dressing, managing fasteners, toileting, bathing, and grooming. It can be used with children from birth to age 7 years, and the information is obtained through parent and teacher interviews, observation, direct assessment, or some combination of the three. The test provides developmental age ranges for individual test items. These can be used to indicate at what level a student is functioning in any of the self-care areas. Present levels of performance are the baseline to measure progress against when the test is readministered. The Brigance inventory can be used with students of varying developmental and cognitive levels, as the testing information is obtained through a combination of direct assessment and caregiver interviews.

Battelle Developmental Inventory. The Battelle Developmental Inventory (Newborg, Stock, Wnek, Guidubaldi, & Suinicki, 1988) has a daily living skills section that examines the child's ability to complete self-care tasks in dressing, grooming, toileting, and eating. It can be used with children from birth to age 8 years, and information can be obtained through parent and teacher interview, observation, direct assessment, or some combination of these. The test provides the evaluator with a standard score, percentile, and age equivalent for the student's skills relative to same-age peers. As it can be administered several ways, it can be used with students of varying developmental and cognitive levels.

PEDI. The PEDI (Haley, Coster, Ludlow, Haltiwanger, & Andrellos, 1992) is a comprehensive clinical instrument that examines key functional capabilities and performance in self-care, mobility, and social function using two subscales. The first consists of functional skills (197 items); the second is caregiver assistance (20 items). It can be used with children ranging in age from 6 months to 7 1/2 years, and information is obtained through parent and teacher interviews, observation, direct assessment, or some combination of the three. This assessment is more appropriate for students functioning at a lower level.

SFA. The SFA (Coster, Deeney, Haltiwanger, & Haley, 1998) measures a student's ability to perform functional tasks and participate in academic and social tasks included in the school day. Designed to be used with students in kindergarten through sixth grade, the assessment can be used with students with varying disabilities. It examines a student's level of participation in six school settings: regular or special education classroom, playground or recess, transportation to and from school, toileting, transitions within the school environment, and snack time or lunch. The test examines the amount of support the child requires to participate in activities in these areas.

In addition, the SFA examines the student's ability to participate in specific school-related functional activities. These include moving throughout the building, managing playground equipment, using classroom materials appropriately, practicing proper hygiene skills, applying self-care skills, displaying functional communication skills, understanding directions, and demonstrating memory of routines and directions. Information is obtained through a questionnaire completed by school professionals. The assessment is criterion referenced and provides a criterion score that indicates at what level the student is functioning currently. It also defines any need for assistance and adaptations and the extent of each student's ability to participate in school activities. An increase in scores indicates an increase in a student's participation in school activities.

Informal Assessments.

Interviews and Checklists. Occupational therapists frequently use checklists and questionnaires when interviewing parents and teachers. These can be used in isolation or in combination with a more formalized assessment. The SCFC also can be used during an interview to determine how a child performs within different contexts. The checklist examines the student's ability to complete a variety of self-care and IADLs expected of the student during a school day, including feeding, dressing, and managing personal belongings and the school environment. The areas of concern are identified by the parents, the student, and the teacher and can help the therapist determine what performance areas to focus on during the evaluation. The results obtained depend on the ability of the parents and the teacher to answer the questions accurately (Shepherd, 2001).

Observations. In addition to interviewing the student's parents or teachers, the occupational therapist also should observe the student participating in those self-care tasks that are of concern. These observations may occur in the natural setting at the time the student is actually performing the tasks (e.g., going to the student's cubby or locker to observe him or her hanging up a coat and bookbag when he or she comes in from the bus). The tasks may be observed in a structured therapy or evaluation session to determine how the child completes them (e.g., having the student put on a button-down shirt over his or her clothes to see if he or she can manage buttons). The therapist identifies the task, has the child perform it, and then observes and documents the child's performance. It is important to consider the context (conditions) that surround the performance (AOTA, 2002).

Observing the student engage in a variety of self-care skills allows the occupational therapist to see how the student initiates and completes a task and document these observations. The therapist then is able to examine what is preventing the student from completing the task. Following this, a baseline can be established for task accomplishments, and the therapist can determine what remediation techniques, adaptations, and modifications may be needed to achieve success and independence. To do this, the therapist needs to develop a task analysis for selected self-care tasks. This will provide intervention to meet the student's individualized needs when determined necessary by the team.

Determining ADL Needs

The following considerations are included to help the educational team look at a bigger picture and consider the student's occupational performance as a component of the assessment. Appropriate components can be addressed, included in the evaluation, and shared with the team by the occupational therapist.

When evaluating a student, there are factors that should be considered in regard to the student's ability to complete self-care tasks during the school day. Is the student motivated to be independent in completing self-care tasks? A student needs to possess the internal drive to want to be independent and not rely on others. To encourage this, the team can use reinforcers for participation.

Is the student able to follow multistep directions? The occupational therapist needs to take into consideration if the child relies on excessive prompting to initiate and complete the task but appears to have the necessary underlying motor ability. If the student needs assistance, use a picture schedule to help sequence the steps and decrease the need for adult support over time.

Does the student have the attention span needed to focus on the task? Is he or she able to visually attend to what he or she is doing (e.g., look at his or her shoes when attempting to tie them)? Just as with handwriting and cutting tasks, a student needs to be able to see (at least initially) what he or she is doing when completing self-care tasks. To help the child focus, only work on one step at a time using repetitions. Use components and tools in contrasting colors to make them easier to see and focus on, and have the child work on the tasks on a table so they are easier to see.

Is the student able to understand directional and spatial terms frequently incorporated into directions? To assist the student, evaluate and teach the concepts needed to complete the task before working on the task itself. This does not have to be done by the occupational therapist; it can be done by the teacher or teacher's aide in the classroom setting. Speech therapists also are a resource for suggestions and can help work on spatial and directional concepts.

Does the student have the needed hand skills to complete the task? If the child needs to refine his or her hand skills, work on a specific fine motor skill in isolation. This can be a preparation activity before it is incorporated into the specific task. Share with classroom staff activities that incorporate the skill needed, such as the pincer grasp, so that the student can work on it throughout the week.

Will the student have the opportunity to practice the self-care tasks during the school day? If this is not the case, the occupational therapist can be working on the skill in isolation to carry over to the days of the week that the student is not seen for therapy. The therapist's services cannot exist in isolation when self-care skills are being taught. The IEP is written to reflect the student's needs. The goals and objectives are the result of identified needs and should be incorporated into the student's daily curriculum, whether the student is in the regular education classroom full-time or in a resource room environment.

The occupational therapist may need to help teachers and parents understand this concept and help them find opportunities throughout the school week to work on the skill with the student. It is critical that the child be given multiple opportunities for exposure. The skill needs to be incorporated into the daily routine. If the team indicates that this is not possible, then the therapist may want to question if the skill really is a priority in terms of the child's IEP.

Is the student functioning at the developmental level that corresponds to average-age norms for learning the task? Unrealistic expectations must not be placed on the student. He or she needs the cognitive ability to problem solve and stay on task when practicing a task to master it. To accomplish this, break down the task into smaller steps (see the section on task analysis later in this chapter).

Using the Evaluation Information

Once the evaluation is completed, the results should be shared with the team. The team can determine if any areas of concern identified by the occupational therapy assessment are affecting the student's ability to benefit from his or her educational program. For example, the student may not be able to button smaller buttons, but he or she does not wear button-down shirts and does not have to change the shirt while at school, so neither of these appear to be a problem. The occupational therapist should be instrumental in facilitating this team discussion.

Determining the Need for Occupational Therapy Services

The team must understand that occupational therapy services, if needed, can be addressed in a variety of ways and do not have to be provided weekly for the child to make progress. It is the occupational therapist's responsibility to discuss with the team the service delivery options available.

Specific occupational therapy service delivery options were defined and discussed in Chapter 1. Examples of such services are discussed here with direct application to self-care issues.

Two types of occupational therapy services are applicable to self-care issues. The first, direct service, can be provided by the occupational therapist to remediate an identified problem. During therapy the therapist can work on a particular skill or task component that is affecting the student's ability to achieve independence in a given task (e.g., child lacks in-hand manipulation skills, which affects the ability to button his or her pants). The therapist also should provide specific activity suggestions that can be done in the classroom. These should incorporate in-hand manipulation skills to reinforce what is being done in therapy.

Consultation, or collaboration, is the second type of service that can be provided. The occupational therapist collaborates with classroom staff and a student's parents on specific techniques and approaches for completing a task, such as using a flip-over approach when putting on a coat. The therapist also can provide suggestions for adaptive equipment, such as using a zipper pull, or modify a method for completing the task so that the student can be independent, such as having the student put a shirt on over his or her head with the buttons already fastened.

Recommendations can be made both for students who are in settings in which self-care skills are worked on daily as a part of the functional curriculum and for students who have access to teacher aide services. The student is observed engaging in the hygiene or grooming routines that are a part of the school day. The therapist then collaborates with the student's teacher and parents to produce recommendations or offer equipment suggestions that will help the student achieve the skill. Whichever method is adopted, the therapist needs to follow up at scheduled times during the school year (e.g., monthly, quarterly) to check on the student's progress and offer further recommendations to the staff.

Considerations for Interventions

Occupational therapists need to understand what is preventing a child from performing a specific task. This requires observation and evaluation of how the child attempts to perform the task compared to what skills are needed for its successful completion. It also requires analysis of the task itself.

Creative Thinking

The task can be broken down into individual steps, and the motor components needed to complete each step can be defined. Intervention techniques appropriate for the task and the child's ability need to be identified. To do this, the therapist must think creatively rather than apply the same intervention techniques to each student for a specific task. The therapist must look at different ways to perform the same task.

The best way to identify different ways to perform the same task is to observe a variety of individuals performing it, yourself included. Observe the function of each hand in terms of type of grasp and how and where the task (e.g., clothing) is being stabilized. Next, consider the child's existing motor abilities. Could the child complete the task if it was modified to allow him or her to use existing skills? For example, Michael's left hand has a much weaker grip than his right hand. As a result, his left hand is unable to maintain a strong enough grasp to pull the left side of his waistband over to the right side to engage the metal slide fastener. Because the grip of his right hand is stronger, he is able to grasp the right side of his waistband and pull it over to the left to engage the metal slide. Using this modified approach allows Michael to engage the metal slide fastener and is more productive than the traditional approach of working to strengthen his left hand.

Consistent Use of Terminology for Directions

Occupational therapists use different cues when teaching the steps to a task. Often the terminology and methods used by an occupational therapist are not consistent with what the student's private therapist, parents, child care provider, teacher, or teaching assistant are using to teach the same skill (e.g., the school-based therapist is teaching the student to tie his shoes using the traditional method, whereas the private therapist is teaching the student using the bunny ear method). All people working on a task with the student must be consistent in their teaching of the skill. Providing a task analysis to describe the steps and the terminology being used to teach the task is an effective approach, as it ensures that everyone is using the same method and terminology with the student. In addition, because the intervention process is focused on changing performance skills, a change in one skill area might influence other interrelated skill

areas. Therefore, there is a need for ongoing review of the outcomes based on the intervention.

Intervention Approaches Specific to Self-Care

As previously discussed, a student's specific self-care needs must be determined and documented on the IEP. Then the need for occupational therapy and the specific types of services required must be determined. The role of the occupational therapist (as a consultant or direct service administrator) helps determine the type of intervention approaches to be used. Smith, Benge, and Hall (1994) identified five intervention approaches therapists may use when there is a problem performing self-care tasks:
1. Reduce the disability,
2. Teach compensation strategies,
3. Modify the task or expectations,
4. Use assistive technology, and
5. Use others for assistance with the task.

Kramer and Hinojosa (1999) discussed using the developmental approach as another intervention technique. A combination of these approaches can help children achieve their self-care goals and objectives.

Developmental Approach

With the developmental approach, the child's developmental and chronological ages are taken into consideration, which is useful when working with younger children with mild disabilities. Intervention is planned according to a typical developmental sequence. Many of the students that occupational therapists serve do not develop skills equal to their same-age peers, nor do they learn skills in the same developmental sequence (Orelove & Sobsey, 1996). As a result, their developmental age may be significantly lower than their chronological age. This must be considered so that intervention can be geared toward specific skills that will increase independence in self-care skills.

There are ways to adapt this approach. For example, the activity can be broken into smaller steps, verbal cues can be modified to ensure that the child understands them, and the environment can be modified to reduce distractions. Determine the best time of the day to have the child work on dressing. It should be at the natural time that the skill needs to be performed (e.g., putting on a jacket before going home). Make sure that any criteria for success are realistic with the child's ability and encourage any achievement. Such positive reinforcement increases motivation and willingness to participate.

Remediation Approach

Shepherd (2001) identified additional approaches that can be used when working on performance skills for self-care task and IADLs. One of these, the remediation approach, is based on information obtained through the evaluation process. It uses the Self-Care Functional Checklist (Appendix 4.1) to identify specific skill components interfering with task acquisition. For example, it is determined that a student is having difficulty buttoning because she is using a lateral rather than pincer grasp. The lateral grasp does not allow for enough manipulation of the button to align it with the buttonhole so that it can be pushed through it. Intervention strategies are designed that work on the development of an appropriate pincer grasp. Remediating the problem in this way can reduce the disability.

Compensatory Approach

With the compensatory approach, alternative techniques are explored, especially if the remediation approach was tried and found unsuccessful. The techniques provide a different method of teaching the same task. For example, if a student is unable to tie his shoes using the conventional approach, then the bunny ear approach can be attempted. If a student is unable to take off a shirt by pulling it over her head first, she can pull her arms out before pulling it over her head.

Task Modification

Modifying the task or the expectations of the task can reduce or eliminate the need for direct intervention. The occupational therapist can be instrumental in identifying the appropriate modifications and sharing them with the team for further discussion. Replacing a button on a pair of pants with Velcro® eliminates the need for the child to have to button. Enlarging the buttonhole can make it easier for a child who displays the ability to complete the buttoning act except for the pushing of the button through the hole. At times it is necessary to discuss with the team the possibility of modifying task expectations. This is especially true if it does not appear that the child is able to perform the task. Modifying the task also can be used if intervention has been tried with minimal to no progress. For example, this approach can be used if the child had an objective to button $1/2$-inch buttons but has not shown any progress because of his inability to manage or manipulate the button even after a variety of strategies and techniques had been tried. At this point, the team may consider discontinuing the goal.

Assistive Technology

The need for assistive technology must be identified in the IEP. Assistive technology is defined in Sec. 300.5 of the Individuals With Disabilities Education Act: an *assistive technology device* is any item, piece of equipment, or product system, whether acquired commercially off the shelf, modified, or customized, that is used to increase, maintain, or improve the functional capabilities of a child with a disability.

As defined, assistive technology aids task performance by providing a device to support a task's completion. The device may be low technology, such as a buttonhook or nonskid material, or high technology, such as an electric page turner. Occupational therapy has a critical role in identifying the need for assistive technology devices and in the selection, modification, or creation of the devices.

When selecting an assistive device, several factors must be considered (Shepherd, 2001). The device must assist in the task without being cumbersome and be acceptable to the child and family so that it is more likely to be used. As such, it also must be practical for the setting in which it will be used, it must be durable, and it must be affordable. To continue to meet the child's needs in the future, the device needs to be expandable, safe, and easily maintained or replaced. Whenever possible, the child should have an opportunity to try the device beforehand to make sure that it is appropriate and will meet his or her needs. The child should be able to complete a specific task more efficiently when using the device than without using it.

Personal Assistance

At times assistance may be required to complete a task. The child always should be expected to complete those steps he or she is capable of performing first, and then assistance can be provided for the remaining steps. For example, engaging the zipper on a jacket is a difficult task. The child may demonstrate the ability to complete all of the steps needed to put on the coat but remains unable to engage the zipper. Once adult assistance is provided to engage the zipper, the child is able to zip it up with no additional help.

Methods of Interventions

After evaluating the student and determining areas of concern and what is contributing to his or her difficulty in completing a self-care task, intervention strategies or modifications need to be developed and implemented to help the student learn to complete the skill. Completion of self-care tasks requires the fine motor components and the ability to perform multiple steps. At times different fine motor components are required for each step.

Task Analysis

A task analysis provides specific information about the child's fine motor abilities and his or her ability to complete each component of a task. The occupational therapist needs to determine what is preventing the child from completing specific steps or skills of a task. There are so many variables to consider when performing a task analysis that it often is difficult to define and separate the fine motor components from the other components (e.g., attention and motivation) interfering with the child's ability to complete the task. At times, it may not be the fine motor components that are affecting the student's inability to complete the task. For example, if a child does not visually attend to the task as he or she attempts to perform it, he or she is not receiving the visual feedback necessary to help him or her determine if he or she is performing the task correctly or if he or she needs to modify the approach. The child may have the appropriate grasp needed to perform the task, but his or her lack of visual attention is preventing him or her from being successful. Once the task analysis is complete, specific strategies can be developed to work on the identified areas.

Chaining Techniques

Chaining techniques can be effective when trying to teach a series of steps needed for task completion. There are two chaining techniques: backward and forward.

Backward Chaining. Backward chaining requires the child to perform only the last step of the task. For example, in shoe tying the occupational therapist or other adult completes all of the steps, including poking the loop through. The child pinches and pulls the laces tight. As this part of the task is mastered, the child then is expected to complete the last two steps of the task. This process continues up through the remainder of the steps until all of them are mastered. Finally, the child needs to be able to generalize the steps learned so that the task can be completed in the correct sequence.

Forward Chaining. Forward chaining begins by teaching the first step of the task. Once this step is mastered, the second step is taught. The tasks continue to be presented in sequential order until all have been mastered. This technique also helps the child learn the order in which the steps are performed.

Assistance During Intervention

Prompting and Cueing

Prompting and cueing provide additional sensory input auditorily, visually, or physically and can be used when a self-care skill is being taught to the child. Verbal prompts provide the least amount of support. When using them, the occupational therapist needs to confirm that the child understands what is being asked so the request can be translated into a motor response. Remember that the initial directive given to the child to indicate the task he or she needs to complete (e.g., "Jimmy, button your shirt") should not be considered a verbal prompt.

If Jimmy does not respond and the therapist states "Find the bottom button, and line it up with the bottom hole," this is considered a verbal prompt. A common tendency is to increase the verbalizations (keep talking) if the student does not respond. It is important to minimize this when trying to get a child to perform. If he is not responding because he is unable to translate the verbalization into a motor response, then he will continue to dis-

play increased difficulty as the verbalizations continue. Verbal prompting also can be used to talk the child through the steps of the task before the child initiates the step. The therapist may say "Cross and pull through" just before the child attempts the first step of shoe tying.

Visual and Gestural Prompting

Visual prompting can be used to produce the correct motor response when a child has difficulty processing verbal information. The occupational therapist might point or gesture toward the button that he or she wants the child to button. Or, when the child has difficulty aligning the zipper so that the shank can be inserted into the base, the shank can be colored with a marker to show the contrast between the shank and the rest of the zipper. The top of the base also can be colored so that the child can line up the pin. A contrasting color should be used to make it easier to differentiate the shank from the rest of the zipper.

Physical Prompting

Students may need physical assistance from the occupational therapist to complete a given task. For example, a student who is asked to complete the steps to shoe tying is unable to poke the lace through the opening. The therapist provides a physical prompt to poke the lace through so that the child can then "pinch and pull it tight" to get practice with that step of the task.

Hand-Over-Hand Assistance

Hand-over-hand assistance is the most restrictive type of prompt used with a child. The occupational therapist physically helps the child complete the task, for example, placing his or her hands over the child's hands to hold each side of the jacket at the bottom by the zipper. The child's hand then is guided by the therapist's hand to push the shank into the slider until it locks in place. The child is not actively participating in the task. However, he or she is able to experience the feeling of engaging the zipper as the therapist guides his or her hand.

Hand-over-hand support needs to be decreased to determine if the child can perform any part of the task him- or herself. If such assistance is needed to complete the entire task, then the team needs to discuss if the task needs to be modified further or discontinued at this time.

Intervention Techniques Specific to Individual Tasks

Finger Feeding

By ages 6 1/2 to 7 months, infants are able to feed themselves a cracker. By 10 months, they further perfect their finger-feeding skills. Infants can reach with one hand to get the food off of the tray and can manage smaller pieces of food. Their ability to release also has matured. Children are able to release larger pieces of food with their wrists held in an extended or neutral position.

Small pieces of food should not be introduced until children are able to grasp and release them. Strips of food, such as a graham crackers, toast, or cookies, should be used initially because they are fairly easy to manage. They are big enough to hold while putting the other end into mouth to take a bite. Smaller round items, such as grapes, hot dog pieces, popcorn, and nuts, should not be used to avoid the risk of choking.

Children will have a difficult time releasing food into their mouths if they have not developed a pincer grasp and continue to use a raking grasp (flexing all the fingers into the palm to grasp the food). The food is not being held in the tips of the fingers but rather is in the palm of the hand. This requires the child to open all of the fingers and push the food into the mouth, which is awkward and inefficient. The child needs to de-

velop a three-finger or pincer grasp so that food can be picked up and held in the fingertips. This makes the release of food into the mouth more accurate and refined. The child also can practice releasing items into a designated location, such as a smaller container, a container with a lid with a hole cut out, and so forth.

To facilitate the three-finger grasp, a variety of small pieces of finger foods can be presented during snack time. If the child is unable to maintain a three-finger grasp, the occupational therapist can flex the child's ring and little fingers into the palm and support the hand in that position as the child attempts to pick up the pieces of food using his or her thumb, index, and middle fingers. Only one small piece of food should be offered at a time, in different orientations. Pieces should be held up off of the table to encourage the finger isolation and wrist extension needed for a three-finger grasp. Food placed directly on the table encourages the child to use the raking grasp to pick it up, as this is easier than trying to isolate the first two fingers to use a three-finger grasp.

This basic technique can be modified as needed. Have the child hold a small object, such as a piece of foam or a cotton ball, with the ring and index fingers to keep those fingers flexed into the palm. These fingers now are isolated and can be used to pick up small pieces of food. The occupational therapist also can try taping the ring and little fingers so they are flexed in the palm as the child is picking up small food items. If the child resists the taping, the therapist can physically hold the ring and little finger flexed into the palm. The choice of food can be modified, too. Use food with more dimension to it so it is easier to pick up (e.g., a thicker piece of cereal or pretzel rod rather than a small piece of potato chip). For more suggestions on developing a three-finger grasp, see Chapter 5 on fine motor functions.

Adaptive Equipment

A Benik splint can be used with children who have spasticity. The splint's purpose is to support the thumb in abduction so that it can rotate down to be used with the index and middle fingers to pick up smaller items. Make sure the child can manage small pieces of food safely in terms of oral motor control. Ask the parents if there is any history of choking with different types and textures of food and if the child has any food allergies. The occupational therapist even may wish to have the parents send in finger foods the child likes or may find the types of finger food the child likes that are appropriate to have at snack time.

Cup Drinking

Multiple components must be considered when working on cup drinking. To address a child's specific needs, the occupational therapist should determine what components the child lacks. Is the child able to grasp and take the cup to the mouth, tip it so the liquids come out, and return it to the table in an upright position?

Before the child can begin learning to handle a cup properly, the proper cup must be chosen. Determine the appropriate size and shape of cup to ensure that it can be held securely and tipped up to get liquid at the bottom without the child having to tip his or her head back into extreme hyperextension. The cup should fit the child's hand and mouth. (Cups with smaller diameters usually are easier for children to manage.) The cup must not be crushable when held or breakable if the child bites the edge. It should have a rolled rim for extra stability if needed and allow for graded control of the liquid flow for a child who has difficulty managing a larger volume of liquids.

Thickened liquids can be attempted to decrease the flow of the liquid so the child has more time to react. If the child is unable to pick up the cup, he or she can try to suck from a straw. Sports bottles that provide long straws and are stabilized by cup holders allow the child to just bend forward to suck from the straw. This allows him or her to be independent.

Depending on the child's ability, the occupational therapist providing the intervention should begin with the appropriate step needed to develop cup drinking. When prompting is needed, the therapist needs to determine the type and amount of prompting required. In general, have the child practice picking up an appropriate size cup (ensuring it fits the size of his or her hand and mouth). Add only a small amount of liquid in the cup initially so that the child has to determine the amount of pressure needed to hold the cup when taking it to his or her mouth.

If needed, place the child's hand around the outside of the cup in the mid-position. Provide tactile input from the cup by pushing it into the palm of the child's hand to increase his or her awareness that the cup is there. If he or she does not grasp the cup automatically, use hand-over-hand assistance to close the hand around the cup. Do this by providing pressure into and around his or her hand. This helps the child create the force needed to maintain the grasp to hold the cup as it is being taken to the mouth.

To get the child to take the cup to the mouth, prompt him or her to appropriately pick up the cup and take it to his or her mouth. Make sure the child keeps his or her wrist in a neutral or slightly extended position with the hand in proper alignment with his or her forearm. Once the cup is at the child's mouth, prompt him or her to tip the cup so that he or she can take a sip. Encourage extension and radial deviation at the wrist. This way his or her head can remain more upright instead of allowing him or her to hyperextend it so that he or she has to take the cup up further to get it to the mouth. Also note that, when the head is hyperextended, it is more difficult to close the airway. This increases the possibility for aspiration of the liquids into the lungs. When there is more liquid in the cup, neither the cup or the head have to be tipped as much, so the determination must be made as to what needs to be controlled: the amount of head hyperextension or the flow and amount of liquid.

Make sure that, when the child puts the cup down, he or she is holding it with all fingers on the side of the cup so that the bottom of the cup is clear. Sometimes a child will place a few fingers on the bottom of the cup to help stabilize it. This makes it difficult to set the cup on the table. Prompt the child to return the cup to the table by providing the needed support so that the cup can be returned in the upright position.

Adaptive Equipment in Interventions

A variety of commercially available cups can be found in the infant department of stores in addition to specific types of cups that can be found in adaptive equipment catalogs. A list of cup types is provided here, with examples of how they can be used. However, it is suggested that readers use the adaptive equipment catalogs for more options. Make sure to control the amount of liquid in the cup and that the cup fits the needs of the student. When a child attempts to drink through a straw, make sure it is developmentally appropriate for his or her age.

Cut-Out and Flexi Cut-Out Cups

This cup is designed so that it can be tipped to reach the liquids at the bottom without having to tip the head back into extreme hyperextension. In general, the larger and taller the cup, the more difficult it is to drink, as it requires that the head be tipped to get the liquids at the bottom.

Flexi cut-out cups are made of a more flexible plastic material that enables the adult to bend the cup. This allows a spout to be formed by the adult that assists in controlling the amount and direction of the liquid given.

Medicine and Spout Cups

Medicine cups are small plastic cups that hold only 1 ounce of liquid. This makes it easier for children to manage, especially preschoolers and students just being introduced to cup drinking.

A variety of commercially available cups have spout tops. The intent of the spout is to decrease the flow of liquid as the child is learning how to drink from a cup. Using a spout top with children who do not have oral motor difficulties is appropriate. However, they are not recommended for children who lack jaw stability or have low muscle tone in the oral motor area. These children may "fix" on the spout for stability by putting their tongues on the outside bottom of the spout. This is not an efficient pattern for drinking. It prevents the lip closure required to create the vacuum needed to manage the liquid. The spout top also is designed to encourage the same patterns used with a nipple (a suckle pattern and tongue protrusion), but the hardness of the cup material means it does not respond like a nipple. This may make it confusing for the child.

Cups With Recessed Lids and Cups With Straws

Cups with recessed lids that go down into the cup have small openings to reduce the flow and amount of liquids. This type of cup encourages proper lip closure.

Children who are unable to hold or lift a cup but who are able to drink from a straw may benefit from a cup or drink bottle with a straw. The cup or bottle can be placed close, enabling the child to bend forward to suck on the straw independently.

Spoons

Children generally attempt to bring a filled spoon to their mouths between ages 12 and

14 months. However, because they lack the ability to laterally move and rotate the wrist effectively, they are apt to turn a spoon over as they take it to their mouths. As children perfect the ability to coordinate the action of the shoulder, elbow, and wrist, movements become more fluid. By 15 to 18 months, they usually can scoop food and bring it to the mouth. Between 2 and 2 ½ years, children are able to hold the spoon in their fingers rather than with a palmar grasp and bring it to the mouth with the wrist supinated in a palm-up position. Children begin to use a fork to stab and shovel food between ages 30 and 36 months (Morris & Klein, 1987).

For an older child still using a palmar grasp on a spoon, the occupational therapist should work on hand separation activities as an intervention separate from feeding. This will develop the hand skills needed to hold the spoon in his or her fingers rather than with the whole hand. (For hand separation activities, see Chapter 5 on fine motor functions.)

Depending on the child's level of independence, begin with the appropriate step needed to develop spoon use. The occupational therapist needs to determine the type of prompt, if any, that is needed.

Grasping the Spoon. Before teaching the child to grasp the spoon properly, provide tactile input from the spoon by pushing it into the palm of his or her hand to increase awareness that the spoon is there. If he or she does not automatically grasp the spoon, use hand-over-hand assistance to close his or her hand around the spoon. Apply pressure into and around the hand to help create the force needed to maintain the grasp to hold the spoon as it is being taken to the mouth. The occupational therapist also can have the child use a palmar cuff. This allows him or her to experience the movement of the spoon being taken to the mouth without having to be concerned about maintaining a grasp on the

spoon. Grasping the spoon can be attempted once the child understands the process.

Loading the Spoon. When loading food on the spoon, the child needs to visually attend to his or her actions so that he or she receives the feedback that the food is on the spoon. Using snack foods such as applesauce and pudding that stick to the spoon when practicing this skill makes the task easier and encourages greater success. If necessary, determine where (e.g., elbow, forearm, hand) to physically prompt the child to assist him or her in scooping the food.

Taking Food to the Mouth. If child is unable to hold the spoon level as he or she carries it to the mouth, the occupational therapist can stabilize the wrist by supporting it on either side as the child takes it to his or her mouth. A backward chaining technique also can be applied in this situation. Using hand-over-hand assistance, take the loaded spoon to the child's mouth a few times. Next, take it to within 3 or 4 inches of the child's mouth and stop, let go, and let him or her take it the rest of the way to the mouth. If support is still needed, the therapist can hold the end of the spoon as the child holds the center of it. Gradually increase the distance until he or she is able to pick it up and take it to the mouth once it is loaded. The therapist should be prepared to provide assistance if the child tilts or tips the spoon as he or she carries it to the mouth.

Inserting Food Into the Mouth. Backward chaining also can be used once the spoon is positioned to make certain that the utensil is carried to the mouth and inserted properly. The type of grasp the child uses affects the type of motion he or she needs to use to angle the spoon so that the tapered front of the spoon points toward the front of the mouth. The therapist needs to support the wrist so that the correct angle can be achieved. The child should be encouraged to take the spoon the rest of the way to the mouth while maintaining the angle. When the child is able to maintain the correct angle, increase the distance, providing prompting as needed to maintain the angle.

Returning the Spoon to the Bowl. Some children drop the spoon as soon as they get the food into their mouths instead of attempting to take it back to the bowl. Because they received an immediate reward, they do not understand that the process is meant to continue. A palmar cuff can be used to prevent a child from dropping the spoon. This allows the occupational therapist or other adult to continue to provide the movement back to the bowl so that the spoon can be reloaded and the process repeated. The intent is to help the child realize that he or she will continue to get food if he or she keeps holding the spoon.

Choosing Effective Spoons. All spoons are not created equal. The correct one can help a child learn more quickly. Its bowl should be shallow to allow the child's upper lip to remove the food and should fit the size of the child's mouth. It should not break if the child bites down on it. This is an important consideration, as most spoons used in schools are plastic and are not very durable. Finally, the length of the handle should be appropriate for the size of the child's hand.

Modifying the Feeding Process. The food used when spoon feeding can affect the success of the process. A child who is having a problem keeping food on his or her spoon may compensate for a lack of control by using one hand to take the spoon to the mouth while stabilizing the spoon with the other hand. Soup, dry cereal or cereal with milk, corn, peas, and canned fruit in a syrup base (e.g., peaches) are foods that are much more difficult for children to manage. Conversely, foods that stick to the spoon allow the child to continue to practice the wrist control needed without becoming frustrated if the food falls

off as he or she attempts to take the spoon to the mouth. Examples of such food include pudding, applesauce, yogurt, oatmeal, mashed potatoes, and macaroni and cheese.

Feeding Evaluation Kit. Many types of utensils and cups are featured in the various adapted equipment catalogs. A feeding evaluation kit that includes a variety of utensils and cups makes the kit more effective when used to assess feeding skills, because specific adapted equipment can be tried as a part of the evaluation. In addition, the occupational therapist can leave a few items for classroom staff to try. This will help determine if a specific type of adapted equipment allows the child to be more successful before recommending it.

Undressing/Dressing Devices

Intervention Strategies. Klein (1983) provides specific dressing and undressing intervention techniques for preschool children, children with developmental delays, and children with physical disabilities. Klein included standard and adapted techniques in addition to modifications and adaptive devices to assist in teaching dressing skills.

Another comprehensive source for interventions is Goldsmith (1999). Goldsmith has developed a packet that contains five individual booklets with pictures and directions that cover the basic dressing skills of buttoning, dressing and undressing, shoe tying, and zippering.

Given that such resources exist, it is not the intent of this section to cover that type of information. Instead, we provide general suggestions and considerations and a process that allows the occupational therapist to develop his or her own individualized intervention techniques.

Occupational therapists should begin by referring to the developmental ages list and the prerequisite skills sections. This will help determine the developmental level, expectations, and components needed for the acquisition of a specific dressing skill. Optimally, when prerequisite skills are present, children are able to independently learn how to dress and undress themselves. It can be assumed that the children receiving occupational therapy services may need additional support, modification or adaptations, or both as they are exposed to dressing tasks.

General Considerations for Dressing and Undressing. As indicated previously, undressing skills typically develop before dressing skills because they require less hand skills refinement. For this reason, begin with these tasks first if the child is unable to do them. For example, if the child cannot manage his or her coat, have him or her begin by working on taking it off first. The size, type of clothing, and a garment's fasteners affect undressing success. Clothing that is easiest to manage includes

- Larger, stretchy garments,
- Loose pullover tops with wide neck openings and short sleeves,
- Loose pants with elastic waistbands,
- Front fasteners that are easy to see,
- Tube socks (no heel to line up), and
- Slip-on shoes (the child can slide his or her feet in without having to hold and manipulate the shoe).

Mark the specific area where you want the child to grab the clothing so that it is oriented correctly when the child puts it on. For instance, a button can be sewn on the inside of the coat beneath the collar. This gives the child a visual cue where to grab the coat so that it is in the correct orientation needed to put on. Remember that it is easier to practice fasteners when the clothing is not on the body. In addition, the clothing must be oriented in the same direction that it would be if it were on the body to ensure that the child uses the correct hands and gets the same visual feedback.

Considerations for Taking off or Putting on Socks. Initially, use a sock that is stretchy and too big, as it will be easier to manage.

- If using a sock that is too big, do not expect the child to put his or her shoe on over it.
- Tube socks do not have a defined heel area; therefore, they are easier to put on, as lining up the heel is generally the most difficult step.
- Make sure the child is in a well-supported sitting position so that his or her arms and hands are free to put on or take off the socks.
- Sit behind or next to the child if assistance is needed; this places you in the same orientation as the child when completing the task.
- Encourage the child to use both hands when putting on or taking off socks; the pull will be more equal and evenly distributed.

Considerations for Taking off or Putting on Shoes. Use a shoe or slipper that can easily be slipped off and on.

- When starting out, remove the laces from tie shoes to make it easier to practice putting them on and taking them off.
- Put a small colored dot on the front inside part of the sole of each shoe with puffy paint or a marker. This helps the child put the shoes on the correct feet by keeping the dots together on the inside. If the child puts the shoes on the wrong feet, the dots will be on the outside.
- For the child who knows right and left, put R and L labels on the inside of each shoe so they are visible to help the child correctly orient the shoes when putting them on his or her feet.
- If the child is standing up when putting on the shoe, he or she may need to stabilize the shoe on another object so that it does not slide as he or she attempts to push his or her foot into it.
- If the child has high-top tennis shoes, then teach him or her to grab each side to pull

them on. If there is a loop on the back of the shoes, the child also can use these to help pull the shoes on.

- With lower-cut shoes, have the child hold each shoe on the bottom and slide it onto the foot.

Considerations for Pulling Pants off and On. At first, use larger pants with an elastic waistband to make the pants easier to remove or put on.

- Use shorts or swimming trunks so the child does not have to manage longer pant legs.
- When the child can manage shorts, move on to lightweight pajamas with long legs. Pajamas have less material to manage than regular pants.
- Once pants are off past the child's knees, he or she can sit down to remove them from his or her feet if his or her balance is not adequate enough to allow him or her to step out of them in a standing position.
- Encourage the child to use both hands when putting on and taking off pants. This ensures that the child's pull is more equal and evenly distributed than if only one hand is used.

Considerations for Taking off or Putting on a Pullover Top. Start the process using a short-sleeved top with a loose-fitting neck.

- Place the shirt front side down on a bed or table so that all the child has to do is pick it up and put it on, as it is in the correct orientation.
- If the child has difficulty removing a top with front buttons, then have him or her unbutton the first two top buttons and remove the shirt over his or her head.
- If necessary, the shirt also can be put on this way, with the buttons already buttoned except for the top ones and cuffs.

Considerations for Taking off or Putting on a Coat. Use the flip-over method for the child who has difficulty positioning the jacket in the correct orientation. Place the jacket face up on a table with the collar toward the child's body. Have the child place both arms in the sleeves and then lift the arms up. This causes the jacket to flip over his or her head into the correct position.

If the child's jacket is a little bigger but not too long, the occupational therapist can try hanging the jacket on the back of the child's chair to orient and stabilize it. Once the coat is hanging on the back of the chair, have the child sit in the chair and put each of his or her arms in its sleeves. When he or she stands up, the jacket goes into the correct position, ready to be fastened. If the chair back is considerably lower than the child's shoulders, have the child place both arms into the armholes and then pull the coat up onto the shoulders.

Gender Differences With Fasteners. It is important to be aware of which side fasteners (e.g., buttons, zippers, snaps) are oriented on the child's clothing. Note that there are differences between boys' and girls' clothing. This affects which hand manipulates the fastener and which hand provides the stability (see Table 4.2).

Considerations for Unfastening or Fastening. The occupational therapist needs to discuss with the team which fastener is most difficult for the child to manage. Then the order that the fasteners are worked on can be prioritized, and the intervention will be more effective and appropriate.

When identifying a task that needs to be developed, such as managing the fastener on pants, the types of fasteners the child has on his or her pants must be identified, as these will need to be managed daily. In the authors' experience, when we charted the types of fasteners one young man wore to school, we found that he had more than five types to manage: a riveted button on blue jeans, a metal slide on khaki pants, a regular button on a different pair of khaki pants, an elastic waistband with a snap on warm-up pants, and a lace lock—a spring-loaded button that

Table 4.2. Gender Differences Using Fasteners

Fastener	Girls	Boys
Buttons (shirts)	Buttons on the left side require use of the left hand to button and the right hand to unbutton.	Buttons on the right side require use of the right hand to button and the left hand to unbutton.
Buttons (pants)	The regular and riveted buttons found on jeans are on the right side.	The regular and riveted buttons found on jeans are on the right side.
Metal slide fasteners for pants	The base is found on the right, with the top part on the left side.	The base is found on the right, with the top part on the left side.
Zippers[a]	The shank on the right side needs to be inserted into the slider on the left side.	The shank on the left side needs to be inserted into the slider on the right side.
Snaps[b]	The base is on the left side, and the top part is on the right side.	The base is on the right side, and the top part is on the left side.

[a]Inconsistencies are seen with adult zippers; the shank is found on the right and left sides for both women and men.

[b]Inconsistencies are seen with snaps on adult clothing for both women and men.

allows the wearer to slide it along the draw-string to tighten warm-up pants. It was decided that the child would wear pants with the same kind of fastener three days a week so that he could practice the type of fastener he was working on while at school. The other two days he wore warm-up pants because he could manage them independently.

Considerations for Unsnapping and Snapping. When working on snapping and unsnapping, first identify the type of clothing that the child needs to be able to snap and the effect it has on his or her ability to function. For example, if the coat has a zipper and then a row of snaps over the zipper, is it necessary to snap them if the jacket is zipped?

- Working on a lightweight jacket with snaps is easier than on a heavy winter jacket; it is easier to align the snaps if the jacket is not too bulky.
- Snaps require a considerable amount of strength; popping small bubble wrap is a very appropriate activity to facilitate the correct position of the thumb and fingers needed for snapping (this activity also provides resistance from the material itself, which improves strength).

- The child who has difficulty aligning and maintaining the alignment to push the snaps together may have more success practicing on a table. This technique, which is entirely different than the way the child needs to learn how to snap, gives him or her a sense of how to align the top and bottom of the snap to engage it. The bottom snap is placed flat on the table with the top snap placed on top of it. When the child pushes down to engage the snap, the table provides the stability and resistance that the child is unable to achieve when holding the snap himself or herself. Once the child can successfully snap on the table, he or she can begin to work on aligning the top and bottom of the snap while holding the item in the correct orientation in his or her lap.
- Modifications can be made to clothing if necessary. Hook and loop fasteners can be used without having to remove the snaps or alter the appearance of the clothing; they can be sewn next to the current location of the top and bottom snap.
- The small size of the bottoms and hips of younger children and toddlers often allow

these children to pull their pants up and down while keeping them snapped. This is not ideal, but it does allow a child to be more independent.

Considerations for Unbuttoning or Buttoning. Buttons with long shanks are easier to manage because they are easier to manipulate. Stretchy fabric is also easier to manage, as it gives more. If a child is experiencing difficulty, there are several options to pursue.

- A collar and cuff button extender can be used especially on cuffs so that they do not have to be unbuttoned. Cuffs are difficult to button because of their location and the thickness of the material. Buttons can be sewn on top of the existing buttonhole so that they appear to be buttoned.
- Hook and loop fasteners can be sewn onto the inside of both shirts and pants and used to fasten it. If a pair of pants has a metal slide as its fastener, then hook and loop fasteners can be sewn next to the existing fastener if it cannot be easily removed.
- Buttons can be sewn on with elastic thread so that there is more give as the child pulls on the button. The buttonholes also can be cut or made larger so it is easier to push the button through. This works especially well with jeans that have a riveted button.

Considerations for Unzipping and Zipping. Developmentally, zipping is one of the more difficult self-care skills to perform. Practicing engaging a zipper is easier on lightweight coats because there is less material, and the zippers are shorter and more flexible. Heavy winter coats typically have bigger, less flexible zippers. In addition, they may be longer, which makes it difficult for the child to reach the zipper. The child may be required to gather the bulky material to attempt to engage the zipper.

Some coats have a double zipper that allows them to be opened from the bottom. It is especially difficult to align both parts of the double zipper to insert the shank into the base to engage it. Coats with elastic along the bottom also are difficult to manage. The child must be able to stretch the elastic enough to bring the two parts of the zipper together and maintain that stretch while trying to insert the shank to engage the zipper. To address the issues listed, modifications can be made to garments or dressing routines. In the fall, it also may be helpful to provide parents with a list of things to consider when shopping for a new winter coat.

- Ski jackets and sports team jackets often are made so that they can be put on over the head, and they do not have full-length zippers that need to be engaged. There is just a short zipper at the top of the jacket to allow the head to fit through the opening.
- The larger plastic zippers used in heavier coats usually are brightly colored. All of the pieces are this color, which makes it difficult to distinguish the parts when trying to engage it. Ask parents for permission to use a permanent magic marker to mark the slide with a contrasting color, which will make it easier to see.
- Zipper pulls can be attached to the zipper tab to make it easier to hold when zipping or unzipping.
- Have the child practice zipping his or her winter coat in the fall before he or she actually needs to wear it.

Considerations for Untying or Tying Shoes. Tying shoes is the most difficult self-care task to accomplish, as it requires many components. If the child is having difficulty with a specific step, consider having him or her practice that step repeatedly in isolation until successful rather than working on each step in succession. If the child requires additional assistance, numerous practical techniques can be applied to the process to help him or her achieve success.

- The child can wear shoes that do not require tying.

- Curly laces can be used so that the child does not have to tie the shoes. These laces provide the ability to tighten the shoe by snugging up the curled lace.
- Different colored shoelaces can be used to provide a visual contrast, or the child can use a stiff ribbon with wire along the edges to practice tying a bow. The wire makes it easier to maintain the shape of the loop as the child practices. He or she also can practice tying a bow with the ribbon around his or her thigh so that it is in the correct orientation but is closer to him or her and easier to manage.
- Models can be made for each step of shoe tying task. Cardboard can be covered with plain contact paper so that it is not a distraction. Two holes are placed in the cover cardboard, and the shoelaces are threaded through the holes. Use different color laces for contrast. Control the length of the shoelaces so that they are easier to manage. Outlines can be drawn to show where to place the laces (e.g., make the X using the appropriate color) so that the child can lay the lace on top of the outline, using it as a visual cue.
- Making marks on the child's own laces with a permanent marker provides a visual cue to help the child know where to grab or align the laces when making a bow. The occupational therapist needs to perform the steps him- or herself to determine what component of the process he or she wants to emphasize and where to place each mark. Marks can be used to indicate where to grab each lace after the first step of crossing and pulling through to help control the size of the loop that the child makes.

Interventions for Hygiene.

Considerations for Handwashing. Practice with colored lotion or antibacterial soap. Have the child cover his or her entire hand; the color of the lotion or soap shows if an area has been missed.

Many children have difficulty performing the rotation component of handwashing that enables them to wash both sides of each hand. Have the child put enough soap on one palm so that, when the palms are rubbed together, enough soap is transferred to the other palm. He or she then can use the palm side of each hand to rub soap on the back of the opposite hand. This eliminates the need to use the rotation component. The child should be encouraged to rinse the soap off by holding his or her hands palm up and palm down under the water.

Interventions for IADLs in the School Environment.

Considerations for Containers and Packages Used in Lunches. If a child is unable to tear open packages commonly found in lunches, the parents can make a cut in the bag so that the child can tear it open. If this approach proves unsuccessful, the parent can put any cookies or chips in a sandwich bag that the child can manage, eliminating the need to tear open the original package.

- Some children have difficulty opening pop-top cans. An opener has been designed that can be used with soda and snack cans. It is, however, important to consider where the opener will be kept to make sure it is available when the child needs it and to reduce the chance of throwing it away. In some cafeterias, the lunch aides carry this opener with them.
- Request that any fruit packed in a container has a lid that either snaps or screws on so that the child can manage independently. To provide the student with practice opening a variety of containers, place classroom or therapy activities inside of containers. The student must open them to get to the activity.

Other Considerations for Lunch Time. Some cafeterias use foam trays with compartments. Heavier items such as milk cartons or fruit can cause a foam tray to become unbalanced, making it more difficult to manage. Plastic trays are easier to use.

Students who buy lunch or extras, such as milk, cookies, or ice cream, may have difficulty managing a wallet along with a tray. Depending on the types of wallet, it can be difficult to get the money out. To alleviate this, if the student purchases the same items each day, the exact amount of money can be placed in a sandwich bag so that he or she either can take the money out or hand the bag with the money in it to the person at the cash register. That way a student does not have to keep track of a wallet or deal with change.

Considerations Using Locks. Managing traditional combination locks can be difficult for some students, especially if the locks are built into the locker.

- Some students can manage a key lock.
- A variety of locks are available commercially that are much easier to open than the traditional combination lock. Some require only that the student line up three numbers in a row to open them. In general, the numbers can be selected and set so that the student can remember the numbers.
- If the child is able to manage a regular combination lock but has difficulty lining up the numbers, highlighting the numbers on the lock makes it easier to find them.

Considerations for Fasteners.

- Parents can make cloth bags to hold activities; these can have a zipper, snaps, or buttons. Students are required to unzip, unsnap, or unbutton the bag to get to the activity and perform the reverse process when putting the activity away.
- Some teachers have art smocks with different types of fasteners to give students an opportunity to practice with them.
- Dressing vests or boards also can be used to practice fasteners. The garment should be oriented so that the child is using the same hand that he or she would use if dressing himself or herself.

- Some teachers have clothing with fasteners in the dress-up or make-believe area of the classroom for children to practice with.

A sample self-care goals form is provided in Figure 4.1.

Completion of the SCFC

The SCFC can be sent to classroom staff to complete before observing or evaluating students. Occupational therapists can use it as a tool to interview the appropriate classroom staff (or parent) to identify areas of performance that may be affecting a student's ability to function in school. If the SCFC already has been completed, the therapist needs to meet with the person who completed it to go over the responses and ask for additional information. Based on these follow-up responses, the therapist should observe or evaluate the areas of concern that have been identified as affecting the student's ability to function in school.

The Interpretation section is included to help occupational therapists summarize and synthesize the information in the SCFC by identifying the components that students lack to perform specific tasks and by listing strategies that can be used to remediate the deficits. The intent is to help therapists integrate the information obtained so that they can identify if specific components are lacking in the child's skill development. If so, and if these were developed, this has a positive affect on many of the areas identified. After completing the observation or direct evaluation, the occupational therapist should go to the Interpretation section at the end of the SCFC to complete the identified information.

In Section 1, the occupational therapist should identify the specific areas of concern that most directly affect the child's ability to function in school. If there are many areas, the therapist can prioritize those that seem to have the greatest impact with input from classroom staff and parents.

1. Student will independently complete _____ out of 5 steps in the shoe tying task analysis _____% for each step (Percent of successful attempts for each step)

2. Student will be able to zip up jacket or coat once zipper is engaged _____% of attempts

3. Student will be able to unzip jacket or coat so zipper comes apart at bottom _____% of attempts

4. Student will independently engage zipper on a variety of coats _____% of attempts

5. Student will line up the top and bottom parts of snap _____% of attempts

6. Student will independently snap the snap on pair of pants. Criteria: _____% of attempts

7. Student will independently snap the snaps on a coat. Criteria: _____% of attempts

8. Student will independently button/unbutton riveted button on his or her jeans. Criteria: _____% of attempts

9. Student will independently button or unbutton buttons on a shirt. Criteria: _____% of attempts

10. Student will properly orient and put on coat using flip-over or traditional method (Circle method used). Criteria: _____% of attempts

11. Student will independently orient and hang up coat on a hook. Criteria: _____% of attempts

12. Student will complete _____ out of _____ steps to manage clothing as a part of the toileting routine. Criteria: _____% of attempts

13. Student will be able to independently access soap/antibacterial lotion from dispenser. Criteria: ____% of attempts

14. Student will independently complete _____ /_____ steps of hand-washing task analysis. Criteria: _____% of attempts

15. Student will manage personal belongings (list specific belongings to collect data on) that are required during the school day (including book bags, folders, art box, locker) _____% of the time

16. Student will manage a combination lock/key lock to open his or her locker _____% of attempts

17. Student will use a 3-finger grasp to pick up small food items and carry to mouth. Criteria: _____% of the time

18. Student will scoop food with spoon and take it to mouth without spilling. Criteria: _____% of attempts

19. Student will stab food with fork and take it to mouth without it falling off. Criteria: _____% of attempts

20. Once spoon or fork is loaded by an adult, the student will take loaded spoon to mouth and take a bite of food. Criteria: _____% of attempts

21. Student will pick up cup, take it to mouth, tilt cup to take a drink, and return it to table so that it remains upright _____% of attempts

22. Student will pick up a cup, take it to mouth, and tilt the cup to take a drink. Criteria: _____% of attempts

23. Student will be able to open containers/packages required at lunch (including Tupperware containers, milk, juice box, pop cans, snack foods) _____% of attempts for each item

Figure 4.1. Sample Self-Care Goals and Objectives

In Section 2, the occupational therapist should list the components that prevent the child from completing the tasks identified in Section 1 to see if common components might be interfering with task completion (e.g., lack of hand separation, lack of wrist mobility needed for spoon feeding and cup drinking). Other factors (e.g., attention issues, inability to understand what is being asked, refusal to perform the task) also should be listed, especially if it appears that the child has the motor components to complete the task.

In Section 3, specific intervention strategies, such as working on hand separation activities to increase supination needed for spoon-feeding, should be listed. The intent of this section is to encourage the occupational therapist to identify specific intervention strategies (or preparation tasks) to address the components identified in Section 2. This is more efficient and effective than having the student practice a task he or she is unable to complete. For example, instead of giving the student small pieces of food during snack time in an attempt to get him or her to use a three-finger grasp, have him or her work on specific intervention strategies needed to develop a three-finger grasp. At the end of the session, give him or her small pieces of food to see if the grasp has changed.

References

American Occupational Therapy Association. (2002). Occupational therapy practice framework: Domain and process. *American Journal of Occupational Therapy, 56,* 609–639.

Brigance, A. H. (1991). *Diagnostic Inventory of Early Development.* North Billerica, MA: Curriculum Associates.

Coster, W., Deeney, T. A., Haltiwanger, J. T., &

Haley, S. M. (1998). *School Function Assessment.* San Antonio, TX: Psychological Corporation.

Gaddes, W. H. (1980). *Learning disabilities and brain function.* New York: Springer-Verlag.

Goldsmith, M. C. (1999). *Teaching dressing skills: Buttons, bows, and more.* Framingham, MA: Therapro.

Haley, S. M., Coster, W. L., Ludlow, L. H., Haltiwanger, J. T., & Andrellos, P. J. (1992). *Pediatric Evaluation of Disability Inventory.* Boston: New England Medical Center Hospital and PEDI Research Group.

Henderson, A. (1995). Self-care and hand skills. In A. Henderson & C. Pehoski (Eds.), *Hand function in the child: Foundations for remediation* (pp. 164–183). St. Louis, MO: Mosby.

Henderson, A., & Pehoski, C. (Eds.). (1995). *Hand function in the child: Foundations for remediation.* St. Louis, MO: Mosby.

Individuals With Disabilities Education Act, P.L. 101-476, 20 U.S.C. §1401 (1990).

Klein, M. (1983). *Pre-dressing skills.* Tuscon, AZ: Community SkillBuilders.

Kramer, P., & Hinojosa, J. (1999). *Frames of reference for pediatric occupational therapy* (2nd ed.). Baltimore, MD: Lippincott Williams & Wilkins.

Morris, S. E., & Klein, M. D. (1987). *Pre-feeding skills.* Tuscon, AZ: Therapy SkillBuilders.

Newborg, J., Stock, J. R., Wnek, L., Guidubaldi, J., & Suinicki, A. (1988). *Battelle Developmental Inventory.* Chicago: Riverside.

Orelove, F., & Sobsey, D. (1996). Self-care skills. In F. Orelove & D. Sobsey (Eds.), *Educating children with multiple disabilities* (3rd ed., pp. 333–375). Baltimore, MD: Brookes.

Shepherd, J. (2001). Self-care and adaptations for independent living. In J. Case-Smith, (Ed.), *Occupational therapy for children* (4th ed., pp. 489–527). St. Louis, MO: Mosby.

Smith, R., Benge, M., & Hall, M. (1994). Technology for self-care. In C. Christiansen (Ed.), *Ways of living: Self-care strategies for special needs* (pp. 379–422). Rockville, MD: American Occupational Therapy Association.

Appendix 4.1. Self-Care Functional Checklist

The intent of the Self-Care Functional Checklist is to help occupational therapists identify the difficulty students have with specific ADLs or IADLs that may affect their ability to function in the school setting, restricting their independence. It is not intended to be used with students who are unable to perform many self-care tasks due to their developmental level. A more appropriate assessment such as the Brigance, Diagnostic Inventory of Early Development, the Pediatric Evaluation of Disability Inventory, or the School Function Assessment can be used for such students.

Student _____

Date of Birth _____

Teacher _____

School _____

Age _____

Therapist _____

Person Completing Form _____

Date _____

Please complete any sections below for which there are areas of concern.

I. Dressing Skills

Yes   No   Does student have difficulty:

___ ___   1a. Putting coat on and taking coat off?

Technique used:
Traditional _____ Flip-Over Method_____

1b. If yes, what type of assistance is needed?_____

___ ___   2. Putting coat on and taking coat off of a hook?

___ ___   3. Pulling sleeves out of coat if they are inside out?

___ ___   4. Putting on art smock or oversized t-shirt or paint shirt? Pull over or front opening? (Circle one)

___ ___   5. Pulling zipper up and down on jacket once engaged?

___ ___   6. Disengaging zipper when pulling it down to take coat off?

___ ___   7. Engaging zipper on a variety of coats? (Is there a difference between student's ability to manage winter coat vs. spring coat, or different types of coats in one season, such as a long coat vs. short coat)?_____

_____

___ ___   8. Managing snaps on a coat?

___ ___   9. Pulling pants and underwear up and down when using restroom?

___ ___   10. Untying and removing shoes?

___ ___   11. Removing shoes when laces are loose?

___ ___   12. Removing boots?

___ ___   13. Putting on shoes?

___ ___   14. Putting on shoes with correct left and right orientation?

___ ___   15. Tying shoes?

If yes, can child complete any steps of shoe tying independently? Please list.

_____

_____

___ ___   16. Putting on boots?

___ ___   17. Managing shoes with hook-and-eye fasteners?

___ ___   18. Managing buttons on shirt?

___ ___   19. Managing buttons on pants?

___ ___   20. Managing snaps on pants?

___ ___   21. Managing riveted buttons on jeans?

Comments:

_____

_____

_____

(continued)

II. Feeding Skills

Yes No Does student have difficulty:

___ ___ 1. Picking up food items and placing them in mouth?

___ ___ 2. Feeding self independently using a spoon?

If yes, what is preventing the child from using the spoon?_____

_____

___ ___ 3. Feeding self independently using a fork?

If yes, what is preventing the child from using the fork?_____

_____

___ ___ 4. Using a knife to spread butter or other spread?

___ ___ 5. Cutting soft foods using a knife?

___ ___ 6. Drinking from a cup?

___ ___ 7. Drinking from a straw?

___ ___ 8. Opening and removing items from lunch bag or lunch box?

___ ___ 9. Opening packages and containers?

If yes, list the containers or packages the child has difficulty opening._____

_____

___ ___ 10. Opening milk cartons or juice boxes?

___ ___ 11. Managing lunch tray, such as putting food items on tray and carrying tray?

___ ___ 12. Managing wallet or change purse to access money to buy lunch?

III. Managing Belongings

Yes No Does student have difficulty:

___ ___ 1. Managing zipper on book bag?

___ ___ 2. Putting items into and taking items out of book bag?

___ ___ 3. Putting book bag on self?

___ ___ 4. Hanging up book bag?

___ ___ 5. Opening art box or pencil case?

___ ___ 6. Getting into desk to take items out?

___ ___ 7. Managing binder/notebook/folders? (if applicable)

IV. Managing School Environment

Yes No Does student have difficulty:

___ ___ 1. Drinking from the drinking fountain?

___ ___ 2. Sharpening pencil using manual sharpener?

___ ___ 3. Managing combination lock (if applicable) and opening locker?

___ ___ 4. Opening classroom, bathroom, building entry doors?

V. Hygiene

Yes No Does student have difficulty:

___ ___ 1. Washing hands independently? (Please check steps student is able to complete):

___ Turning faucet on or off

___ Obtaining soap and applying to hands

___ Rubbing hands together

___ Rinsing hands thoroughly

___ Obtaining paper towels

___ Drying hands thoroughly

Comments:_____

_____

_____

_____

___ ___ 2. Wiping face independently?

___ ___ 3. Blowing nose? (Please check if student is able to complete the following items):

___ Wipes nose using tissue

___ Blows nose on request

___ Initiates getting a tissue to blow nose

(continued)

For Therapist's Use Only

Interpretation of Results:

1. Identify the specific areas of concern (e.g., student unable to drink from regular cup):_____

   _____

   _____

   _____

   _____

   _____

2. What performance components are interfering with the student's ability to perform the identified skills
   (e.g., in-hand manipulation skills, 3-finger grasp, tilting the cup to drink)?

   Dressing: _____

   _____

   _____

   _____

   Feeding:_____

   _____

   _____

   _____

   Managing School Belongings and School Environment: _____

   _____

   _____

   _____

   Hygiene: _____

   _____

   _____

   _____

3. What intervention strategies will be used to remediate the skill deficits? _____

   _____

   _____

   _____

   _____

   _____

Developed by Lynne Pape, MEd, OTR/L, and Kelly Ryba, OTR/L

Hand Skills Needed for Fine Motor Tasks in the Classroom

5

Hand function in a school-based setting is critical because classroom skills are measured primarily by motor output. Each of the following tasks contain fine motor performance skills:

- Work that requires cutting, coloring, and gluing;
- Art projects;
- The playing of musical instruments;
- The manipulation of small items like math cubes;
- The management of the computer (e.g., mouse, keyboard);
- The management of personal belongings; and
- The performance of self-care tasks.

Effective use of the hands to perform or engage in daily activities depends on a complex interaction with a variety of other performance components. Development of hand skills does not occur in isolation (Exner, 2001). The complexity of hand skill use is illustrated by the length of time needed to develop and perfect the skills. Whereas the variety of grasps needed to perform tasks are present during the first year of life, the ability to manipulate objects with the efficiency and precision of an adult continues to develop and improve throughout late childhood and early adolescence (Case-Smith, 1995).

Visual skills play a major role in the development of hand function. The eyes drive the hands. Visual–perceptual and visual–motor skills provide feedback to guide the hands when performing tasks and during interaction with objects. A correlation also exists between a child's cognitive ability and hand skills development; cognition influences the development of hand skills. In addition, cultural and social factors (e.g., gender, socioeconomic status, role expectations) may affect the development of hand skills (Exner, 2001).

Occupational therapists in school settings frequently are called on to evaluate students because of concerns with fine motor performance skills as identified by difficulty with task completion in the educational setting. Although a variety of fine motor assessments are available, the intent of the evaluation process should be to use a variety of assessment tools and strategies, including information provided by the parents and teachers, to gather relevant functional and developmental information. Assessment tools and strategies need to assist the educational team in directly determining the child's educational needs.

The fine motor assessments currently available do not provide data regarding the student's performance and level of competence in the classroom setting. Standardized fine motor assessments require further application and inferences by the occupational therapist if the performance on the test is to be related to performance in the classroom (Clark & Coster, 1998). For example, there is an item in the fine motor subtest of the Bruininks–Oseretsky Test of Motor Proficiency (Bruininks, 1978) that measures response speed. It requires the child to stop the response speed stick with his or her thumb as it is being dropped. Attempting to relate this task to the student's performance in the classroom is very difficult.

School-based occupational therapists must be able to gather data and information to perform an effective assessment that will help educational teams achieve a comprehensive picture of the student's fine motor performance in the educational setting. This information is considered by the team to help determine if fine motor difficulties are affecting the student's ability to benefit from the educational program.

The complexity of hand skill development does not allow this chapter to discuss all of the components that affect this process. The focus is on hand skill development, assessment, and intervention.

Foundation of Fine Motor Skills

The development of refined fine motor skills is necessary for students to perform a variety of tasks required in schools. When students lack the skilled and precise movements needed to function, knowledge of how the central nervous system affects development is helpful when evaluating the areas of concern.

Pehoski (1992), in reviewing neurophysiology literature, discussed two premises important for understanding the central nervous system's control over precision movements of the hand. Whereas it generally is accepted that upper extremity development proceeds from proximal to distal, one premise challenges that concept. This premise puts forth the idea that it is not one motor system that develops proximal to distal but rather two systems. One controls the distal hand and finger movements; the other controls the postural and more proximal hand movements. Therefore, to develop controlled reach and manipulation, the upper extremity must depend on two groups of descending fiber systems. Lemon (1990) indicated that skilled manipulation relies on the corticospinal track, whereas reach primarily relies on pathways that originate from the mid-brain and brainstem. In the second premise, ac-

cording to Pehoski (1992), skilled hand function depends on sensory feedback that might be different for the hand than for the trunk and shoulder girdle (postural control).

Nine-month-old infants are able to use a pincer grasp that involves the thumb and finger tips; however, it is not until around age 4 years that children have the ability to use the hands skillfully for more refined tasks such as buttoning. Several studies have indicated that this development may be related to the maturation of the neural structures that support skilled hand use.

Existence of Two Motor Systems

To understand the importance of the descending motor pathways, Kuypers (1981) has conducted research to show that two fundamentally different motor systems exist. One arises from the brainstem structures, which are believed to relate to posture and proximal control. The other arises from cortical structures (primary motor cortex), which are believed to relate to distal control.

Kuypers (1981) stated that Group A, or medial brainstem pathways, is related to the maintenance of erect posture, integration of body and limb movements, and coordination of body and head movements. Group B, or lateral brainstem pathways, provides independent flexor-biased movements of the extremities, especially in the distal parts. The corticospinal tracts provide precision and speed and, especially in primates, the ability to isolate individual movements as exemplified by finger movements. Corticospinal fibers need to make direct contact with the motor neurons of the hands to produce controlled precise movements. A comparison of the shape of squirrel monkey's hand and fingers to that of the rhesus monkey demonstrates this need. The hands and fingers of the two types of monkeys are almost identical. The difference, as indicated by Lawrence and Hopkins (1976), is that the squirrel monkey has no direct cortical motor connections, so it is only able to grasp small objects by using total finger flexion. The rhesus monkey has direct cortical connections and, subsequently, the ability to manipulate objects with precision.

Muir and Lemon (1983) further demonstrated the importance of the primary motor cortex in the precision use of the hand. The authors trained a monkey to squeeze two levers, one that required a precision grip and another that needed a power grip. The responses from the hand were recorded using an electromyograph. The primary motor cortex neurons were found to be more active during the fractionation of muscles required for discrete movements, such as movements of individual fingers (precision grasp). In the power grip, the monkey produced a general contraction of all the digits, and the neurons were not as active. Clough, Kernell, and Phillips (1968) found that cortical stimulation produced the greatest response in the intrinsic muscles of the hand. This is not surprising, as the intrinsic muscles are important for precision movements of the hand and fingers; the extrinsic muscles are responsible for the force (power grip).

It also has been observed that the primary motor cortex is related to the initiation of willed or learned motor responses as opposed to instinctual motor responses. Hoffman and Luschell (1980) found that, during goal-directed, learned movements, the discharge of motor cortex neurons increased compared to the number discharged during instinctual movements (e.g., using a pincer grasp to pick up a small piece of food vs. using a pincer grasp to pinch someone). Cortically induced, or learned, movements tend to involve the need for long-term training. Occupational therapists can devise treatment interventions to work on the development of more refined, precise movement. This is discussed more specifically in a later section on intervention.

When a learned or willed movement occurs that requires small, precise movements, sensory feedback is provided to assist in the control and modification of the movement. Without this feedback regarding the hand's movements, smooth, efficient performance is seriously affected.

Sensory Motor Integration and Feedback

When small, precise movements occur, the sensory feedback generated travels back to the primary motor cortex, which activates the contracting muscles (Pehoski, 1992). Evarts (1981) discussed the role of somatosensory feedback to the motor cortex in controlling movements. Therefore, loss of sensory feedback from either a peripheral injury or a lesion in the primary sensory cortex affects everyday hand function. Evarts also suggested that sensory information, such as that from the muscle spindle receptors, provides feedback to help correct for small errors. The intrinsic muscles of the hand are the most innervated with muscle spindle receptors (Cooper, 1960). These receptors contribute to skilled hand use by coordinating the forces between extrinsic and intrinsic muscles, rapidly correcting for errors, and providing stability for the digits.

Several factors affect the hand's ability to manipulate objects skillfully. The fingers need to be able to move independently of each other to perform precise, controlled, and efficient tasks. This is not possible if the hand does not receive adequate sensory information about the movement of the fingers and objects within the fingers.

Eliasson (1995) described how the sensory information of an object is integrated with the motor processing to achieve smooth, coordinated movements of the hand. The proprioceptive system provides information about the positions of the limbs both when they are static (limb position sense) and when they are moving (kinesthesia). The receptors are in the tendon organs, muscle spindles, and skin. The tendon organs provide information about the strength of a muscle contraction, and the muscle spindle is responsible for small changes in a contraction. Although not fully understood, it appears that the muscle spindle may be important for force regulation during grasping. The tactile system as a whole helps discriminate between different shapes and textures and provides feedback to the central nervous system to help regulate the force of the muscles during grasping and holding of objects.

Johansson and Westling (1984) found that, when adults use a pincer grip to pick up and lift small objects, the force controlling the grip and the force providing the lift occur at the same time. So when the object is picked up, the force of the grip is adequate to maintain the hold on the object. The change in force for different textures (e.g., silk vs. wood) appears to be related to tactile input so that the grip force can be adjusted to maintain a balance.

Small children also can use tactile and proprioceptive feedback to adjust these forces during the static phase before an object is picked up. However, the final phase, when the object has been picked up and is being held in the air, is not developed until the teenage years (Forssberg, Eliasson, Kinoshita, Johansson, & Westling, 1991). Tactile discrimination itself occurs early in development. One-year-old children can recognize dissimilar objects that differ in texture and shape and use different ways to explore them. Children's nervous systems still are immature, but there is early interaction between somatosensory signals and motor output. It is not until at least age 4 years that children begin to perform skills that depend on precision handling. These skills continue to improve until about ages 8 to 11 years (Koh & Eyre, 1988).

Giuliani (1991) stated that the execution of movement is controlled by two types of mechanisms. Sensory information initiates coordination of the movement and plays a direct role in a closed-loop, or feedback, mechanism. Initial skill acquisition, especially one that requires discrete and complex movements, uses this type of mechanism. It also is used in the development of skills that need hand–eye coordination.

The second type of mechanism is the open-loop, or feedforward. This mechanism may use the sensory information prior to movement and evaluate the movement once it is completed, but the sensory input does not change the motor output during execution. The feedforward mechanism is used with rapid or well-learned movements (Giuliani, 1991).

Both of these mechanisms are used in the development of motor control. Initially, the infant performs new skills slowly and deliberately, using the feedback process to reinforce the skills. With practice, the skill comes to be performed automatically without the sensory feedback, using a feedforward mode of execution (Alexander, Boehme, & Cupps, 1993).

Movements of the hand, like any other movement, require sensory feedback. Tactile feedback helps regulate the force of the grasp needed to pick up and move an object without its slipping as it is being moved. The proprioceptive system provides feedback regarding the position of the arm and hand at rest and during movement. In addition, the primary sensory cortex assists in developing motor memories that allow for efficient motor execution. Therefore, sensory feedback is critical for the development and ongoing monitoring of skilled function in the hands.

Haptic Perception

The importance of sensory feedback in the development of precision movements has been discussed. As the hand performs everyday activities such as zipping a jacket, it also depends on its ability to process and perceive additional information needed to achieve the task. The hand needs to be considered a perceptual, or information-seeking, organ (Stilwell & Cermak, 1995).

Haptic perception (active touch) helps infants begin to process the information needed to learn about the characteristics of objects (Ruff, 1980). The development of active touch deals with the retrieval, analysis, and interpretation of the tactile properties (e.g., size, shape, texture) to assist in the identification of objects through manual and in-hand manipulation (Gibson, 1962). Haptic perception often is referred to as the ability to recognize common objects and shapes through touch. However, it is important to be aware of the fact that the hand also is used to obtain information about textures, weight, hardness, size, and spatial orientation (Stilwell & Cermak, 1995).

Around ages 4 to 6 months, infants' mouths are the source of haptic information. The mouth can gain information about the size, shape, and texture of objects before the hands are developmentally able to do so. As infants develop, the hands become a perceptual system that participates in their construction of knowledge as they begin to manipulate objects (Hatwell, 1987). For Gibson (1962), the process of tactile scanning includes a combination of feedback from tactile, kinesthetic, and proprioceptive sensations.

Vision plays a key role in the development of haptic perception. Rochat (1989) noted a major link between vision and haptic exploration and suggested that refined object manipulation is more likely to occur when infants look at the objects as they manipulate them. This indicates the need for infants to see their hands during object manipulation. Haptic manipulation is important in the early learning of object characteristics. Ruff (1980, 1982) indicated that, as infants look at the objects they are manipulating and see them from different viewpoints, they are learning about the objects' properties. This is important for the development of object recognition (form constancy) so that the object can be recognized in different orientations or in any context. In addition, the infant acquires tactile and kinesthetic information about the object.

Around age 6 years, children are able to explore objects with their hands without needing to use their vision. This allows them to more efficiently manipulate objects and perform daily tasks without relying on their vision for feedback. This is critical for the accomplishment of self-care tasks, especially when a task is not being performed in the child's visual field (e.g., buttoning a button on the back of the body).

Impact of Cognitive Abilities

Fine motor manipulation skills depend on the interaction of cognitive and motor abilities. Limitations in either of these areas may influence the development and performance of the other.

In specific developmental assessments, motor performance scores often are dependent on the child's cognitive ability to understand the directions and replicate the task. The motor component is less important. For example, if a child can pick up and stack three cubes but is unable to duplicate a three-cube bridge, he or she does not get credit for his or her motor abilities, because that specific task requires more perceptual and cognitive performance than motor.

Lidz (1987) defined *cognition* as the capacity by which a person acquires, organizes, and uses knowledge. It is considered to include multiple classes of mental capacities such as attention, perception, memory, reasoning, problem solving, and language (Glass & Holyoak, 1986). Some have argued that it also needs to include higher level processes such as imagining, creating, planning, categorizing information, conceptual thinking, and using symbols (Exner & Henderson, 1995).

A *motor skill* is composed of the precisely executed and organized movement sequences used to accomplish a specific goal. Three fundamental characteristics of motor performance—goal direction, proficiency, and organization—are identified in this definition. The goal-directed component differentiates skilled movement from other movement, as it requires planning and memory.

The second characteristic that distinguishes motor skill is *proficiency,* or the quality and accuracy, of the movement (Fitts & Posner, 1967). Finely coordinated movement requires sensory feedback as the movement is being performed. This ensures that adjustments that require perception and cognition can be made (Sugden & Keogh, 1990).

Third, skilled movements always include an organized sequence of activities (Fitts & Posner, 1967). Daily activities such as dressing, eating, and writing require a sequence of actions that needs to be executed quickly, efficiently, and with minimal effort (Connolly, 1973). Problem solving, planning, strategy acquisition, and learning are necessary for sequential, organized movements (Exner & Henderson, 1995).

Planning, problem solving, sequencing, organizing, and learning all require cognition. Difficulty with any of these is seen when working with children who have cognitive deficits. These difficulties must be considered and be put into perspective when working on fine motor skill acquisition so that realistic expectations can be defined.

Basic Cognitive Processes

The characteristics of motor performance and the cognitive components that are critical to the development of motor skills already have been discussed. Attention, perception, memory, and thinking are the aspects of cognition specifically involved with motor skills.

Attention

Attention is a basic component of all cognitive activities. Klein (1976) noted that new motor skills could be acquired only when attention is focused on the skill. Both simple and complex motor skills require the regulation of attention for their development. Attention is used the most during the initiation of movement and when learning a new movement. As the skill becomes more automatic there is less need to attend to the task.

When working on the acquisition of specific fine motor tasks, it is critical to document the frequency needed to redirect a student back to the activity. This information should be included in the daily notes and represented in the data when reporting the student's progress.

Perception

Perception allows us to acquire information about places, objects, and events (Gibson & Spelke, 1983). Perceptual–motor and perceptual–conceptual functions both are essential for skilled hand use.

Perceptual–motor function provides the monitoring of movement that supplies the feedback necessary to attain precise movements. When people reach for objects, they are not aware of the movement adjustments made to grasp the objects because perceptual–motor control is unconscious (Exner & Henderson, 1995).

Perceptual–conceptual systems also function within the environment. They assist in deciding what to do and in what sequence, based on perceptual knowledge of objects, places, and events. Perception depends on obtaining information about the environment. Movement sequences are planned based on this information (Gibson & Spelke, 1983). Understanding and using the perceptual knowledge of objects requires language (e.g., being able to label the object as a ball) and the cognitive ability to plan the movement sequences.

Memory

All of our knowledge is stored in *memory,* but that storage only lasts varying amounts of time. Long-term memory is relatively permanent. Short-term memory remains only for a brief time after information is processed. Long-term and short-term memory are critical to the development of fine motor skills. Both allow people to store and use past information to assist in the recalling of concepts and the categorizing of knowledge, reasoning, problem solving, and planning. Occupational therapists show children how to perform specific skills that use knowledge or memory. As children learn the skill, they store that knowledge in their memory so that they are able to recall it when needed (Exner & Henderson, 1995).

When working with students with known cognitive deficits, it is not uncommon to see that, by the end of a session, they appear to understand the components needed to perform a specific skill. However, by the next session, the occupational therapist often will note that it is necessary to begin the process over again. It is critical to document the lack of ability to acquire and maintain the skill. This all should be included in daily documentation and progress notes.

Thinking

According to Exner and Henderson (1995), *thinking* is classified as a higher order mental process that acts on knowledge encoded and stored in memory. Organization of the knowledge base into conceptual categories and the use of knowledge in reasoning, problem solving, goal selection, and planning are included in these mental processes. Knowledge is organized through thinking. It is used for the selection of a goal, the selection of a plan of action, the prediction of consequences for that action, and judgment of the monitored outcome (Exner & Henderson, 1995).

The need to depend on memory for making predictions and judgments often is very difficult for some of the students with whom occupational therapists work and affects the students' ability to acquire and generalize fine motor skills.

Using Processes in Interventions

When designing intervention strategies, it is important to select activities that are appropriate for a child's cognitive ability and developmental level. This motivates the child to try the activity and be successful enough to continue doing it. When activities are too difficult for students, they often become frustrated and may refuse to participate.

It is important to break a task down into specific parts when providing intervention so that each step can be taught. Do not attempt or expect to expose the child to the whole task. This step is especially important when working on self-care tasks, such as dressing and managing fasteners.

Therapy documentation needs to reflect the effect of each cognitive component on the acquisition of fine motor skills. Documentation of the student's behavior, including frustration and refusal to participate, is critical. This information can be used to modify intervention strategies or goals. It can be applied during discussions of the appropriateness of working on tasks that require higher level cognitive abilities than some students are capable of using.

Reach, Grasp, and Release Development

Engaging in play and education requires the ability to explore, manipulate, and perform activities of daily living and other school-related tasks that depend on the development of hand skills. Primitive and reflexive hand function evolves into efficient manipulation skills within the first year of an infant's life. It is imperative that occupational therapists understand how children develop the foundation needed for specific functional skills. This information is used when evaluating specific hand functions and functional skills within the school setting. It also can assist the therapist when identifying and developing interventions.

Newborn

Upper Extremity Development. Newborns display random upper extremity movement in combination with reflex activity. When in a supine position, the asymmetrical tonic neck reflex is elicited by the head turning to the side. Functionally, this results in the hand being within infants' visual field; however, newborns do not attend to their hands. When prone, infants' legs are flexed up under the stomach, causing the majority of their weight to shift forward through the head and upper extremities.

Hand Development. Infants' hands usually are closed in a fisted position with the thumb inside the palm. The grasp reflex is present and is elicited when an object comes in contact with the palm. Newborns have no ability to voluntarily release an object that is in the hand. The object either is dropped inadvertently as the arm is randomly moved away from the body and the grasp reflex relaxes or an adult must remove it. Newborns are unable to reach or grasp an object with intent or in response to a stimulus (Erhardt, 1982). If newborns make contact with an object, that contact is secondary to random movement.

Early Infancy (0–3 Months)

Upper Extremity Development. By age 3 months, infants are able to push up from a prone position to lift their head. This enables them to visually scan their environment. With this movement, infants are receiving proprioceptive and kinesthetic cues that are beginning to be integrated into their body scheme. These cues contribute to functional control of the upper extremity (Colangelo, Bergen, & Gottlieb, 1976). Infants are unable to reach out because of a lack of shoulder stability and an inability to laterally shift their weight to free their arm, so they explore their environment with their mouth.

In a supine position, the head and arms are held in midline, and the fisted hands can be brought to the mouth. The increase in midline control provides the support needed for improved visual skills, such as convergence and midline visual regard. Infants now begin to observe their hands. As infants focus on specific objects, there is movement in the arms and hands that illustrates the connection between the visual and motor systems. The visual system is a powerful motivator that encourages reaching. Three-month-olds may activate both arms to swipe at objects. At this age, the upper extremity displays flexion in the elbows and extension in the wrist and hand during reaching (Erhardt, 1990).

Hand Development. At age 2 months, infants retain an object briefly when it is placed in their hands. The object is released without voluntary control, because there is still an influence from the grasp reflex. Two-month-olds also can clutch and scratch their blanket, which increases the tactile input into their hands. By age 3 months, infants are able to sustain a voluntary grasp when contact is made with an object. When approaching an object, the wrist is in flexion, ulnar deviation, and the thumb is adducted. The thumb is not actively involved; the ulnar, or central, fingers are used for grasping (Alexander et al., 1993).

Middle Months (4–6 Months)

Upper Extremity Development. Four-month-olds are able to push up on more extended arms from a prone position and are beginning to shift their upper body weight to the side when propped on their forearms. As weight is shifted over the forearm to the ulnar side, radial deviation of the wrist is reinforced. This prepares the hands for a more efficient grasp pattern. In a supine position, the child reaches with a more consistent symmetrical approach. When reaching, the elbows are extended and can briefly be held in space while contact with an object is made (Erhardt, 1982).

At age 5 months, infants are able to reach

from a prone position when their weight is shifted to one side, which frees the other side to reach out. This is the beginning of isolated control of each shoulder. This control is needed to achieve the unilateral reaching that manifests at approximately age 6 months. When propping the upper body on extended arms, the increased weight-bearing through the hands lengthens both the long finger flexors and the intrinsic musculature of the palm and thumb, which in turn provides additional tactile and proprioceptive input.

Five-month-old infants still use the bilateral reaching pattern but are beginning to grasp objects with one hand. Later, this single hand is joined by the other hand, which indicates the beginning of a unilateral reach that will develop within the next month. Sensory input from the flexors and the musculature prepares the hand for increased use of its radial side, including the thumb. At age 6 months, infants continue to reach forward with one arm, further developing isolated control of one shoulder girdle from the other (Alexander et al., 1993).

Hand Development. When 4-month-old infants reach for an object, the hand tends to remain open with the thumb held close to the palm. Infants display variety in the grasping pattern depending on the object's size, shape, and orientation. At this age, the grasp consists of active finger flexion into the palm without involvement of the thumb. Release continues to be involuntary.

Five-month-old infants use a symmetrical palmar grasp. They actively hold the object in the palm by flexing their fingers against the base of their thumb. There is more contact with objects, and they are beginning to bring them to their mouth for additional exploration. They can lift their arms up against gravity and are beginning to transfer objects from one hand to the other, initially taking them to the mouth with one hand and then grasping them with the other. They are beginning to release their grip by opening the hand

away from objects supported externally by an adult (Alexander et al., 1993).

At age 6 months, there is better wrist stability, which allows for more refined movement. The palmar grasp with the thumb abducted continues to be used to grasp smaller items; however, a radial–palmar grasp now is being used to grip larger objects that fit into the palm. The radial–palmar grasp occurs when the fingers press the object against the radial side of the hand and the opposed thumb (Erhardt, 1982). Six-month-olds are able to release an object through a two-stage transfer: The object first is picked up with one hand, and then it is transferred to the other hand. This requires concentration and effort, and infants are still unable to voluntarily release an object in space.

Pre-Toddler (7–9 Months)

Upper Extremity Development. At ages 7 to 9 months, children are able to reach in all directions and can raise their arms high enough to visually explore objects from a variety of spatial orientations. Their hands and eyes are more coordinated. Both work together, directing children's reaching by allowing them to better judge the distance and position of an object in relation to their body. This is the beginning of *praxis,* or the ability to plan and execute a sequence of movements to achieve an end result. Praxis depends on children's ability to interpret and reproduce kinesthetic cues and is related to tactile input. It is the tactile input that provides children with the feedback that he or she has successfully grasped the object (Colangelo et al., 1976).

Hand Development. Opportunities to move on all fours, with weight shifting into the palms, help children to develop balance reactions within the hand and reinforce the palmar arches (Boehme, 1988). At age 7 months, the radial–palmar grasp is being mastered. Objects are held in the palm supported by the first two fingers and the thumb. The beginning of supination is seen. Children are able to turn an object over to visually explore the other side.

The radial–digital grasp emerges at age 8 months. This grasp allows children to hold an object with the fingertips and to stabilize it with an opposed thumb (Erhardt, 1982). The visible space between the thumb and fingers indicates that the palmar arches are active. By age 9 months, children are able to achieve better distal control—the result of increased wrist stability as it moves from a neutral position to an extended position.

Continued weight bearing through the ulnar side of the hand as children hold objects while they creep helps develop the dissociation between the ulnar and radial sides of the hand. The two sides begin to work independently. This allows the development of the three-finger grasp and isolated pointing of the index finger. Such dissociation is critical, as it allows the development of the skilled side of the hand (the thumb, index finger, and middle finger) to support tool use.

A raking grasp, in which children use their fingers to rake small pieces into the palm, also is seen around age 7 months. The lateral pinch (thumb is adducted on the side of the index finger) develops by age 8 months. At age 9 months, an inferior pinch emerges, in which children hold an object between the thumb and the middle joint of the index finger. By the end of this stage, children can manipulate and explore all aspects of an object. This helps develop a sense of object permanence (Alexander et al., 1993).

Toddler (10–12 Months)

Upper Extremity Development. For toddlers, reaching is no longer compulsive but instead is rather deliberate. Toddlers are able to focus their undivided attention on a toy. They no longer need to look back and forth continually between their hand and the toy, and they are able to reach forward with intent. They can accommodate their hand to the size of the object for which they are reaching.

Toddlers' use of their arms has progressed from the bilateral and associated movements seen in infancy to a unilateral, or one-side, use. They have developed the capacity to inhibit the movements of their extremities. Skilled use of the hand also has developed in a unilateral fashion. Both hands may be active at the same time, but only one is functional and attended to by the toddler. Hand function generally is *ipsilateral,* which means that toddlers tend to use their right hand to interact with objects on the right side of the body and the left hand to work with objects on the left side. Crossing the midline is not often seen at this point (Colangelo et al., 1976).

Hand Development. By the end of this stage, children's hands have become efficient and functional. The fingers function better because the wrist is more stable. A pincer grasp is present; the thumb is able to neatly oppose the index finger. They now can hold an object between the distal pads of the thumb and index finger. The ability to inhibit movement of the other three fingers allows the index finger to be isolated for poking.

During this time, children may begin to demonstrate a hand preference. Children will hold an object with one hand and manipulate it with the preferred hand. Coordinated bilateral hand function begins at the end of the first year. Children have a sense of what is happening on both sides of the body at the same time and are able to coordinate these actions. Initially, bilateral skills consist of one hand functioning as a stabilizer as the other functions as a manipulator. More sophisticated bilateral skills that require different actions from each hand, such as shoe tying, do not appear until much later (Colangelo et al., 1976).

Toddlers manipulate objects by pushing, pulling, squeezing, and rotating them with both hands and enjoy toys with movable parts and observable actions. They have mastered the three-jaw chuck grasp, which involves holding an object between the thumb and first two fingers. This grasp, however, is insufficient for smaller objects. The pincer grasp is used to meet this need. By age 12 months, children can pinch by using the finger tips and thumb; with practice, greater thumb rotation is attained. Ten-month-old to 12-month-old children finger feed with more proficiency than younger children. At age 12 months, children begin to have the fine motor control needed for independence in the world (Alexander et al., 1993).

The interplay between the finger flexors and extensors allows toddlers to release objects with control. Previously, although flexor tone in the hand predominated, it lacked grading (the ability to control the movements). Therefore, grasp was accomplished by total flexion of the fingers. Release generally occurred through relaxation of the finger flexors. Toddlers can activate extensors in the hand on purpose to release objects into a container (Colangelo et al., 1976).

The Second Year

After the first year, further refinement occurs in previously developed grasp patterns, and additional, more sophisticated patterns emerge. Case-Smith (1995) described the increase in hand skills from ages 12 to 18 months. Children use these skills in more complex play activities because they now have a much better understanding of the functional purpose of objects and so are able to use them for their intended functions. In addition, they are using more than one object, which further results in more advanced bilateral skills.

Objects can be held with the fingertips when the hand is relatively static. Manipulation of objects continues to be performed by transferring them from one hand to the other. Children remain unable to manipulate them within just one hand. The ability to pick up and hold two objects in the same hand promotes individual finger movements and the continued dissociation of the two sides of the hand.

Between ages 12 and 15 months, increasing control of the intrinsic muscles may be seen. Children now are able to manage flat objects, such as cookies and crackers. This increased control affects the hand's ability to release. The ability to stack up to three cubes can be accomplished because children are able to stabilize the arm in space while maintaining mobility of the hand and fingers. This increased stability allows the wrist to move independently, which promotes tool use. Objects, such as a spoon or marker, are held with a static grasp. Movement occurs at the proximal joints (e.g., shoulder, elbow, wrist), but children are unable to manipulate the objects within their hand.

By the end of the second year, children can use this increased stability of the arm and the increased mobility of the hand to perform even more complex skills. The improved accuracy in placement and release of cubes allows 2-year-olds to create a six-cube tower. They are able to release the cubes with graded individual movement of the finger extensors. This increased mobility contributes to further refinement of tool use. Tasks that require more precise movements are performed using a pincer grasp, whereas the palmar grasp is used for those that require power (Case-Smith, 1995). Although studies are limited in this area, it appears that the ability to the use the power grasp needed to pound with a toy hammer develops in most children between ages 18 months and 3 years (Exner, 2001).

In-hand manipulation begins to develop at age 2 years. Children demonstrate finger-to-palm translation; they are able to pick up smaller objects and move them from their fingertips to their palm. They also are able to pick something up and turn it around in their hand using simple rotation, although they generally will use an external surface or both hands to accomplish this.

These skills continue to mature during the third year of life. Palm-to-finger translation and complex rotation are not used efficiently until children are ages 4 to 4 ½ years (Pehoski, Henderson, & Tickle-Dengen, 1997). Children continue to increase the speed of their in-hand manipulation tasks through age 6 years. As these skills mature during the preschool years, children begin to engage in activities that require control and the subtle movement of tools for writing, drawing, and brushing teeth (Case-Smith & Berry, 1998).

Within the first two years, the development of hand skills has gone from a reflexive grasp to a whole-hand grasp to sophisticated individualized manipulation. Multiple factors have contributed to this process. The postural control and proximal stability of the arm have resulted in increased hand control and children's ability to integrate tactile, proprioceptive, and visual feedback to increase movement precision. With increased cognition, children have developed more complex play schemes, which incorporate the functional use of objects and tools. Knowledge of this progression of fine motor development is necessary for occupational therapists to possess, as it is the basis from which hand function develops.

Tool Use

Fine motor development also includes children's ability to use tools. Tools serve as extensions of children's hands and allow children to perform more complex tasks. Connolly and Dalgleish (1989) defined *tool use* as "a purposeful, goal-directed form of complex object manipulation that involves the manipulation of the tool to change the position, condition, or action of another object"

(p. 895). Children use tools to accomplish many play, self-care, school, and work tasks.

Tool use begins to be seen once children master the foundation skills of reaching, grasping, and releasing, typically during the second year. Children's ability to perform in-hand manipulation skills, to position tools within the hand once they are picked up, determines the development of tool use. Cognition is a key factor in the acquisition of skills in which tools are used.

Connolly and Dalgleish (1989) emphasized that children need to know what they want to do with a tool (the intention of the task) and how to accomplish it (the operational aspect). This process requires cognitive skills to perform the intentional component and motor skills to perform the task that uses the tool.

The amount of exposure and opportunity children are given to use a tool affects their ability to perfect its use. If the parents are reluctant to allow their child to use a spoon during mealtime because they are concerned about the mess, the child has less opportunity to practice the skill. If the skill is to become functional and efficient for daily use, practice is necessary. Practice and repetition allow the child to reduce the amount of attention needed to complete the task so that it becomes automatic and can be performed faster with increased accuracy. The tool itself requires only one hand to hold it, but its use typically requires the assistance of the other hand to perform a completely different task. For example,

- When brushing the teeth, one hand holds the toothbrush while the other applies toothpaste.
- When cutting, one hand holds the scissors while the other manipulates the paper.
- When eating, one hand holds the spoon while the other stabilizes the dish.
- When using a knife for cutting food, one hand must hold and guide the knife while the other stabilizes the food, either with another tool or the hand itself.

Skilled use of the spoon, fork, and knife can require up to four years to develop.

Upper Extremity Components in the Development of Hand Function

The Shoulder

The shoulder is the most mobile of all the joints. It is able to move within three planes in space. As the most proximal joint of the upper limb, it allows the arm to reach forward in front of the body, up above the head, around to the back, out to the side, and around in a circle. Such movement is critical to reaching and often is where movement to position the hand begins. Activities such as combing hair or putting on a jacket cannot be performed without shoulder movement. The shoulder, in combination with the scapula, provides the stability needed to support the arm to allow for distal function.

The Elbow

The elbow is the intermediate joint of the upper extremity. It connects the upper arm and the forearm. As a result of movement at the shoulder, the elbow provides the movement needed so that the forearm can position the hand close to or away from the body. For example, when the elbow is extended and the forearm or hand is pronated, the elbow enables the hand to grasp objects and tools. With flexion at the elbow and supination of the forearm, the hand can bring those objects or tools or food to the head or mouth.

Forearm Rotation

Rotation is the movement of the forearm around its longitudinal axis, or pronation–supination (Kapandji, 1982). This allows the hand to be placed in any position to grasp or support an object. Rotation involves the elbow flexed at 90° and resting against the trunk of the body. *Pronation* occurs when the palm faces down and the thumb points medi-

ally toward the body. *Supination* occurs when the palm faces up and the thumb points laterally away from the body. *Neutral rotation* occurs when the palm faces the body medially and the thumb points up in neither pronation or supination.

The forearm's ability to pronate–supinate is critical for hand orientation control. It allows the hand to assume the optimal position for grasping. Combined with shoulder and elbow movement, it also allows the hand to reach to any part of the body and plays an essential role in all actions of the hand during work. Pronation–supination permits the hand to rotate an object, such as a screwdriver. When the forearm is pronated, the hand is slightly tilted toward the ulnar side in an attempt to bring the thumb and the index and middle fingers into line with the axis of the hand's rotation. In supination, the hand is tilted toward the radial side and favors a supportive grip to carry objects. The development of supination is critical to a child's fine motor success. Controlled use of the radial fingers and thumb depends on forearm supination (Kapandji, 1982).

The Wrist

The wrist is the most distal joint of the upper extremity. It allows the hand to assume optimal positions for *prehension,* the grasping and manipulating of objects. Movements of the wrist, combined with pronation and supination, permit the hand to be oriented in any angle to grasp or hold an object.

For the wrist to be in a functional position, it must be extended 40° to 45° and is in slight ulnar deviation to 15°. The finger flexors are in their most advantageous position here because they are shorter than when the wrist is neutral or flexed. This optimal position allows for both a power grasp and precision movements. When the wrist is extended, the thumb is able to oppose the other fingers. However, when the wrist is flexed, the efficiency of the flexors is only a quarter of what it is when the wrist is extended (Kapandji, 1982).

The Hand

The hand performs many movements, but its essential function is prehension. The fingers, combined with an opposable thumb, create unlimited prehension opportunities for the hand. The hand is not only a motor organ; it also is a sensory receptor that provides vital feedback for its own performance. This feedback is essential for *stereognosis,* which is the ability to identify objects by touch alone. It allows the hand to use texture, weight, temperature, and shape to identify objects without using vision (Kapandji, 1982).

The Thumb

Hand function relies on the thumb. It is an essential component that acts as a stabilizer in the radial palmar and digital grasps, the pincer grasp, and the lateral and power grasps. The thumb functions dynamically and provides movement, which is seen in the dynamic tripod grasp. Its ability to oppose allows it to move into the hand to work with the fingertips during the performance of a variety of tasks and the maintenance of the web space. Opposition of the thumb is present in most hand activities. The thumb also is a critical component for in-hand manipulation. Without the thumb, the hand loses most of its capabilities (Kapandji, 1982).

The Arches of the Hand

For the hand to grasp, it must change its shape to accommodate the object being grasped. When grasping a larger object, the hand becomes cupped as its bones form three types of arches: transverse, longitudinal, and oblique.

The two transversely oriented arches go across the palm. The four longitudinal arches go down the length of the palm from the wrist up through the fingertips. The four oblique

arches go diagonally across the hand. Each of these three types of arches is formed by the thumb during opposition with the other fingers (Boehme, 1988).

The Transverse Arches. The two transverse arches form the hand into a cup. They create a concave surface in the palm by bringing the ulnar and radial borders of the hand toward each other. The proximal transverse arch is found in the middle of the palm. It provides stability and is reasonably fixed. The distal transverse arch passes through the metacarpal heads (the knuckles) at the distal end of the palm and provides mobility.

The Longitudinal Arches. The longitudinal arches begin at the wrist. They fan out from there and follow along the metacarpal bones and phalanges to the fingertips. Concave on the palmar surface (Kapandji, 1982), the longitudinal arches allow the grading of finger movements and can flatten or cup themselves to accommodate objects of various sizes.

The Oblique Arches. The oblique arches link the thumb to each fingertip for opposition. The most important oblique arch is that which links the thumb and index finger because this movement is frequently used when grasping smaller objects. The intrinsic muscles are responsible primarily for the changes in the configuration of the arches. As such, they are essential for fine motor function, especially manipulation and tool use.

Extrinsic and Intrinsic Muscles of the Hand

Two muscle groups are responsible for hand movement. The *extrinsic* muscles are found in the forearm, and the *intrinsic* muscles are located in the hand. These muscle groups must work together to create the stability and mobility needed to perform a wide range of fine motor tasks. The function of the hand depends on the synergy of many muscles that manipulate the wrist and the fingers. The wrist muscles are very important because they stabilize it and prevent unwanted movement. This allows the fingers to maintain the position needed to produce tension and prehension. The function of the hand and wrist muscles is synergistic. They work together to provide a functional grasp, release, and skilled manipulation (Benbow, 1995).

When there is normal resting tone in the extrinsic and intrinsic muscle groups, the wrist and digital joints are in a balanced position. The forearm is in the midposition, the wrist is in extension and the fingers are in slight flexion, and the hand is in its optimum functioning position (Strickland, 1995).

Components of Hand Function

The following components are necessary for efficient use of the hand, and they must work together to provide the stability and mobility that allows precise movement. They provide the foundation for higher level skill development, such as in-hand manipulation. It is critical that the functions of the following components be understood so that their impact on hand function can be determined.

Muscle Tone

The hand's muscle tone provides its underlying stability. With increased tone or spasticity, there is decreased mobility and flexibility. With decreased tone, there is decreased joint stability.

Wrist Stability

A grasp is stronger when the wrist is extended. Stability of the wrist allows finger movements at the best mechanical advantage for range and control. To maintain such stability in extension, which is needed for precise distal function, the wrist flexors must work antagonistically with the extensors. This provides co-contraction of both muscle groups and maintains the wrist in a functional position (Benbow, 1995).

As previously noted, the functional position of the wrist is achieved when the wrist is in 40° to 45° extension and 15° of slight ulnar deviation. The ulnar deviation provides stability to the ulnar fingers and aligns the hand so that the radial fingers and thumb can work more effectively. With the wrist in extension, the thumb can oppose the fingers to achieve tip-to-tip prehension.

Lack of stabilization in wrist extension affects the abduction and rotation of the thumb, the arching of the hand, and the isolation of intrinsic motor control. Children with inadequate wrist stability may compensate by flexing their wrists to get bone-on-bone stability. With the wrist in flexion, the thumb cannot fully oppose to meet the index finger at the tip. In-hand manipulation cannot occur biomechanically because the thumb and fingertips do not meet (Case-Smith & Berry, 1998).

The Palmar Arches

The palmar arches enable the hand to
- Support the hand in a functional position,
- Grade finger movement by changing the hand's configuration,
- Cup the hand to form a concave surface in the palm,
- Shape the hand to accommodate objects of various sizes,
- Oppose the thumb to each finger, and
- Move objects within the hand against the palmar surface (Bridgeman, 2002).

In-Hand Manipulation

In-hand manipulation occurs when one hand is used to adjust an object for more effective placement in that same hand before use, placement on a surface, or release. The object remains in the hand and usually does not come in contact with a surface (Exner, 2001).

This type of manipulation builds on the biomechanical components that enable a child to demonstrate precision grasping patterns. To develop efficient in-hand manipulation, the child first must demonstrate

- Active control of supination, wrist stability, and control in slight wrist extension;
- Thumb opposition and tip-to-tip prehension;
- Isolated thumb and radial finger movement (intrinsic muscles);
- The ability to control small degrees of flexion and extension at the metacarpal–phalangeal (MCP) joints (intrinsic muscles); and
- Separation of the radial and ulnar sides of the hand, with the ulnar fingers providing stability to the hand and the radial fingers demonstrating individualized movements (Case-Smith & Berry, 1998).

Three basic patterns of in-hand manipulation have been identified: translation, shift, and rotation. Such manipulation includes five basic types of patterns: finger-to-palm translation, palm-to-finger translation, shift, simple rotation, and complex rotation.

Each of the in-hand manipulation skills may occur in isolation or while a child is simultaneously stabilizing one or more objects in the same hand. The ulnar fingers stabilize the object, and the radial fingers perform the in-hand manipulation. The stabilized object usually is held in the central, or ulnar, part of the palm. When stabilization of an object within the hand occurs during in-hand manipulation, the skill is named and the phrase "with stabilization" is added (e.g., "simple rotation with stabilization"). An example of the palm-to-finger translation with palmar stabilization is the holding of several coins in one hand and the use of palm-to-finger translation to move only one coin to the pads of the fingers while retaining the grasp on the other coins (Exner, 1992).

The following information on in-hand manipulation is compiled from Exner (1990, 1992, 1995, 2001).

Finger-to-Palm Translation. The object is grasped at the finger pads or the fingertips and then is moved into the palm. Finger-to-palm translation is used when picking up a coin or key from a surface and moving it to the palm. It usually is seen in children between ages $1\frac{1}{2}$ and 2 years. Finger-to-palm with stabilization is seen between ages 3 and $3\frac{2}{5}$ years.

Palm-to-Finger Translation. Palm-to-finger translation, which is more difficult than finger-to-palm translation, is used to complete such tasks as moving a coin from the palm of the hand out to the fingertips for placement into a vending machine or piggy bank. It is seen in children ages 2 to $2\frac{2}{5}$ years. Palm-to-finger translation with stabilization is seen in children ages 5 to $5\frac{2}{5}$ years.

Shift. Shift occurs when an object is moved or adjusted by the finger pads in a linear direction. The fingers usually are extended, and the thumb moves in controlled opposition, extension, and flexion. There is alteration of the thumb and of finger movement. Such alteration may be used to make final adjustments to an object's position after it has been picked up. Examples of shift are seen when moving a coin from the finger pads to fingertips and when adjusting a pen in the hand so that the fingers and thumb are closer to the tip. This skill also is used in buttoning, fastening, and lacing. The ability to shift an object using in-hand manipulation does not develop until between ages 4 and 5 years.

Simple Rotation. Simple rotation occurs when an object is turned or rolled 90° or less between the pads of the fingers and the pad of the thumb. The rotation may occur only between the index finger and thumb, such as when winding up a toy. If more fingers are used, they typically act as a unit. The fingers are held in adduction, and the thumb is held in opposition. Examples are unscrewing a small bottle cap, turning a dial, and picking up a small peg from a surface and putting it into a pegboard. It also is used when adjusting a puzzle piece by turning it slightly to orient it correctly so that it will fit into its proper space. Development of simple rotation is seen in children ages 2 to 2 ½ years.

Complex Rotation. Complex rotation involves the single or repeated turning of an object around its axis (end over end) either 180° or 360° using only finger and thumb movements. The fingers move independently of one another. The object usually is stabilized alternately by the fingers and thumb. When the thumb stabilizes the object, the fingers move it; when the fingers stabilize it, the thumb moves it. An example of complex rotation is using the eraser end of a pencil and then returning it to a lead down position. Another example is turning a paper clip so that the opposite end can be used for placement on a piece of paper. Complex rotation with a small peg is seen in children ages 2 ½ to almost 3 years. Complex rotation with palmar stabilization is seen in children ages 6 to 6 ½ years.

Hand Separation

The separation of the two sides of the hand provides the stability that allows for mobility. The ulnar side of the hand is referred to as the power side and includes the ring and little (pinkie) fingers. It provides stability for the hand and power for grip. The hand's radial side is called the skilled side and includes the thumb and the index and middle fingers. This side is necessary for skilled, fast, and precise movements that incorporate the fingers and thumb in opposition, such as turning a bolt on a screw (Benbow, 1995).

Thumb Opposition to Maintain Web Space

An open web space is a critical component of such skilled hand movements as a functional pencil grasp. It allows the mid-range flexion and extension of the MCP joints that occurs in handwriting. Created by the opposition of the thumb and the index finger, maintaining an opened web space is dependent on the hand arches, separation of the two sides of the hand, and the hand's intrinsic muscles.

Evaluation or Screening Process

Requesting an evaluation or screening for a student who has fine motor concerns usually begins with some type of referral. The educational team, psychologist, classroom teacher, special education teacher, or the parents may initiate such a referral. Depending on its format, specific areas of concern may be listed, such as "the child has difficulty managing fasteners" or "the child has difficulty in art class with projects that require cutting and coloring." This information gives occupational therapists an idea of the concerns being presented. The therapist then can contact the individuals who initiated the referral to get more background information to begin the evaluation process.

A screening can determine if further assessments or interventions are needed (American Occupational Therapy Association, 1999). The method of evaluation needs to be based on the student's specific needs. Various tools and strategies should be used to gather functional information about those fine motor abilities relevant to the student's performance in the school setting. Such a combination of techniques can gather information that assists the team in determining if the child has difficulty performing the fine motor tasks necessary for him or her to benefit from his or her educational program.

A functional-based assessment provides more specific information in relation to the daily requirements that the student is expected to perform than does a formal assessment. Scores from formal assessments or norm-referenced tests do not provide information regarding the student's ability to function within a curriculum or school environment. These types of tests require inference by the occupational therapist to relate the student's performance on the test to performance in the classroom (Clark & Coster, 1998).

Components of the Evaluation

The intent of the Individuals With Disabilities Education Act is that any evaluation must include a variety of methods to gather information. Occupational therapists first must get to know a student's developmental background to determine how best to approach the evaluation process. This can be accomplished by contacting the person who initiated the referral or the primary person with information about any fine motor concerns.

Next, the occupational therapist can review the student's work samples to determine how much support the child was provided to complete the task. It is important to find out if interventions have been tried. When looking at work samples, such as cutting or art projects, it often is helpful to look at the work of other classmates for comparison.

After the occupational therapist has reviewed the student's work samples, he or she can interview the parents and classroom personnel. This provides insight into the child's performance of tasks common to both the home and school. The authors have created a Functional Education Checklist (FEC; see Appendix 5.1) that examines tasks the child is expected to accomplish during the school day. Using this checklist gives the therapist an opportunity to learn about the child's ability to perform functional tasks such as using a dominant hand consistently, using tools, using two hands together, writing, managing personal belongings, managing self-care and eating skills, and managing gross motor skills within the school environment.

This checklist not only identifies areas of concern, it also helps the occupational therapist focus on priority areas that need to be evaluated. It eliminates the need to evaluate certain areas such as self-care if no concerns

were identified on that section. When discussing areas of concern identified on the FEC with classroom staff, asking open-ended questions is often more helpful than giving them choices to explain the possible reason for the difficulty.

The child also needs to be observed actually performing the tasks that are of concern, at the time they naturally occur during his or her day. This allows the occupational therapist to gather information about the setting and the task. Studying the setting provides additional information about how the child performs in different context areas.

Once all areas of concern have been identified, each should be evaluated directly. This should be done at a separate time in an isolated area so that the student does not feel self-conscious. Watching the student perform each task gives the occupational therapist an opportunity to gather information about what is preventing him or her from being successful. For example, even though the child can open and close a pair of scissors and make consecutive cuts, he or she is unable to stay on the line when asked to cut. Observation shows that the child is unable to stay on the line because he or she does not look at the paper while cutting. In this case, the problem does not appear to be related to a fine motor difficulty but rather to attention issues.

Interventions During the Evaluation Process

Interventions also can be tried during the evaluation process. For example, if a student is pronating his or her hand when cutting, the occupational therapist may provide a physical prompt to get him or her to stabilize the upper arm against the trunk. This should get his or her hand into a more neutral thumbs-up position. Such information can be included in the evaluation results and shared with the team.

If global concerns exist about the student's ability to perform bilateral tasks, the occupational therapist can identify those tasks that need to be accomplished daily, such as managing his or her bookbag, cutting with scissors, stirring, opening containers, and stabilizing the paper when writing. The classroom staff can provide insight into which activities make up this daily routine. Next, the student needs to be observed performing these specific tasks to identify areas of difficulty within each task.

A write-up should be completed for those tasks evaluated. This should describe what affected the student's ability to complete the tasks and the effect this has on his or her ability to function in the school setting. For example, if there are specific concerns about the student's ability to cut out complex shapes, the occupational therapist can examine his or her ability to grasp and position the scissors in his or her hand and on his or her fingers. The therapist can observe how the student holds the paper with his or her assist hand (e.g., hand pronated, in midposition) if the student manipulates or turns the paper while cutting and if he or she is attending visually to the task. The student's ability to stay on the line while cutting out the shapes also should be documented, and a description of each component observed should be included.

Evaluation of Specific Hand Function Components

As has been indicated, it is necessary for occupational therapists to observe and assess directly all of the fine motor performance concerns identified by the team. According to Benbow (1995), children with dysfunctional hands typically show symptoms of a lack of neuromuscular maturity. Low muscle tone affects the hand's internal stability. The wrist lacks stability, and the digits lack controlled flexion, extension, and rotation critical for

hand function. The arches of hand often are flat, and there is lack of separation between the radial and ulnar sides of the hand.

To determine what is affecting the overall function, each component should be evaluated, including muscle tone, wrist stability, palmar arches, hand separation, thumb opposition, the ability to maintain an open web space, and in-hand manipulation.

This evaluation should be done in addition to looking at the specific tasks the child is having difficulty completing, such as managing fasteners. Identifying specific components, such as wrist stability and hand separation, that are absent during attempts to carry out this task assists the occupational therapist in finding appropriate intervention techniques. Developmental hand activities can be used to prepare and strengthen the hand in preparation for using it to perform the more global task of managing the fasteners.

Other Areas to Consider

The occupational therapist also may also choose to observe or evaluate the following areas in combination with examining the specific areas of concern identified on the checklist or through other methods.

Postural Control in Sitting. The student's position at his or her desk needs to be evaluated. Many times, the desk height, chair height, or both are not appropriate for the student's height and size across context areas (e.g., classroom, resource room, art room, music room).

The correct position when sitting on a chair at a desk is with the feet supported on the floor with the ankles, knees, and hips at a 90° angle. The desk's height should be approximately 2 inches above the height of the student's elbow when it is bent to 90°. The arms should be held forward slightly (approximately 30°) from the trunk. If the student tends to sit on his or her feet when at the desk, this usually indicates that the desk is too high or that the chair is too low for him or her to work comfortably. The student also should be able to sit independently, maintain sitting without propping head on hands, and be able to make the necessary postural adjustments when sitting on the chair.

Hand Configuration. When evaluating hand configuration, the occupational therapist must
- Describe the student's muscle tone,
- Note the stability of the joints (e.g., hyperextension of the distal joints when holding a pencil or applying pressure),
- Describe the shape of the hand at rest (e.g., flat),
- Consider the student's ability to oppose the thumb to each finger, and
- Observe the student's joint flexibility and ability to shape his or her hand around objects of different sizes.

Sensory Processing. In observing a student's sensory processing ability, the occupational therapist should note the student's reaction to being touched and consider his or her tactile discrimination. This is the student's ability to
- Identify objects by touch alone,
- Explore objects using his or her whole hand or individualized finger movements, and
- Indicate where he or she has been touched.

The therapist also should note the student's
- *Proprioception,* or ability to look at his or her hands while he or she is reaching, grade his or her movements, and identify where body parts are in space without vision, and
- *Haptic perception,* or ability to identify an object's properties (e.g., size, shape, texture, weight, spatial orientation).

Reach. The range of motion for both upper extremities can be evaluated functionally. However, the ability to reach up above the head and around to the back are more critical for self-care tasks than are other movements. In terms of fine motor skills, the ability to reach forward, out to the side, and across the body's midline is important. A student needs to be able to reach to obtain objects.

The occupational therapist should note the proximal stability needed to reach and maintain a grasp on objects in space when the arm is not supported. In addition, the therapist can observe the position of the hand when the student is reaching. This can help determine if he or she is able to accommodate and orient his or her hand correctly to grasp the object.

Grasp. To evaluate the various grasps the student uses and his or her ability to dissociate the two sides of the hand to use its skilled side, the occupational therapist must observe
- Handedness—use of both hands during the same activity (e.g., uses left and right to pick up blocks),
- Hand switching during an activity (e.g., uses the right and left hands to color),
- Hand preference for tool use,
- Spontaneous use of the nonpreferred hand,
- Ability to stabilize objects,
- Specific grasp used to efficiently perform a task,
- Wrist's position to determine sufficient wrist stability to use the fingers efficiently, and
- Ability to oppose the thumb and maintain an open web space.

In-Hand Manipulation. The occupational therapist needs to observe a student's ability to perform all of the components of in-hand manipulation with and without stabilization, including
- Finger-to-palm translation,
- Palm-to-finger to translation,
- Shift
- Simple rotation,
- Complex rotation, and
- All the these (except shift) with stabilization.

The occupational therapist must determine if in-hand manipulation skills are required for a specific task and any difficulties that affect the child's ability to complete the task. It also is important to note any attempts to modify a task or compensate for the lack of the skill, such as putting a pencil in his or her other hand to turn it over and then transferring it back to the writing hand when he or she needs to erase.

Release. Occupational therapists should determine if students being evaluated possess the ability to release a variety of different-sized objects under different conditions. Does a student need to stabilize the object on a support surface to be able to release it, or can he or she release it in space? The therapist then needs to document the type of release required to perform the specific task.

Bilateral Skills. Students should be evaluated to determine if they are able to perform tasks that require the use of both hands either working cooperatively or performing different tasks independently of one another. The occupational therapist needs to list the bilateral skills a student uses during his or her daily routine. As discussed previously, these may include managing his or her bookbag, stabilizing the paper for writing and cutting, managing fasteners, and performing other similar tasks. How does the student stabilize an object (e.g., a container) when grasping it and when not grasping it (e.g., stabilizing the paper when writing)? Does he or she use both hands together to perform the same task? Or does he or she use one hand to manipulate and the other to stabilize? Any specific bilateral skills needed to perform a specific task should be noted.

Tool Use. The occupational therapist can evaluate a student's ability to use such tools as scissors, writing utensils, eating utensils, pencil sharpeners, and rulers. If an area of concern requires tool use, then the therapist can evaluate the specific tool needed to perform the task.

Motor Planning. The occupational therapist must determine if the student is able to

- Plan and execute a novel movement that requires fine motor skills;
- Initiate and complete a classroom or art project that requires multiple steps;
- Use a variety of tools, such as a compass or ruler;
- Begin a task after given a directive;
- Complete each step of the task without asking for additional assistance; and
- Initiate the task without looking to see what other students are doing.

Formal Assessments

Many types of assessments can be used to evaluate fine motor skills, depending on specific needs. Some include a fine motor component; others look at the support the student needs to participate in the educational setting. As previously discussed, if test results yield developmental scores, the occupational therapist should not use the scores in isolation to recommend intervention but instead should consider how performance on the assessment items affects the student's ability to function in the context of the educational setting. The following assessments can be used in combination with other evaluation techniques to supplement information on fine motor functioning.

Diagnostic Inventory of Early Development

The Diagnostic Inventory of Early Development (Brigance, 1991) examines a student's performance in a variety of fine motor tasks in the areas of grasp, hand–eye coordination, use of tools (e.g., scissors, rulers), completion of puzzles, prewriting skills, bilateral skills, and school-related tasks (e.g., folding paper, using a pencil sharpener). In addition, the self-help skill area includes tasks that require fine motor skills. The assessment can be used for children from birth to age 7 years or for older students who are functioning in that range.

Occupational therapists can obtain background information through interviews with the parents and teachers, observation, direct assessment, or a combination of these. Because the information is being obtained through direct assessment and caregiver interviews, the Brigance can be used with students of varying developmental and cognitive levels.

The test looks at specific tasks related to school function and provides developmental age ranges for individual test items. These can be used to indicate at what level a student is functioning in the fine motor areas. Baseline information obtained from the assessment can be used to indicate present levels of performance and, when readministered, to measure progress, comparing the new results to those of the initial assessment.

Battelle Developmental Inventory

The Battelle Developmental Inventory (Newborg, Stock, Wnek, Guidubaldi, & Suinicki, 1988) evaluates tool use through a limited number of specific items. It can be used for children from birth to age 8 years, yet because of the various ways in which it can be administered, it can be used with children of varying developmental and cognitive levels.

Information can be obtained through interviews with the parents and teachers and through observation, direct assessment, or a combination of these. The test provides the evaluator with a standard score, percentile, and age equivalent for the student's skills in relation to same-age peers.

Pediatric Evaluation of Disability Inventory

The Pediatric Evaluation of Disability Inventory (Haley, Coster, Ludlow, Haltiwanger, & Andrellos, 1992) is a comprehensive clinical instrument that examines key functional capabilities and performance using two subscales: functional skills (197 items) and caregiver assistance (20 items). It can be used

with children ranging in age from 6 months to 7 ½ years. In general, it is appropriate for students who function at a lower level, as it looks at a student's ability to perform functional skills and the amount of assistance provided by the caregiver. In addition, it documents the modifications made to allow the child to participate in the task, whether to the task itself or through the use of equipment.

Information can be obtained through interviews with the parents and teacher, through observation or direct assessment, or through a combination of these. Hand skill components are included in the self-care domain, but there are not specific components that relate to the functional fine motor tasks required in the school setting.

School Function Assessment

The School Function Assessment (Coster, Deeney, Haltiwanger, & Haley, 1998) measures a student's ability to perform functional tasks and participate in academic and social tasks included in the school day. It is designed for use with students of varying levels of disability in kindergarten through sixth grade. The test examines a student's level of participation in six school settings (regular or special education classroom, playground or recess, transportation to and from school, toileting, transitions within the school environment, and snack time or lunch). It looks at the amount of support the child requires to participate in activities within these six areas. A student's ability to participate in specific school-related functional activities also is assessed, such as the manipulation of objects, the use of various materials, written work, eating, and tool use.

Information is obtained through a questionnaire completed by school professionals. This criterion-referenced assessment provides a criterion score, which indicates at what level the student currently is functioning. It notes any need for assistance and adaptations and can measure changes in the student's performance. Higher scores indicate increased participation in school activities and overall progress.

Erhardt Developmental Prehension Assessment

The Erhardt Developmental Prehension Assessment (Erhardt, 1982) measures fine motor prehension in newborns and children up to age 15 months. Because 15 months is considered the period of prehension maturity, the test can be used as an approximate norm for assessing older children and children with developmental delays or motor impairments. In addition, the pencil grasp and drawings of children from ages 1 to 6 years also can be evaluated.

This assessment examines involuntary arm–hand patterns, voluntary movements, prewriting skills, and drawings. Information is obtained through direct assessment, and scores are based on the presence or absence of normal grasp patterns and the identification of gaps in skill sequence, significant delays, and the need for intervention. These scores are transferred to a scoring sheet to estimate each hand's developmental levels and can be used to establish objectives and treatment interventions and to document progress.

Bruininks–Oseretsky Test of Motor Proficiency

The Bruininks–Oseretsky Test of Motor Proficiency (Bruininks, 1978) assesses motor functioning in children ranging in age from 4 ½ to 14 ½ years. It is composed of a Short Form and a Complete Battery. The Short Form consists of 14 test items and can be used as a screening tool of general fine and gross motor proficiency.

The Complete Battery provides individual measures of fine motor and gross motor skills and a comprehensive index of the child's overall motor proficiency. Comprised of 46 test items divided into 8 subtests, this component assesses running speed and agility, balance, bilateral coordination, strength, upper limb coordination, response speed, visual–motor control, and upper limb speed and dexterity. The Complete Battery takes on average 45 to 60 minutes to administer; the Short Form can take between 15 and 20 minutes. This assessment is norm-referenced and provides standard scores for individual subtests and standard scores, percentiles, and stanines (standard scores that range from a low of 1 to a high of 9, with 5 being average) for each of the composite scores. Age equivalents for each of the eight subtests also are provided.

Peabody Developmental Motor Scales

The Peabody Developmental Motor Scales (Folio & Fewell, 2000) is a norm-referenced and criterion-referenced assessment that asseses the motor skills of children from birth to age 6 years. It is composed of six subtests:
* *Reflexes* measures a child's ability to automatically react to environmental events;
* *Stationary* measures the child's ability to sustain body control within his or her center of gravity and retain equilibrium;
* *Locomotion* measures the child's ability to transport his or her body from one base of support to another;
* *Object manipulation* measures the child's ability to throw, catch, and kick balls;
* *Grasping* measures the child's ability to use his or her hands and fingers; and
* *Visual–motor integration* measures the child's ability to integrate and use his or her visual–perceptual skills to perform complex eye–hand coordination tasks.

This evaluation takes approximately 45 to 60 minutes to administer. Results can be used to estimate a child's motor competence relative that of his or her peers. The test provides standard scores; scaled scores; percentiles; and fine motor, gross motor, and total motor quotient scores. Its authors also have written a motor activities program of 104 activities designed to developmentally target the skills within the six subtests.

Miller Assessment for Preschoolers

The Miller Assessment for Preschoolers (Miller, 1988) is a standardized test that consists of 27 test items arranged into five Performance Indices: Foundations, Coordination, Verbal, Non-Verbal, and Complex Tasks. The Performance Indices assess a student's developmental status across different content domains, such as behavior, motor, and cognition. Each performance index falls into one of three types of developmental abilities: sensory and motor abilities, cognitive abilities, and combined abilities. It is designed to identify children ages 2 years and 9 months through 5 years who have developmental delays.

The sensory and motor abilities component consists of the Foundations and Coordination Indices. Items in the Foundations Index examine a child's basic motor skills and awareness of sensations. Areas assessed include the child's sense of position and movement, sense of touch, development of basic components of movement, and sensory integration and neurodevelopment. Items in the Coordination Index simultaneously examine the child's sensory and motor abilities, including complex gross motor tasks, fine motor tasks, and oral motor tasks.

The cognitive abilities area consists of items found in the Verbal and Non-Verbal Indices. The Verbal Index includes items that examine the child's memory, sequencing, comprehension, association, and expression in a verbal context. The Non-Verbal Index measures the child's memory, sequencing, visualization, and performance of mental manipulations not requiring spoken language.

Combined abilities items are found in the Complex Tasks Index. This index measures the child's sensorimotor abilities in conjunc-tion with his or her cognitive abilities.

The test takes about 25 to 35 minutes to administer and provides normed scores expressed as percentiles for the child's total score and for the scores within the individual performance indices. The assessment also offers a Behavior During Testing Checklist. The occupational therapist can complete this while administering the assessment to document any atypical or abnormal behavior. The data collected on this checklist can be used as supplemental information to the evaluation process. Abnormal behavior during the assessment may indicate that the total score is not indicative of the student's true sensory, motor, or cognitive capabilities that are secondary to his or her behavior.

Providing Intervention

Many resources exist that provide specific suggestions for fine motor interventions, including activities. In this chapter, intervention is approached as a way to

- Help occupational therapists synthesize the information presented to structure the treatment session,
- Identify factors that need to be considered when providing intervention,
- Emphasize the need to provide interventions for treating specific hand components, and
- Provide activities to work on the development of specific components of hand function.

Structuring the Treatment Session

The information provided in this chapter offers guidance for developing interventions to address the needs of a child who is having difficulty with refined hand movements. The intent is to apply these guidelines to provide rationale for specific intervention strategies and approaches that should be considered when structuring a treatment session.

Additional suggestions are provided to help occupational therapists structure specific interventions in terms of sequencing them in order of implementation. Selection of appropriate objects to facilitate specific grasps and how to position and present objects also is discussed.

Developing Proximal Stability and Distal Function. The central nervous system has control over the hand's precision movements. The following considerations need to be incorporated when providing intervention for a child with poor hand skills that result in difficulty with refined hand movements. These considerations are based on the research studies presented in this chapter.

Traditionally, occupational therapists have provided intervention based on the premise that fine motor skills develop in a proximal–distal progression. Recently, however, research has been presented that indicates that there actually are two separate motor systems, one that controls the hand's precision movements and a second that controls postural and proximal movements.

If a child has poor proximal stability and poor hand skills, therapeutic interventions directed toward working on both areas should not be approached sequentially but rather simultaneously. Activities to improve shoulder stability need to be done at the same time that intervention specific to the development of precise hand skills is being provided.

Exercises to improve shoulder and scapula stability can include weight-bearing, compression, and traction types of activities. Flexing the arms at the shoulder to at least 90° and extending at the elbow while performing such activities is important. Some suggestions for specific activities include

- Working in a prone, propped position with the elbow positioned directly below the shoulders with the forearms bearing the weight

- Working from a position on all fours, having the child pick up cards, beanbags, balls, and other similar objects and putting them into a container, alternating hands
- Extending the arms out to the side and making arm circles
- Having the child make chalk circles of various sizes on the blackboard.

If the child lacks shoulder stability, then it is appropriate to provide external stability proximally so that distal function can occur more efficiently. Have the child stabilize his or her arms against his or her trunk or rest his or her forearm on the edge of a table. This will allow him or her to work on hand skills that require more precise movements without waiting for shoulder stability to occur.

It has been discussed that hand skill manipulation depends on the corticospinal pathway, which originates in the primary motor cortex. Evarts (1981) has suggested that cortically controlled movements are learned and require the child to pay attention to his or her movements as he or she practices activities so that learned responses can be developed. Children who have fine motor difficulties typically avoid participating in fine motor activities. As a result, they receive less exposure and the practice that is essential for the development of the skills.

Developing Cortically Controlled Movements. Development of cortically controlled movements requires long periods of training. The occupational therapist must be able to treat the specific areas of weakness through the use of activities that will engage the child and maintain his or her attention. The child needs opportunities to practice specific tasks that require the hand to perform goal-directed activities. It is the therapist's responsibility to find activities that are of interest to the child and appropriate for the development of a specific hand skill.

Sensory information is critical to learning and refining movements. It provides the information needed to adjust and correct a movement and updates the motor program for its correct execution the next time that it is needed. The development and ongoing monitoring of the majority of skilled hand functions requires sensory feedback. The tactile system assists in discriminating between different textures, shapes, and surfaces. It also offers feedback to the central nervous system to help determine how much force is needed when grasping an object. The information the proprioceptive system provides about the static position of the extremity and movement of the extremity is critical to grading movement (Eliasson, 1995).

Providing Sensory Input to Develop Sensory Feedback. The occupational therapist needs to be aware of how a child uses sensory feedback for motor output. Providing activities that require use of different kinds of sensory feedback helps the therapist understand how the child uses sensory information to assist in manipulation. Having the child perform tasks without using his or her vision separates the visual feedback from the sensory feedback.

If it appears that the child has difficulty using sensory information, the occupational therapist can incorporate sensory input into the intervention program or help the child develop strategies to compensate for inefficient sensory feedback. Providing practice and repetition of a specific task is an appropriate intervention strategy to make up for a less-efficient feedback system.

Cognitive development affects the development of fine motor skills. A child's ability to maintain the attention needed to engage and practice movements and skills is critical to the development of precision hand skills. Children with cognitive delays have difficulty sustaining attention to the task and understanding the directions and steps required to perform a task.

Addressing Cognitive Delays. When working with a child with cognitive delays, it is important to use task analysis to break tasks into specific steps so that each step can be taught individually. It also is important to select activities that are at the child's developmental level. This increases the child's opportunity for success when performing them. If the child is successful, this may motivate him or her to continue to interact further with the activity and provide him or her with the necessary repetition and practice needed to improve fine motor manipulation abilities.

Sequencing Interventions for Implementation

When planning interventions for fine motor treatment, the occupational therapist must consider how to break down the steps and in what order to provide the interventions. Exner (1995) discussed the following sequence of activities that focuses on fine motor concerns that may be included in a treatment session. These can be taken into consideration, depending on the goals for a given session, to help the therapist determine the order in which to implement specific interventions.

The Child's Position. The position that the child will use when working on an activity, for example, sitting versus prone, needs to be determined so that appropriate activities can be selected based on the position. Sitting is the most commonly used position, especially in school settings, as it is in this position that the child most often must function. As indicated previously, the height of the work surface is critical to ensuring the optimum position for the upper extremity. Exner (1995) recommended that the forearm and hand be positioned in slight supination (30°–45°) to allow the child to use his or her thumb and radial fingers more efficiently and be able to visually attend to the activity.

Using a prone position also is an option because it provides an opportunity to work on shoulder stabilization. In addition, it provides the forearm stability needed to work on supination, grasping, in-hand manipulation, and bilateral tasks. Activities that can be performed within a small area should be selected because this position prevents working in wide ranges of movement.

Postural and Proximal Control. Postural and proximal control also need to be considered before beginning specific fine motor tasks. A position that provides the necessary postural control in terms of head and trunk stability is critical. Proximal control and stability are necessary to promote distal function, and the most stable position for the arm is that in which the humerus is adducted to the side of the trunk with the elbow flexed to 90° and, if necessary, the forearm stabilized on the work surface. This allows the hands the freedom to work on more refined hand skills.

Working on Isolated Hand Function. Isolated hand function can be addressed once the position and proximal control have been provided. As indicated earlier, the need to have the hand positioned in slight supination (30°–45°) is important when working on fine motor tasks that require use of the radial fingers and thumb. Techniques that encourage active supination (Exner, 1995) include presenting items in a vertical orientation, presenting objects diagonally to the child's body (beginning at 60° to the side), and positioning objects in front of the child's shoulder. Presenting objects to the child diagonally encourages the pattern of external rotation with supination. Gradually decreasing the angle allows the child to work on reaching in front of his or her body while still encouraging the same pattern of external rotation with supination. To encourage forward reaching, position the object in front of the child's shoulder rather than at the child's midline. This decreases the potential for using internal rotation and pronation that may occur when objects are presented at the midline.

Working on Grasp Development. Depending on the type of grasp being worked on, the occupational therapist needs to determine the most appropriate size and type of object to use. Other characteristics of the object also need to be considered, such as its shape, the material that it is made of, and its weight. The size of the child's hand should be factored into the equation as well. If the child's hand is small, a larger object may provide more stability because it does not require the amount of control that a smaller object does.

It is critical to select activities that are interesting to the child, as fine motor intervention cannot be done to the child by the occupational therapist. As discussed previously, the child must be actively involved and attend to the task. Therefore, the activity must interest and motivate him or her to continue to interact with it.

Development of the grasp pattern that uses metacarpophalangeal flexion with interphalangeal extension is critical because it requires use of the intrinsic muscles and is typically the position or pattern seen after a child has completed the manipulation of an object. Begin by working on the grasp in a more stable position before expecting the child to reach and grasp. It is possible to grade the amount of stability provided within a treatment session and vary the presentation in terms of the amount of support. The following ways to present objects to the child are listed from the most stable position to the least (Exner, 1995):

- Grasping from the therapist's fingers;
- Grasping from the therapist's palm;
- Grasping from the table, with the object close to the child's body in front of the

shoulder and then further from the body in front of shoulder;

- Grasping from the table, with the object further from the child's body and near his or her midline;
- Grasping the object off of the surface area and positioning it to facilitate external rotation and forearm supination.

Working on Voluntary Release. Voluntary release depends on graded finger extension along with wrist stability with finger extension. The quality of the release is affected by the quality of the grasp. Many of the considerations listed for working on grasping can be applied to releasing, such as size and weight of the objects.

If there is lack of proximal stability, the child can use humeral adduction to stabilize the upper arm against his or her trunk. The child also can use the support surface to stabilize his or her forearm and the hand holding the object. The child releases by extending the fingers away from the object stabilized on the support surface.

Using Functional Activities to Integrate Skills

Integrating skills through functional activities is the final, yet necessary, strategy to include in the intervention process. The occupational therapist needs to use activities during the child's treatment session that he or she is expected to perform during the school day. Also important is involving critical individuals in the child's life, such as parents and teachers. This ensures that the child is given the opportunity to practice using activities in a variety of settings.

The ongoing aspect of direct intervention requires the occupational therapist to evaluate a child's needs continuously. Creating a balance between the need for direct intervention and the need for the compensatory strategies or adaptations should be considered when determining what is needed to as-

sist the child in acquiring and achieving the ability to use fine motor skills to accomplish daily life tasks. As a school-based therapist, collaborating with classroom staff and the parents is as important as providing direct intervention. Recommendations and suggestions can be provided through such collaborations that ensure that the child is given opportunities to practice the skills within multiple settings.

Using Fine Motor Kits

Fine motor kits can be used to reinforce the skills being worked on in therapy and to give the child additional opportunities to work on specific skills. They provide specific fine motor activities, and the child can use them throughout his or her day. Basically, a variety of individualized activities are put together in a container for the child. The activities selected give him or her the opportunity to work on specific, needed skills, such as hand separation and use of thumb opposition.

If the child is capable of performing the tasks alone, then the teacher usually allows him or her to do so when done with his or her work. If a child needs guidance to use the objects appropriately, the activities can be done only when there is staff support present. Directions for how to perform each activity need to be provided in the kit, and it also is helpful to demonstrate the tasks to any staff who will be supervising. When selecting activities, make sure that they are appropriate for the classroom setting so that the other students are not disturbed. Activities cannot make noise, and objects should be stable enough that they will not roll or fall off of the student's desk.

Developing Specific Hand Function Components

The following strategies should be used as preparation activities to develop hand function necessary to perform the functional task identified through the evaluation process, for example, working on the in-hand manipulation skills needed for buttoning. During the treatment session, the occupational therapist would work on activities, such as pushing cards through a slot and holding coins with a three-finger grasp and pushing them into putty, that incorporate the use of shift needed to work buttons. At the end of the session, the therapist then should have the child practice buttoning as stated on his or her IEP objective to collect data and document his or her performance on the daily note (sample IEP objectives can be found in Appendix 5.2).

Wrist Extension

Wrist stability is necessary to develop precision grasping. Wrist extension provides the stability needed for efficient muscle function and positions the hand to allow the thumb to oppose or rotate downward. This permits smaller objects to be picked up and supported between the pad of the thumb and the pad of the index or middle fingers. The following activities assist in developing wrist extension.

Use of a Vertical Surface. The occupational therapist should provide activities that require the child to work with his or her arms and hands moving against gravity in an upright position. This promotes wrist extension and the development of the arms and shoulders. It is very important to position the activity so that the child has to reach out and up. In this way, the hand is encouraged to position itself in extension. If the activity is positioned too low, below his or her reach, it will encourage wrist flexion.

Painting at an easel encourages the child to fill in a defined area using short strokes. Moving the paintbrush up and down gives him or her more opportunities to use wrist extension. The occupational therapist also can have the student use the easel to write or color, if it has a paper pad or a chalkboard or both.

Activities can be placed in a vertical orientation by using a tabletop easel to promote wrist extension. The easel may need to be elevated to get the appropriate wrist extension. Peeling the plastic pieces off of a Colorforms (Colorforms, Inc.) sheet promotes wrist extension if the student is encouraged to pull them off from the top. Placing items on the board also promotes wrist extension. Felt boards and flannel boards can be used similarly. Pegboards, especially rubber ones, work well in when oriented vertically (i.e., attach the pegboard to the wall). Lite-Brite (Milton Bradley Co.), because of its shape, is already in a vertical orientation. In addition to encouraging wrist extension, the movement needed to insert the pegs promotes the finger flexion and extension needed for the formation of letters in handwriting. Similarly, Geoboards positioned vertically assist in finger strengthening and wrist extension.

Paper Scrunching. With the forearm in pronation on the table, have the child put his or her hand into a plastic freezer bag with scraps of paper about the size of a gum wrapper (~3" x 1"). Have the child grab one piece of paper at a time and crumble it into a ball. Continue to do this until all the paper inside the bag is scrunched. You may want to put a small activity or specific treat, such as a piece of wrapped hard candy that requires the use of forearm stabilization to open, in the bag so that when the child is done, he or she can either have the treat or do the activity.

Palmar Arches

The development of the palmar arches is critical to the development of precision movements. The arches allow the hand to shape itself around objects. The following activities assist in developing the hand's palmar arches.

Squeezing a Ball. Have the child hold his or her hand so that the palm is up. Place a foam or textured (for sensory input) ball on the palm and encourage him or her to hold it. After his or her hand is shaped around the ball, have him or her squeeze it two or three times.

Tennis Ball Activity. Cut a slit into the center of a tennis ball. Have the child hold the ball within one hand and squeeze it to open the slit. Finally, have him or her place small objects, such as coins and beads, inside.

Hand Cupping. When the child is done squeezing the ball, ask him or her to keep the hand palm up with the ball in it. Then remove the ball, but have the child keep his or her hand cupped in the same position that it was in when he or she was holding it. Gradually put small items into the hand one at a time, encouraging him or her to keep it cupped so that the items do not fall out.

Play Dough. Place enough play dough on the child's palm to cover it. Encourage him or her to squeeze it just using that hand. This will require him or her to cup the hand to activate his or her fingers. Then ask the child to make a ball, having him or her cup both hands to form it.

Ball Rotation. Have the child hold two balls that will fit in a cupped palm in his or her palm and rotate them within the palm.

Dice. The occupational therapist should introduce this activity once the child can maintain his or her hand in the cupped position. Have the child cup both hands and place a pair of standard size dice in one hand. Have him or her place the empty hand over the top of other one at a 90° angle so that the dice are enclosed. Then have the child shake the dice, encouraging him or her to keep both hands together so that the dice do not fall out. Use of the dice can be incorporated into classroom activities such as counting or playing a board game.

Bubble Wrap. The bigger bubbles work best when using bubble wrap. Have the child position his or her hands in wrist extension while using a three-finger grasp to pop the bubbles by placing the index and middle fingers on top of a bubble and applying pressure upward with the thumb until the bubble pops.

Jars. Occupational therapists can use jars of various sizes to store fine motor ma-nipulatives used during treatment sessions. Opening of a jar can become part of the intervention; a child then performs the activity inside. Therapists also can have the child hold the jars in a horizontal orientation to encourage wrist extension.

Hand Separation Activities

The ability to separate the hand is necessary to the development of the skilled use of the thumb and the index and middle fingers. The ring and little fingers provide stability by flexing into the palm. The following items and activities assist in developing skilled hand use. Also, if the child is having difficulty keeping the ring and little fingers flexed into his or her palm, he or she can be given a small object to hold using these fingers.

Spray Bottles. The occupational therapist should use spray bottles that require squeezing a trigger to activate. Have the child squeeze the trigger with his or her first two fingers while holding the bottle with his or her thumb and ring and little fingers. The spray bottle can be used to erase completed work on the chalkboard, to spray hands, wipe off tables, and water plants.

Stringing Beads on Lacing Cards. Stringing beads using a plastic craft string rather than thinner cotton string makes it easier to manage.

Coins or Buttons. Place buttons or coins through a small slit in the lid of a coffee can or margarine tub or into a bank. The container can be oriented vertically so that the child has to use wrist extension to stabilize the hand to put the object through the slit. The student also can be asked to turn the items over and sort them. Each of these tasks requires the use of the skilled side of hand.

Tweezer Scissors. Tweezer scissors are designed with two loops like scissors but with blunt ends and are used like tweezers. Have the child hold a pair of tweezer scissors like scissors, with the thumb and middle fingers placed in the loops. Once the child is gripping them properly, ask him or her to pick up a variety of smaller objects and place them in a designated area. This activity can be used to work on such educational skills as counting and one-to-one correspondence. The child should try to use the tweezer scissors in a thumbs-up position if at all possible. Try to keep the child from pronating his or her hand when he or she picks up objects. To keep the hand in the proper position, the items the child picks up need to be placed to allow him or her to do so.

Clothespins. Make sure the child uses a three-finger grasp when he or she grabs the clothespins. The clothespins can be marked with numbers, letters, colors, or other learning material that the child can use as part of a file folder activity. The occupational therapist can have the child's name written on the edge of the folder; the child then can select the letters in his or her name, placing them on top of the letters written on the folder.

Snack Foods. Students should be provided with individual small pieces of finger foods, rather than a whole cookie or cracker, at snack time. This encourages use of the skilled side of the hand in a three-fingered grasp to pick up the pieces individually.

Golf Tees. The child can push golf tees into a thicker piece of Styrofoam, holding the tees with a three-finger grasp and pushing them in until they are flush with the piece of Styrofoam.

Pieces of Chalk or Crayons. Use small pieces of chalk or crayons. The smaller size facilitates a three-finger grasp because the child only has a small area to grasp.

In-Hand Manipulation

In-hand manipulation is used to turn, rotate, and manipulate small objects within the hand. This is the last skill to develop and depends on the development of the previous skills discussed. Allow children to develop the various in-hand manipulation skills before expecting them to use them "with stabilization."

To work on in-hand manipulation, a child needs to be able to grasp objects with the pads of the fingers and thumb opposition, isolate the index finger (at least), and be able to separate each hand. If these components are not present, the child lacks the intrinsic muscle control needed.

If the child has the components needed, it also is important to consider at what age specific in-hand manipulation skills develop so that those worked on are appropriate for the child's developmental level.

Activities can be used to work on a variety of in-hand manipulation skills, or multiple activities can be used to work on one specific type of in-hand manipulation. Have the student pick up small objects with his or her thumb, index, and middle fingers and move them from the fingertips into the palm to "hide" them. It may be necessary to teach the concept through demonstration before having him or her perform it alone.

One by one, have the student move small objects from his or her palm to his or her fingertips. This can be done during snack time by making it into a game to see how many small pieces of snack he or she can pick up and hold in his or her hand without dropping them. Then have the child take them out one at a time so he or she can eat them. This also can be done when working on counting or money skills. The student can pick up coins or other small objects and count and sort them as he or she brings them to the fingertips to drop them into the designated area.

Have the child grab a marker or pencil at its top. Show him or her how to "walk" his or her fingers down toward the point. To add a slightly competitive element, the child can race the occupational therapist to see who reaches the point first.

Stringing beads also works on in-hand manipulation. When the child picks up a bead, he or she has to manipulate it in his or her hand to orient the opening (hole) to be able to insert the string. The child could even make his or her own beads. Using clay or putty, have him or her make small balls by rolling pieces between the pads of the thumb and index finger. When the ball is made, the student can use a blunt object, such as dull pencil, to poke out the center of the ball to create a bead.

Using index cards, color a spot on one of the four sides. Alternate between four different colors. Place all of the cards, colored side down, in a pile. Have the child pick them up one at the time and turn them over using finger movements instead of supination. Holding each card between the pads of his or her fingers and thumb, have him or her rotate it so that the color spot is on top. Next, have him or her place the cards in piles that are sorted by color. This is a good activity to prepare for manipulating the paper when cutting.

Thumb Opposition

Thumb opposition is needed to maintain an open web space. In addition to many of the other activities already presented to work on thumb opposition, these also may be helpful.

- *Creasing paper:* Have the child fold tagboard or construction paper and crease it using the pads of the index finger and the thumb.
- *Closing plastic freezer bags:* Have the child line up the seams or zipper sides and press them together using the pads of the thumb and the fingers.
- *Using a strawberry huller:* Have the child use a strawberry huller to pick up small items. Using items that can be compressed, such as peanut packaging material or a porcupine ball, have the child squeeze each one while holding it with the huller to provide additional resistance.
- *Pushing items through a resistive surface:* Make a design using push pins. The child also can push toothpicks into modeling clay or pick-up-sticks into a Styrofoam block presented on a vertical surface.

Bilateral Hand Skills

Initially, an infant uses both hands together to perform the same task. A toddler begins to stabilize objects with one hand while the other hand performs the task. The ability of the hands to perform two different tasks at the same time comes later. The need to develop bilateral hand skills is important because most activities require the use of both hands to accomplish them. Many school-based tasks, including removing the top from a marker, opening the book bag and taking out a folder, unzipping and removing a jacket, and stabilizing the paper when writing or cutting, require one hand to hold or stabilize an object while the other hand manipulates or performs the task.

To encourage bilateral hand use, have children use blocks that fit together. Initially, use rigid containers or objects because they are easier to hold. Later, increase the difficulty by having the child hold objects that are more flexible and less stable and that require the active use of the stabilizing hand to keep the item open, such as holding the book bag open while removing a folder and holding a paper or plastic bag open while putting an item in or taking one out.

Have each child hold a container while putting small items in it. When playing in the sand, have children each hold a bucket and use a shovel to fill it.

References

Alexander, R., Boehme, R., & Cupps, B. (1993). *Normal development of functional motor skills.* Tucson, AZ: Therapy SkillBuilders.

American Occupational Therapy Association. (1999). *Occupational therapy services for children and youth under the Individuals With Disabilities Education Act* (2nd ed.). Bethesda, MD: Author.

Benbow, M. (1995). *Neurokinesthetic approach to hand function and handwriting.* Albuquerque, NM: Clinician's View.

Boehme, R. H. (1988). *Improving upper body control: An approach to assessment and treatment of tonal dysfunction.* Tucson, AZ: Therapy SkillBuilders.

Bridgeman, M. (2002). *The fine motor olympics manual.* Framingham, MA: Therapro.

Brigance, A. H. (1991). *Diagnostic Inventory of Early Development.* North Billerica, MA: Curriculum Associates.

Bruininks, R. (1978). *Bruininks–Oseretsky Test of Motor Proficiency.* Circle Pines, MN: American Guidance Service.

Case-Smith, J. (1995). Grasp, release, and bimanual skills in the first two years of life. In A. Henderson & C. Pehoski (Eds.), *Hand function in the child: Foundations for remediation* (pp. 113–135). St. Louis, MO: Mosby.

Case-Smith, J., & Berry, J. (1998). Preschool hand skills. In J. Case-Smith (Ed.), *Occupational therapy: Making a difference in school system practice* (pp. 2–46). Bethesda, MD: American Occupational Therapy Association.

Clark, D., & Coster, W. (1998). Evaluation/problem solving and program evaluation. In J. Case-Smith (Ed.), *Occupational therapy: Making a difference in school system practice* (pp. 2–46). Bethesda, MD: American Occupational Therapy Association.

Clough, J. F. M., Kernell, D., & Phillips, C. G. (1968). The distribution of monosynaptic excitation from the pyramidal tract and from primary spindle afferents to motoneurons of the baboon's hand and forearm. *Journal of Physiology, 198,* 145–166.

Colangelo, C., Bergen, A., & Gottleib, L. (1976). *A normal baby the sensory–motor processes of the first year.* Valhalla, NY: Blythedale Children's Hospital.

Connolly, K. (1973). Factors influencing the learning of manual skills by young children. In R. A. Hinde & J. Stevenson-Hinde (Eds.), *Constraints on learning* (p. 361). London: Academic Press.

Connolly, K., & Dalgleish, M. (1989). The emergence of a tool-using skill in infancy. *Developmental Psychology, 25,* 894–912.

Cooper, S. (1960). Muscle spindle and other muscle receptors. In G. H. Bourne (Ed.), *The structure and function of muscle* (pp. 255–257). New York: Academic Press.

Coster, W., Deeney, T. A., Haltiwanger, J. T., & Haley, S. M. (1998). *School Function Assessment.* San Antonio, TX: Psychological Corporation.

Eliasson, A. (1995). Sensorimotor integration of the normal and impaired development of precision movement of the hand. In A. Henderson & C. Pehoski (Eds.), *Hand function in the child: Foundations for remediation* (pp. 40–53). St. Louis, MO: Mosby.

Erhardt, R. P. (1982). *Developmental hand dysfunction: Theory, assessment, and treatment.* Tucson, AZ: Therapy SkillBuilders.

Erhardt, R. P. (1990). *Developmental visual dysfunction models for assessment and management.* Tucson, AZ: Therapy SkillBuilders.

Evarts, E. V. (1981). Role of motor cortex in voluntary movements in primates. In J. M. Brookhart & V. B. Mountcastle (Eds.), *Handbook of physiology, section I, volume II, motor control, part 2* (p. 1103). Bethesda, MD: American Physiological Society.

Exner, C. (1990). In-hand manipulation skills in normal young children: A pilot study. *OT Practice, 1,* 63–72.

Exner, C. (1992). In-hand manipulation skills. In J. Case-Smith & C. Pehoski (Eds.), *Development of hand skills in the child* (pp. 35–45). Bethesda, MD: American Occupational Therapy Association.

Exner, C. (1995). Remediation of hand skill problems in children. In A. Henderson & C. Pehoski (Eds.), *Hand function in the child: Foundations for remediation* (pp. 197–222). St. Louis, MO: Mosby.

Exner, C. (2001). Development of hand skills. In J. Case-Smith (Ed.), *Occupational therapy for children* (4th ed., pp. 268–306). St. Louis, MO: Mosby.

Exner, C., & Henderson, A. (1995). Cognition and motor skills. In A. Henderson & C. Pehoski (Eds.), *Hand function in the child: Foundations for remediation* (pp. 93–110). St. Louis, MO: Mosby.

Fitts, P. M., & Posner, M. T. (1967). *Human performance.* Belmont, CA: Brooks/Cole.

Folio, M. R., & Fewell, R. R. (2000). *Peabody Developmental Motor Scales* (2nd ed.). Austin, TX: Pro-Ed.

Forssberg, H., Eliasson, A. C., Kinoshita, H., Johansson, R. S., & Westling, G. (1991). Development of human precision grip I: Basic coordination of force. *Brain Research, 85,* 451–457.

Gibson, E. J., & Spelke, E. S. (1983). The development of perception. In P. H. Mussen (Ed.), *Handbook of child psychology* (Vol. 2, p. 58). New York: Wiley.

Gibson, J. (1962). Observations on active touch. *Psychological Review, 69,* 477–491.

Giuliani, C. (1991). Theories of motor control: New concepts for physical therapy. In M. Lister (Ed.), *Contemporary management of motor control problems: Proceedings of the II STEP Conference* (pp. 29–35). Alexandria, VA: Foundation for Physical Therapy.

Glass, A. L., & Holyoak, K. J. (1986). *Cognition* (2nd ed.). Reading, MA: Addison-Wesley.

Haley, S. M., Coster, W. L., Ludlow, L. H., Haltiwanger, J. T., & Andrellos, P. J. (1992). *Pediatric Evaluation of Disability Inventory*. Boston: New England Medical Center Hospital & PEDI Research Group.

Hatwell, Y. (1987). Motor and cognitive functions of the hand in infancy and childhood. *International Journal of Behavioral Development, 10*, 509–526.

Hoffman, D. S., & Luschell, E. S. (1980). Precentral cortical cells during a controlled jaw bite task. *Journal of Neurophysiology, 44*, 333–348.

Johansson, R. S., & Westling, G. (1984). Role of glabrous skin receptors and sensorimotor memory in automatic control of precision grip when lifting rough or more slippery objects. *Experimental Brain Research, 56*, 550–564.

Kapandji, I. A. (1982). *The physiology of the joints. Vol. 1: Upper limb* (rev.). New York: Churchill Livingstone.

Klein, R. M. (1976). Attention and movement. In G. E. Stelmach (Ed.), *Motor control issues and trends* (p. 80). New York: Academic Press.

Koh, T. H., & Eyre, J. A. (1988). Maturation of corticospinal tracts assessed by electromagnetic stimulation of the motor cortex. *Archives of Diseases of Children, 63*, 1347–1352.

Kuypers, H. G. (1981). Anatomy of the descending pathways. In J. M. Brookhart & V. B. Mountcastle (Eds.), *Handbook of physiology, section I, volume II, motor control, part I* (pp. 107–137). Bethesda, MD: American Physiological Society.

Lawrence, D. G., & Hopkins, D. A. (1976). The development of motor control in the rhesus monkey: Evidence concerning the role of corticomotoneuronal connections. *Brain, 99*, 235–254.

Lemon, R. N. (1990). Contributions to the history of psychology: LXVII Henricus (Hans) Kuypers F.R.S. 1925–1989. *Perceptual and Motor Skills, 70*, 1283–1288.

Lidz, C. S. (1987). *Dynamic assessment.* New York: Guilford Press.

Miller, L. J. (1988). *Miller Assessment for Preschoolers*. San Antonio, TX: Psychological Corporation.

Muir, R. B., & Lemon, R. N. (1983). Corticospinal neurons with a special role in precision grip. *Brain Research, 261,* 312–316.

Newborg, J., Stock, J. R., Wnek, L., Guidubaldi, J., & Suinicki, A. (1988). *Battelle Developmental Inventory.* Chicago: Riverside.

Pehoski, C. (1992). Central nervous system control of precision movements of the hand. In J. Case-Smith & C. Pehoski (Eds.), *Development of hand skills in the child* (pp. 1–11). Rockville, MD: American Occupational Therapy Association.

Pehoski, C., Henderson, A., & Tickle-Degnen, K. (1997). In-hand manipulation in young children: Translation movements. *American Journal of Occupational Therapy, 51,* 719–720.

Rochat, P. (1989). Object manipulation and exploration in 2- to 5-month-old infants. *Developmental Psychology, 25*, 871–874.

Ruff, H. A. (1980). The development of perception and recognition of objects. *Child Development, 51,* 981–992.

Ruff, H. A. (1982). Role of manipulation in infants' responses to invariant properties of objects. *Developmental Psychology, 18,* 682–691.

Stilwell, J. M., & Cermak, S. A. (1995). Perceptual functions of the hand. In A. Henderson & C. Pehoski (Eds.), *Hand function in the child* (pp. 55–80). St. Louis, MO: Mosby.

Strickland, J. (1995). Anatomy and kinesiology of the hand. In A. Henderson & C. Pehoski (Eds.), *Hand function in the child: Foundations for remediation* (pp. 16–39). St. Louis, MO: Mosby.

Sugden, D., & Keogh, J. (1990). *Problems in movement skill development*. Columbia: University of South Carolina Press.

Appendix 5.1.
Functional Educational Checklist

Student Name _____   Date of Birth _____

School _____   Grade _____

Teacher _____   Date _____

Person Completing Form _____   Therapist _____

I. Attention/Behavior/Motivation

Comments:

_____

_____

Yes   No   Does student have difficulty:

__ __   1. Concentrating on and attending to classroom tasks?

__ __   2. Actively participating in classroom activities?

__ __   3. Following directions (single and multi-step)?

__ __   4. Initiating work after directions have been given?

__ __   5. Completing tasks on time?

__ __   6. Organizational skills, such as organizing desk, cubby, or locker?

Comments:

_____

_____

II. Hand Use

Yes   No   Does student have difficulty:

__ __   1a. Using a consistent hand when completing activities?

1b. Does student appear to be right-hand dominant or left-hand dominant? (circle one)

__ __   2. Using classroom tools, such as scissors, when completing tasks?

__ __   3. Using both hands together to complete a task, such as stabilizing paper while cutting or writing, zipping a coat, placing items in a book bag, or carrying items?

__ __   4. Picking up/manipulating small objects, such as math cubes and other classroom manipulatives or food items?

III. Visual–Motor Skills/Handwriting

Yes   No   Does student have difficulty:

__ __   1. Drawing prewriting shapes (e.g., vertical line, horizontal line, circle, cross, diagonal line, square, X, and triangle) needed for letter formation?

__ __   2a. Forming uppercase and lowercase print letters and numbers when a model is provided?

__ __   2b. Forming uppercase and lowercase print letters and numbers independently?

__ __   3a. Forming cursive uppercase and lower-case letters when a model is provided (if applicable)?

__ __   3b. Forming uppercase and lowercase letters in cursive independently (if applicable)?

__ __   4. Keeping letters a consistent size when writing and keeping letters within the lines of grade-appropriate paper?

__ __   5. Providing spaces between letters and words so that they are readable?

__ __   6. Accurately copying information from the chalkboard to paper?

__ __   7. Accurately copying information from a paper positioned on the student's desk?

__ __   8. Erasing information completely after making a mistake?

__ __   9. Completing written work within a designated time frame?

(continued)

___ ___ 10. Writing so that it is readable by others?

___ ___ 11. Effectively using a computer to complete written assignments?

Comments:

_____

_____

IV. Self-Care Skills

Yes No Does student have difficulty:

___ ___ 1. Managing a coat (e.g., putting on or taking off, hanging up)?

___ ___ 2. Putting items into or taking items out of a book bag?

___ ___ 3. Putting supplies into or taking supplies out of desk or locker?

___ ___ 4. Engaging zipper on a variety of jackets and zipping up jacket?

___ ___ 5. Managing other fasteners, such as buttons, snaps, zippers, on clothing?

___ ___ 6. Tying shoes?

___ ___ 7. Blowing nose?

___ ___ 8. Washing hands?

___ ___ 9. Using restroom independently?

Comments:

_____

_____

V. Eating Skills

Yes No Does student have difficulty:

___ ___ 1. Picking up and bringing finger foods to the mouth?

___ ___ 2. Using utensils?

___ ___ 3. Drinking from a cup?

___ ___ 4. Drinking from a straw?

___ ___ 5. Opening packages or containers?

___ ___ 6. Opening milk cartons or juice boxes?

Comments:

_____

_____

VI. Managing School Environment and Mobility

Yes No Does student have difficulty:

___ ___ 1. Drinking from a drinking fountain?

___ ___ 2. Using a pencil sharpener?

___ ___ 3. Managing a combination lock (if applicable) and opening a locker?

___ ___ 4. Managing lunch money and a wallet?

___ ___ 5. Carrying and placing food items on a lunch tray?

___ ___ 6. Opening and closing classroom, bathroom, and building entry doors?

___ ___ 7. Keeping up with peers when walking to desired location?

___ ___ 8. Navigating around obstacles, such as uneven sidewalks, curbs, or playground equipment, without falling?

___ ___ 9. Managing stairs (if applicable)?

___ ___ 10. Managing getting on and getting off the school bus?

Comments:

_____

_____

VII. Gross Motor Skills

Yes No Does student have difficulty:

___ ___ 1. Sitting or standing unsupported independently?

___ ___ 2. Completing simple gross motor tasks, such as jumping, hopping, running, and skipping?

___ ___ 3. Walking or running without tripping or falling?

___ ___ 4. Managing playground equipment?

___ ___ 5. Using gross motor equipment, such as jump ropes, balls, bats, or racquets?

___ ___ 6. Participating in group activities or games in physical education class?

Comments:

_____

_____

Created by Lynne Pape, MEd, OTR/L, and Kelly Ryba, OTR/L

Appendix 5.2.
Sample IEP Objectives for Hand Function

I. Bilateral Hand Skills

1. When given a task that requires two hands, student stabilizes the activity with one hand and performs it with the other hand. Criteria: _____% of opportunities.

   Because many tasks during the school day require students to use both hands (e.g., stirring, zipping a coat, managing fasteners, shoe tying, cutting, writing, managing a book bag), list the tasks that will be focused on in treatment. This data will be collected and included in the objective.

2. With _____ (degree of assistance) student uses non-preferred hand as an assisting hand during bilateral activities _____% of the time.

3. When given a bilateral task with an initial demonstration, student initiates and completes it. Criteria: _____% of attempts.

II. Cutting

1. Student picks up and positions scissors correctly within his or her fingers (e.g., thumb in small hole, fingers in large hole) _____% of attempts.

2. Student uses both hands in a thumbs-up approach when cutting with scissors and holding the paper _____% of the time.

3. Student snips edge of paper _____ times when using scissors _____% of attempts.

4. Student cuts a straight line remaining within 1/4 of an inch of the line and starting and stopping at designated points _____% of attempts.

5. Student cuts out a variety of shapes that require changes in direction (e.g., curved lines, circles, squares, triangles) and remains within 1/4 of an inch of the line so that all parts are recognizable _____% of attempts.

6. Student stabilizes paper with hand held in a thumbs-up position _____% of attempts.

7. Student stabilizes and turns the paper when cutting around shapes that require changes in direction, so that all parts are recognizable ____/____ attempts, or _____% of attempts.

8. Student holds ruler in place with assisting hand while making pencil line with dominant hand _____ out of _____ times.

9. Student cuts with scissors with dominant hand while other hand assists by turning paper _____% of the time.

III. Coloring

1. Student colors a shape or picture, remaining within the lines. Criteria: No more than _____ deviations _____% of attempts.

2. Student colors in a shape or picture, completely filling the entire space. Criteria: _____% of attempts.

3. Student independently stops coloring when shape or picture space is completely filled. Criteria: _____% of attempts.

4. When coloring, student uses wrist movements to vary the direction of strokes rather than turning the paper. Criteria: _____% of the time.

5. Student colors an area not larger than 2 inches using only finger movements, with the wrist and hand stabilized on the support surface. Criteria: _____% of the time.

6. Student grades pressure applied when coloring so as not to break the crayon or wrinkle or rip the paper. Criteria: _____% of the time.

IV. Arm and Hand Skills

1. Student purposefully uses surface to assist in the release of an object _____ out of _____ times.

2. Student uses controlled release of an object above a _____ (size) container with wrist extension, _____ out of _____ times.

3. Student is able to stabilize elbows in extension grasping objects in space _____ out of _____ times.

4. Student can release a small object from a pincer grasp with wrist extension _____ out of _____ times.

5. Student can hold an object between opposed thumb and pads of fingers with no palm involvement _____ out of _____ times.

(continued)

6. Student initiates and completes an activity using the same hand consistently _____% of the time.

7. Student can point or poke with index finger, keeping all other fingers flexed _____% of the time.

8. Student is able to pick up _____ (number) of small pegs, one at a time, and move them to the palm of the same hand _____ out of _____ times.

9. Student can hold and move a coin or chip from the palm to the fingertips of the same hand ___ out of _____ times.

10. Student can reposition pencil from writing position to erasing position, using only one hand ___ out of _____ times.

V. Motor Planning and Sequencing

1. Student completes a _____ (number)-step activity as demonstrated (e.g., packing a book bag, completing an obstacle course, folding a towel).

2. Student completes a specific _____ (number)-step activity following verbal directions (e.g., packing a book bag, completing an obstacle course, folding a towel).

3. Student completes a specific _____ (number)-step activity with only initial directions (e.g., packing a book bag, completing an obstacle course, folding a towel).

4. After being given the initial directive, student completes a specific _____ (number)-step activity (e.g., packing a book bag, completing an obstacle course, folding a towel).

Created by Lynne Pape, MEd, OTR/L, and Kelly Ryba, OTR/L

Developing a Process to Address Handwriting Concerns

6

Students with difficulty writing are frequently referred to occupational therapists working in school-based settings. Written output, or handwriting, is required daily for a variety of school-related tasks. Students compose stories, copy spelling words, perform math calculations, answer questions in a written format, take notes during class, and complete written examinations. Outside of school, children also need to be able to write efficiently to do homework, sign a card or write a thank you note, take telephone messages, write a list, or leave a note. If a student has difficulty performing the mechanics of handwriting (e.g., forming letters efficiently), then higher level writing components (e.g., organizing thoughts to compose an answer) also may be affected.

When there is a problem with handwriting performance, it is important for occupational therapists to identify which components of the process are being affected. If the student is able to write the uppercase and lowercase letters of the alphabet in isolation so that they are legible and can copy words from a paper or the blackboard with no difficulty, yet his or her daily work is difficult to read, then the therapist needs to help the team determine where the process is breaking down.

This chapter provides school-based occupational therapists with an approach to use when dealing with handwriting concerns. Determining *why* the student is having difficulties and *what* is preventing him or her from being successful with written output or handwriting can be a very difficult process. Information included here is based on acquired experience of handwriting issues encountered by the authors when serving multiple school districts.

A variety of items are discussed in this chapter to help occupational therapists develop a process to use when addressing handwriting concerns. They are encouraged to understand how handwriting is taught to students in traditional classrooms and to students in special education classes within the school districts they serve. They need to determine if there is a specific curriculum used for either print or cursive. Performance components included in the handwriting process also are covered. Knowledge of these increases a therapist's awareness that handwriting requires more than fine motor skills and that other areas can affect handwriting.

Use of the Handwriting Teacher Questionnaire (see Appendix 6.1) developed by the authors will help occupational therapists define specific handwriting concerns. Handwriting evaluations, the need for occupational therapy support, and how to establish measurable objectives are presented. Intervention programs for handwriting are shared, along with discussion of which programs work best in addressing certain issues. The use of assistive technology to augment handwriting, including specific devices and software options, also is discussed.

Handwriting Facts

Handwriting adds a unique, personal touch in a time when computers, faxes, and e-mail are the norm. Handwriting adds intimacy to a letter and reveals details about the writer's personality. Throughout history, handwritten documents have sparked love affairs, started wars, established peace, freed slaves, created social movements, and declared independence. Although it sometimes gets lost in the ocean of digital technology, handwriting still remains a constant in communication. With each phone message jotted down, each note secretly passed in class, and each memo quickly written in a meeting, the printed word remains important.

According to the Writing Instrument Manufacturers Association, illegible handwriting and other handwriting-related issues cost the United States more than $200 billion each year in lost time and money:

- Phone calls are made to wrong or non-existent numbers.
- Packages are delivered on the wrong dates or to the wrong addresses, or they contain the wrong items.
- Mailings are delayed or never received because postal employees cannot make out the addresses.
- Each year, up to $95 billion in tax refunds cannot be delivered because of unreadable addresses on the tax forms.
- At their 1994 conference, the American Medical Association found prescriptions and medical records to be major health hazards; the health of at least 1 in 10 Americans is endangered by a physician's handwriting.

Groff (1961) has documented that at least 1 out of every 3 school teachers writes so illegibly that students have trouble reading assignments, notes on the blackboard, or corrections on written work. In addition, it has been shown that better handwriting results in as much as a full letter grade higher for similar or identical work.

To explain why illegibility affects society to such a great extent, Gladstone (2002) further indicated that handwriting instruction averages only 5 to 10 minutes a week, with little or no instruction after Grades 3 or 4. Teacher training no longer includes any instruction in the teaching of handwriting. From the 1930s to the 1950s, handwriting instruction began disappearing from the course lists of teachers' colleges. Today, such training is not even offered—let alone required—in most top colleges. Graduates no longer have to demonstrate competence in teaching handwriting. This means that today's teachers received their own final lessons in handwriting at about ages 7 or 8 years—and they received those lessons from teachers who themselves had their own final training and evaluation in handwriting at that age. Graham and Weintraub (1996) also found that only 36% of teachers indicated that they received formal training in handwriting instruction in their undergraduate coursework.

Handwriting in the School Setting

McHale and Cermak (1992) studied the types of fine motor activities that school-age children perform in the classroom setting and the amount of time used to complete them. They found that between 31% and 60% of the day's activities require fine motor skills. Paper-and-pencil tasks account for 85% of the time spent on fine motor tasks. The remaining percentage is spent handling manipulatives. So it is conceivable that children could spend between one-third to one-half of their day performing paper-and-pencil tasks while at school. A breakdown in this process significantly affects the child's ability to function within the classroom setting and, ultimately, affects the written material used to convey what the child knows.

The importance of handwriting has been documented in terms of the frequency that it is used throughout a student's daily routine. The consistency of its use is apparent, but the method of how it is taught is not consistent. Graham (1992) found that, in some classrooms, handwriting is taught systematically using either a specific handwriting curriculum or materials developed by the teacher. There was no formal instruction on handwriting taught in other classrooms. Instead, practice and instruction were provided sporadically on an individual or as-needed basis.

Depending on a district's requirements or lack thereof, students may be exposed to a variety of handwriting methods as they progress through elementary school. Most students are able to learn handwriting regardless of what approach is used. In a study by Graham and Weintraub (1996), it was found that students were able to copy letters when given a model without having formal instruction in how to form the letters. Others, however, benefit from a systematic approach that reinforces letter formation so that they are able to write more efficiently.

Several studies have attempted to determine the prevalence of handwriting difficulties. Alston (1985) and Rubin and Henderson (1982) found that an estimated 12% to 21% of school-age students experienced some form of handwriting difficulty. For students attending urban-area schools, such estimates were as high as 44%. They also found that boys are more likely to have handwriting difficulties than girls (see Alston, 1985; Ruben & Henderson, 1982).

Understanding How Handwriting Is Taught

Occupational therapists providing services in a school-based setting must understand what the handwriting expectations are at each grade level, beginning at preschool, for both the traditional classroom population and the special education population. As noted, it also is important to be aware of how the district provides instruction in the area of handwriting and if it is based on a specific district-wide curriculum.

The authors of this text provide occupational and physical therapy to multiple school

districts and therapy services to more than 800 students. We have encountered a wide range of approaches to handwriting instruction among various districts, most notably at the kindergarten level. Most do not have a formal curriculum that is used when teaching handwriting, especially printing.

In one district, all kindergarten classes meet in one building, yet there are differences among the teachers as to how the students are exposed to or taught handwriting. One teacher starts at the beginning of the alphabet and shows her students a "letter of the week," pairing it with the sound of the letters. Another groups letters into families based on how the letters are formed and then pairs them with the sound of the letters. Teachers do not have a formal curriculum, so each uses his or her own terminology when describing how to form letters.

In another district, the kindergarten teachers decided to use a phonics approach when exposing students to the letters. Each letter is presented in the order that it is introduced in the phonics program so that students learn its sounds and also are exposed to writing it.

There are different ways to find out what the handwriting expectations are for each grade level. In addition to talking to staff directly, it can be helpful to look at the content standards or course of study for specific expectations. Report cards may indicate grade-level expectations, particularly at the lower grades. For example, in one school district, the kindergarten language arts (writing) course of study indicates that students will demonstrate increased use of uppercase and lowercase letter formation and correctly write their own names. Under the math course of study, it states that students will count and write the numeral that relates to a number of objects in a set of 10 or less. Yet, a kindergarten report card from a different district indicates that students will print their names, identify uppercase and lowercase letters, and print the alphabet but does not indicate that they will write numbers.

When occupational therapy services are being provided to support handwriting objectives in those grade levels in which handwriting is being formally taught, occupational therapists must know the type of instruction used and who is providing it. There must be a consistency in the approach by all involved. This is discussed in more depth later.

Handwriting Expectations

Because there is so much variety in how handwriting is taught, it is important to gather as much information as possible. A description of what our agency typically finds at each grade level is provided. In addition, specific questions are listed to assist school-based occupational therapists in making sure that they are aware of the expectations and the method in which handwriting and letter formation are being approached.

Preschool

Research has indicated that readiness to begin writing should be based on a child's ability to copy geometric forms (Weil & Amundson, 1994). This typically does not occur until the second half of the kindergarten school year.

The Ohio Department of Education in the Language Arts Academic Content Standards for pre-kindergarten states that students will print the letters in their own name and other meaningful words with assistance, using mock letters, conventional print, or both. These content standards are based on what most children should be able to accomplish by the end of preschool.

To address this area and in preparation for kindergarten, some preschools for children with special needs will have students trace over laminated copies of their first name. The difficulty is that students usually are not monitored as they do this, so correct letter formation is not being emphasized, but it is not developmentally appropriate to ask students to do so at this age anyway. Most students typically trace in a left to right progression, but they do not always trace the letters using correct formation, as they have not had sufficient exposure in how to do so. They may trace letters from bottom to top and segment them as they trace them (i.e., trace a line and then go back and add another part to it).

Overall, this is a difficult area to address. A broad level of ability may be demonstrated among students in the preschool classroom. Some may be able to write their names correctly, whereas others will be unable to do so.

Before implementing the content standards in Ohio, preschool teachers began exposing students going on to kindergarten to basic paper-and-pencil tasks in the second semester of their final year in preschool. Teachers typically had students write their names on their art projects, initially tracing over dotted lines and then copying them from a model. They also provided activities that gave students a chance to practice the pre-writing shapes and lines, such as using a diagonal line when matching pictures on a worksheet or tracing dotted circles that were part of a picture and then coloring them.

Questions to Ask.
- What are the curriculum expectations for handwriting in the preschool setting?
- How are these expectations incorporated into a student's daily routine?
- Are there different expectations for students of different ages?
- Is there an attempt to provide direct instruction regarding handwriting?
- How is occupational therapy expected to support these expectations?
- How is letter formation taught (continuous stroke or ball and stick)?

Kindergarten

Depending on the individual school district, a variety of methods may be used to expose kindergartners to handwriting. At the beginning of the school year, most districts expect students to write their names on the line at the top of a paper or worksheet. If the space is too small, students can turn their papers over and write on the back. The expectation is that kindergartners will write their names using an uppercase letter for the first initial and lowercase letters for the rest of the name. Some districts do not expect kindergarten students to write their last names until the second semester.

Kindergarten teachers sometimes will have students use a spiral notebook to practice writing. Even though the pages are lined, the teachers do not expect students to keep their letters on a line or between two lines. One district expects students to be able to write all of the uppercase and lowercase letters by the end of the year; by the second semester, students are copying sentences projected onto a screen by an overhead projector.

Other districts expose their kindergartners to a letter each week. Students are expected to practice writing the uppercase and lowercase versions of the letter and to be able to say the sounds for that letter.

Some kindergarten teachers teach handwriting to the entire class systematically. The number of students in their classrooms makes it is difficult for them to provide individualized feedback as the students are forming letters. During a handwriting lesson, many students in such classrooms may be observed beginning their letters from the bottom even though the teacher put a mark at the top of the line to indicate where to begin. Teachers are able to assist only a few students at a time. The rest of the students are left practicing incorrect letter formation.

Questions to Ask.

- What is the expectation for handwriting in kindergarten? When are students exposed to letter formation, and when are they expected to master it?
- Is a specific curriculum used by all kindergarten teachers in a school or district? If

so, how is letter formation taught, as a continuous stroke or ball and stick? Continuous stroke formation uses a single stroke to form all the lowercase letters except f, i, j, k, t, x, and y. The ball and strick approach uses multiple lines when forming lowercase letters, requiring the child to pick up the pencil when forming some letters.

- Is handwriting taught to the whole class at once or to small groups so that the teacher can better instruct students on the formation of their letters?
- Are students using lined paper and, if so, what type?

First Grade

Typically, printing is taught in first grade. The methods may vary depending on a teacher's level of comfort and experience and the existence of a formal curriculum. Worksheets, not workbooks, generally are used when teaching printing because they allow each letter to be emphasized individually. Handwriting may be incorporated into the language arts program so that students are exposed to letter formation while they are using it for specific assignments.

Questions to Ask.

- What is the expectation for handwriting in first grade?
- How long does it take to teach all of the uppercase and lowercase letters?
- Is there a specific curriculum used by all of the first-grade teachers?
- If there is not a specific curriculum, do teachers present the letters in the same order during instruction? Do they use consistent terminology when they refer to the lines on the paper or when forming the letters? If so, how is letter formation taught, as a continuous stroke or ball and stick?
- Is handwriting taught to the whole class at once, or in small groups so that the teacher can better instruct students on the formation of their letters?

- Are students using lined paper and, if so, what type? Do all of the teachers use the same type of paper?
- Do the students have letter strips on their desks, or are there models available within the classroom?
- What are the specific expectations for students in special education who receive occupational therapy?
- Are these students in the classroom during handwriting instruction? Is individualized attention provided to make sure that they are forming their letters correctly?
- What is the role of the special education teacher or the occupational therapist in the area of handwriting?

Second Grade

Some teachers spend the beginning of the second grade quickly reviewing letter formation. The focus of the majority of the year is using print as a part of students' daily assignments. In some districts, cursive writing is introduced toward the end of the year.
Questions to Ask.
- Are letter formations reviewed?
- Is remediation provided for students with difficulty printing? If so, by whom?
- What is the role of the special education teacher?
- Is cursive introduced?

Third Grade

Cursive is introduced to most students in the third grade. School districts generally use workbooks when teaching cursive. Students are taught all of the uppercase and lowercase cursive letters within a 6-week to 8-week period. The lowercase letters are introduced first. Once these are mastered, the uppercase letters are presented.

Depending on the setting, once formal instruction has been provided, students may be required to use cursive for specific tasks, such as spelling tests or essays. At the same time they are being taught how to write in cursive, students also are being exposed to reading it. This is important for occupational therapists to understand, because even if some students do not use cursive, they do need to be able to read it. By fourth grade, most assignments and board work are done in cursive.
Questions to Ask.
- What is the expectation for handwriting in third grade?
- How much time is allotted to teach all of the uppercase and lowercase letters?
- Is a specific curriculum being used to teach cursive?
- Are workbooks being used as a part of the curriculum?
- Do teachers use consistent terminology for letter formation?
- How and when are the connectors taught if they are not presented as part of the individual letters?
- Is handwriting taught to the whole class at once or in small groups so that the teacher can better instruct students on the formation of their letters?
- Are students using notebook or lined paper? If so, what type? Do all of the teachers use the same type of paper?
- Do the students have cursive letter strips on their desks, or are there models available within the classroom?
- What is the expectation for using cursive after the students are exposed to formation of all of the letters?
- Do students have a choice when they use cursive, or are there assignments that must be done in cursive?
- Are assignments and board work written in cursive?
- What are the specific expectations for those students in special education who are receiving occupational therapy?
- Are these students in the classroom during handwriting instruction?

- Are all students in special education exposed to the entire cursive alphabet?
- If not, what is used to determine the level of exposure?
- Are all students given an opportunity to learn how to write their names in cursive so that they have a functional signature?
- Is individualized attention provided to make sure each student is forming their letters correctly?
- What is the role of the special education teacher or occupational therapist?
- Is there a different or modified handwriting curriculum for students in special education?

Fourth Grade

By fourth grade, most formal handwriting instruction has been provided. At this point, the demand for written output has increased in proportion to an increased volume of work. Students are expected to use handwriting to communicate and as a method of showing the teacher what they know.

Questions to Ask.

- Are students expected to use cursive for all written work?
- Do students have the option to print if it is more legible?
- If a student has difficulty with cursive, is remediation provided? If so, by whom?

Performance Components Needed for Handwriting

Students use handwriting to communicate facts, ideas, thoughts, and feelings. At the same time, it provides the teacher with a mechanism to evaluate what a student has learned.

Students with specific disabilities may have difficulty mastering—or be unable to master—all of the components needed to use handwriting to communicate. It is important that occupational therapists understand all of these components. Because letter formation requires use of the hands, many people assume that handwriting is primarily a fine motor task. Parents or teachers frequently believe that a child's fine motor difficulties are the source of his or her handwriting problems. However, the fine motor component is just one small part of what is needed for students to be able to use writing to express their ideas.

Prewriting Skills

Before a child is exposed to handwriting, specific prewriting skills should be present. Vreeland (1998) has indicated that most children have developed the prewriting skills needed for letter formation by the second half of the kindergarten year. Starting handwriting instruction before a child has mastered these prewriting skills may cause poor writing habits, a dysfunctional pencil grip, and overall discouragement (Alston & Taylor, 1987).

The Developmental Test of Visual Motor Integration (VMI) is one assessment used to predict readiness for writing. A student's score is based on the ability to copy the first nine figures as stated by Beery (1982): vertical, horizontal, circle, plus sign, right and left diagonal lines, square, X, and triangle. In 1989, Beery revised that statement, saying instead that handwriting should not be addressed until the child can copy the oblique cross (X) that typically occurs at 4 years, 11 months, as it requires that the child draw the diagonal lines required to form many letters.

Studies have found significant relationships with VMI scores as predictors of handwriting performance accuracy (Maeland, 1992; Sovik, 1975). Weil and Admundson (1994) found a significant difference between performance on the test and the ability to copy letters. This verified that kindergarten students should be ready for handwriting instruction during the latter part of the year.

In 1994, Tseng and Murray determined that the VMI was the best predictor of handwriting legibility. Tseng and Cermak (1993) reviewed ergonomics and perceptual–motor components and agreed that the nine basic prewriting shapes should be mastered before handwriting is introduced. Cornhill and Case-Smith (1996) also reviewed studies and conducted their own testing that indicate that visual–motor integration abilities were related significantly to handwriting success. Students identified as having good handwriting scored higher on tests that measured motor accuracy, visual–motor integration, and in-hand manipulation (Maeland 1992; Sovik 1975; Tseng & Murray, 1994).

As indicated, prewriting skills are handwriting's foundations. By the latter half of kindergarten, most students have developed these necessary skills (Weil & Admundson, 1994). For those students with disabilities, however, this may not be the case. It is imperative that the occupational therapist educates the team as to the components needed as precursors before beginning handwriting. In this way, the educational team can determine how to approach the teaching of these skills. Students classified as mentally retarded or with multiple disabilities might never achieve all of the prewriting components; however, expectations are that they will be exposed to handwriting as a part of the curriculum.

Vreeland (1998) compiled a list that includes the following handwriting prerequisites.

Hand Dominance. Hand dominance develops as a result of the ability to coordinate the two sides of the body. Between ages 4 and 6 years, a child typically shows a hand preference when using tools and when performing fine motor tasks. This preference encourages consistent hand use so that skills can be developed for those tasks that require precision.

Crossing Midline and Bilateral Integration. Students need to be able to cross the midline of their bodies when forming specific

letters and when writing across a page. They also need to be able to stabilize the paper while writing with the other hand. Students who have difficulty with bilateral integration may continue to switch hands during activities because of their inability to cross their midlines.

Functional Pencil Grip. A student needs an efficient, functional grasp that allows the controlled movements needed for letter formation. Schneck and Henderson (1990) identified the dynamic tripod and the lateral tripod as common functional pencil grips. The tripod grasp is formed by three fingers functioning together; the dynamic quadropod is formed by four fingers functioning together. Schneck (1991), however, also looked at the grips of students who had good handwriting and those who had poor handwriting. She found that proprioceptive and kinesthetic feedback affected handwriting legibility more than did pencil grip alone.

Expanding on Schneck's findings, Tseng (1998) developed a comprehensive pencil grip classification. Her findings supported those studies that found the lateral tripod and dynamic quadropod equal to the dynamic tripod in legibility, speed, or both. Dennis and Swinth (2001) examined the influence of pencil grasp on the handwriting legibility of fourth-grade students during both short and long writing tasks. They found that the type of grasp used did not affect legibility as much as the length of the writing task. They also found the lateral quadropod to be a functional pencil grip.

Koziatek and Powell (2003) looked at how the type of pencil grip affected the handwriting speed and legibility of fourth-grade students. The Evaluation Tool of Children's Handwriting, discussed later in this chapter, was used to determine legibility. Photographs were taken of students' pencil grips as they wrote. The researchers found that four main pencil grips were used among the 99 students observed: 38 students used the dynamic tripod, 18 students used the dynamic quadropod, 22 students used the lateral tripod, and 21 students used the lateral quadropod. Use of any particular grip did not affect legibility.

The literature now supports the use of these four types of mature pencil grips. As shown, studies also have indicated that use of any of these did not affect handwriting legibility or speed. School-based occupational therapists must be aware of this research as they evaluate students with handwriting difficulties. Achieving the perfect dynamic tripod grasp may not be necessary for those students able to functionally use one of the three other types of recognized grasps.

Understanding of Directional and Spatial Terms

Students must be able to recognize right from left and apply this information to external objects. They must be able to discriminate the letters and numbers needed to read and write. Finally, they must be able to translate verbal directions, such as "Start at the top and make a straight line down," into motor responses.

Ability to Copy Lines and Shapes. As discussed, there is a correlation between the ability to copy the first nine shapes on the VMI and the ability to form letters. The ability to copy the shapes is a prerequisite for learning letter formation.

Ability to Use Eyes and Hands Together. A child must be able to attend to tasks visually. Visual feedback and guidance to the hands is essential for motor output in terms of letter formation, placement, and alignment. The eyes drive the hands when writing, because early letter formation is not automatic.

Ability to Maintain an Upright Posture. The student must be able to maintain the adequate sitting posture needed for writing. There needs to be head and trunk stability to allow arm and hand mobility.

Orientation to Print. As indicated, students must be able to discriminate between letters and numbers. They also need to be able to identify letters. This is critical for the development of visual memory so that there is meaning to what is being copied or written.

Additional Performance Components

Learning to write requires motor, sensory, perceptual, and cognitive skills. These skills must be integrated into the writing process. To understand the complexity of the skills required for handwriting, it is important to discuss the following additional performance components and their contribution to the handwriting process. Vreeland (1998) grouped these components into sensory–motor, cognitive, and psychosocial areas.

Postural Control and Stability. Upper extremity control depends on the external stability of the head and trunk. Proximal control of the upper extremity also is necessary to provide a stable support base for the control of the distal joints (Benbow, 1995). Students who have difficulty with postural control and stability may stabilize, lean, or prop their heads on their arms.

Body and Spatial Awareness. Internal body awareness allows the perception of movements and the position of body parts (proprioception) without relying on visual feedback. It assists in the development of laterality, or a child's internal awareness of the left side and right side. It also aids in directionality, the child's external awareness of left and right on himself or herself and on others and the realization that there is a right and left side to objects. It allows the child to monitor the position, movement, speed, and force of his or her writing. It provides a foundation for bilateral integration in the ability to across midline. Motor planning also relies on body awareness and proprioceptive feedback.

Students with poor body awareness may need to visually monitor their hands when performing a fine motor task, especially handwriting. Difficulty with motor planning requires a child to think about the specific movements needed for letter formation. He or she has difficulty forming and retrieving the motor memory of the letters. As a result, he or she may make the same letter three or four different ways. He or she may write slowly because of the need for the visual feedback. His or her handwriting has not reached the level of being automatic (Cermak, 1991).

Levine (1985) has indicated that some students who have poor handwriting have inadequate somatosensory perception (poor feedback about the position of the hand and fingers). A student may have problems in finger identification or in knowing the precise position of his or her arm and hand. He or she may position his or her head close to the paper to visually monitor what the hand is doing because of inadequate processing of somatosensory information. In addition, he or she frequently may attempt to adjust the pencil within his or her hand or grasp the utensil tightly to provide more feedback.

Visual–Motor, Visual–Perception, and Attention. Visual–motor ability enables the student to copy shapes, symbols, letters, and numbers. Ocular motor control allows the eyes to move and work separately from the head. This permits the child to efficiently look up at the board or at a paper on his or her desk when writing or copying. It allows the eyes to guide the hand movements needed for writing.

When beginning to print, the hand's output depends on the input and ongoing guidance of the visual system (Benbow, 1995). The student needs to visually monitor the point of his or her pencil to control stroke length and angle and to know where to intersect the lines. When writing in cursive, visual control becomes secondary to proprioceptive feedback. Various visual–perceptual components are needed for both printing and cursive to provide feedback about where to place words on the paper or on the writing line and to space words and letters properly. Visual discrimination is needed to perceive the differences between letters and numbers.

Fine Motor Components. In addition to the pencil grasp discussed previously, there are other fine motor components that affect a student's ability to manage a pencil. Benbow (1995) discussed the importance of wrist and hand function as it relates to handwriting. Wrist stability is necessary, as is the ability to oppose the thumb to the index finger to maintain a stable and open web space, stable palmar arches, and the ability to separate the two sides of the hand. For more specific information on these components, please refer to Chapter 5 in this book.

The student needs to be able to perform the in-hand manipulation needed to manage the pencil. Translation is required to position and adjust the pencil within the hand. Complex and simple rotation are necessary to pick up the pencil from the support surface and position it within the hand and to be able to rotate it to be able to erase.

Exner (1992) has identified three aspects of fine motor control that affect handwriting. The first is isolation of finger movements, which is needed to support the pencil grasp and to monitor discrete movements. The second is the grading of movements. This also is needed to support the pencil grasp and to provide fluid movements. Finally, proper timing of movements is needed to control the rhythm and flow of writing.

Cognitive Components. The effect of cognition on skill development has been discussed throughout this text. Lidz (1987) defined *cognition* as the capacity by which a person acquires, organizes, and uses knowledge. Cognition also includes multiple classes of mental capacities, such as attention, perception, memory, reasoning, problem solving, and language (Glass & Holyoak, 1986).

Amundson (1992) indicated that cognitive information contributes to a student's overall handwriting dysfunction. Occupational therapists need to consider the student's attention span, memory (visual, verbal, and motor), and sequencing of events and items during assessments of conceptual skills.

Evaluating a student's level of cognition through an ability or IQ test often is required when determining if a student has a disability. Specific disabilities identified in the Individuals With Disabilities Education Act (IDEA) that may include cognitive deficits are mental retardation, autism, traumatic brain injury, or multiple disabilities. To assist in identifying realistic expectations, occupational therapists need to be aware of a student's ability level.

Psychosocial Components. Students who have difficulty writing may have self-concept or self-esteem issues as a result. They may lack the interest and motivation to write and resist tasks that require handwriting. They also may provide short answers or phrases when writing and rush through their work, not taking the time to go back and review it. This can affect overall legibility. If asked to go back and redo an assignment, a student may become very frustrated and act out.

A child's occupational performance includes self-care, work, and play activities. For the school-age child, work includes educational activities such as reading, writing, and calculation. Functional written communication is used both at school and at home, so the child must to be able to convey information to others in a legible manner (Admundson, 2001). The acquisition of handwriting skills requires the integration of the sensory, motor, perceptual, and cognitive abilities that have been discussed. The occupational therapist needs to consider these performance components when evaluating a student's writing ability and when presenting information to the team regarding possible intervention strategies.

The Referral Process

Oliver (1990) and Reisman (1991) have identified problems with handwriting as one of the most common reasons for occupational therapy referrals. In one study, Reisman (1991) found that those students referred to occupational therapy for handwriting concerns were appropriately referred based on their handwriting evaluation scores when their scores were compared to those of other groups. In another study by Hammerschmidt and Sudsawad (2004), a questionnaire was used to identify why elementary school teachers refer students with handwriting difficulties to occupational therapy. The reason most frequently chosen was because the student did not improve with classroom assistance alone. Illegible handwriting was identified as the most frequently seen problem with these students. These studies indicate that teachers are making appropriate referrals to occupational therapy based on test scores and when classroom interventions or assistance did not improve the students' handwriting.

Gathering Background Information

The occupational therapist can contact the person initiating the referral or the primary person who has information regarding a student's handwriting issues. Collecting such information also is an opportunity to determine what, if any, intervention strategies have been attempted. The therapist needs to define the exact concerns of the individual making the referral so that they can be addressed through the evaluation process. The handwriting checklists developed by the authors can be used when gathering information.

Reviewing Work Samples

The occupational therapist can review a student's work samples to find out how much support was provided to the child while completing the task. It is important to determine if an intervention has been tried. Looking at a variety of work samples such as copying from the board, worksheets that require writing in a designated area, and math papers that require lining up the numbers in correct columns provides information about the child's performance in the classroom setting. The therapist also should compare a work sample that required the student to organize and compose thoughts (the writing process) to a sample that required only copying (the writing mechanics). In addition, it is often helpful to look at other classmates' work for comparison.

Interviewing Parents and Classroom Personnel. Interviewing the parents and classroom personnel provides insight into the child's handwriting performance at home compared to school. Use of the Handwriting Teacher Questionnaire (Appendix 6.1) to structure the interview helps the occupational therapist obtain consistent information from all teachers and school staff. The handwriting questionnaire either can be given to a teacher to complete before meeting with the therapist, or it can be completed during the meeting.

Use of this questionnaire helps teachers focus on other areas, such as reading ability and letter awareness, that can be contributing factors to the handwriting difficulties. The information gathered not only identifies areas of concern but also helps the occupational therapist focus on priority areas that need to be evaluated. When discussing specific handwriting concerns with classroom staff, asking open-ended questions is often more helpful than offering choices to explain the possible reasons for a difficulty.

Observing the Student in a Natural Environment. Observing the child actually writing in the classroom setting also is helpful, because the occupational therapist can gather information about the setting as well

as the task. Looking at the setting provides insight into how the child performs in different areas. If his or her handwriting performance in the classroom is significantly different than during a formal evaluation, then the therapist may discover the reason for this. For example, in the classroom, the child may rush through his or her work and correct mistakes by writing over them instead of erasing them.

Assessing Directly Identified Concerns. After identifying all areas of concern, it may be necessary to perform a handwriting evaluation. This evaluation will provide specific data to help determine what is affecting the student's ability to write.

Providing Interventions During the Handwriting Evaluation. The occupational therapist can use the handwriting evaluation as an opportunity to try interventions. For example, he or she may have the student write on a variety of types of paper to determine if the width of the lines on the paper improves legibility.

Formal Handwriting Evaluations

A variety of commercial evaluations are available that can help occupational therapists assess handwriting concerns.

Evaluation Tool of Children's Handwriting

The Evaluation Tool of Children's Handwriting (ETCH; Admundson, 1995) measures the handwriting legibility and speed of students in Grades 1 through 6. It evaluates both print and cursive handwriting. Items tested include the writing of the alphabet in lowercase and uppercase, numeral writing, near-point copying (copying from a paper on the desk), far-point copying (copying from the board), print-to-cursive transition, dictation, and sentence composition. It is a criterion-referenced assessment that indicates legibility percentiles for each of the items and overall legibility scores for letters, words, and numbers.

Minnesota Handwriting Assessment

The Minnesota Handwriting Assessment (Reisman, 1999) measures the legibility, formation, alignment (placement on the line), size, and spacing for near-point copying of students in Grades 1 and 2. It is a norm-referenced test that looks at handwriting quality and speed or standard and D'Nealian styles of print. It also can be used to monitor handwriting progress.

Children's Handwriting Evaluation Scale for Manuscript Writing

The Children's Handwriting Evaluation Scale for Manuscript Writing (Phelps & Stempel, 1987) measures the handwriting speed and quality of students in Grades 1 and 2. Using a near-point copying task, this norm-referenced test evaluates letterforms, spacing, rhythm, and overall appearance.

Children's Handwriting Evaluation Scale

The Children's Handwriting Evaluation Scale (Phelps, Stempel, & Speck, 1984) assesses the cursive writing of students in Grades 3 through 8. Using near-point copying of short paragraphs, this norm-referenced test measures letterforms, spacing, rhythm, and overall appearance.

Denver Handwriting Analysis

The Denver Handwriting Analysis (Anderson, 1983) is a criterion-referenced tool that evaluates the cursive handwriting of students in Grades 3 through 8. It measures near-point copying, far-point copying, writing the alphabet from memory, print-to-cursive transition, and dictation. A time limit that differs per grade also is assigned to each task.

Test of Legible Handwriting

The Test of Legible Handwriting (Larsen & Hammill, 1989) evaluates the handwriting legibility of students in Grades 2 through 12. Essays written by the students are evaluated,

and a score is determined by matching each sample to one of the three scoring guides, which are descriptors or samples of handwriting. Examples are provided for both print and cursive. Raw scores are converted to standard scores or percentiles. The sum of the standard score also can be converted to a composite legibility quotient.

Evaluation of Handwriting Performance

Ziviani and Elkins (1984) developed a method for assessing printing ability in children ages 7 to 14 years. Each student's handwriting ability was evaluated based on legibility components, such as formation, spacing, alignment, size, and speed.

The Evaluation Process

In this section, the evaluation process is defined. Specific steps for the occupational therapist to use are provided.

Taking into consideration all of the areas previously discussed, formal or informal testing can be used to evaluate a student's handwriting. However, such evaluations should include each of the following domains of handwriting: legibility, speed, and ergonomic factors.

Amundson (1992) described the domains of handwriting as those tasks required of the student in the classroom, including the writing of uppercase and lowercase letters, number writing, far-point copying, near-point copying, print-to-cursive transition, dictation, composition, and endurance.

The ETCH, developed by Amundson (1995), evaluates each of these. While the following factors and considerations are specific to the ETCH, they also are relevant to other handwriting assessments that evaluate similar components.

Writing Letters and Numbers

An occupational therapist must determine if a student writes the uppercase and lowercase alphabet and numbers without a model. This helps determine if the student has a visual memory for letters and numbers and can write them automatically. Timing the student provides further information. If the child needs to verbalize the alphabet to write the letters and must start at the beginning each time he or she writes a letter, this increases his or her time and should be documented.

If there is a question about the student's efficiency when writing in cursive, then having him or her write the uppercase and lowercase alphabet in both print and cursive while timing each task provides valuable information when the times are compared. A major discrepancy in time between print and cursive helps the team determine if writing in cursive is a viable option. The team also learns which letters the child can write, as it is not uncommon to find that students who struggle with cursive frequently are unable to form all of the uppercase cursive letters, as they are not used as often.

Far-Point and Near-Point Copying

The occupational therapist should ask the student to copy a sentence from a model hung on the wall (vertical far-point copying) and copy another sentence from a paper on the desk (horizontal near-point copying). While the student is performing this task, the therapist should observe how frequently the student looks at the model. The therapist may want to make a hash mark on a letter each time the student looks up or circle letters or words when the student writes them together. This helps determine if the child is able to chunk letters together to read and write them as individual words or if he or she needs to look at the model for each individual letter. Looking at the model frequently increases the time needed to copy the sentences.

Observing this task and the time it takes the student to complete it also helps the occupational therapist determine why the student writes slowly when he or she copies. For instance, if the student forms letters correctly when he or she writes and writes legibly, yet takes considerable time to copy the sentences, any delays and difficulties may not be because of problems with the mechanics of handwriting.

Dictation

A student also should be able to write words dictated to him or her by the occupational therapist. This is an opportunity to evaluate the student's ability to process information auditorily and translate it into a written format.

Print-to-Cursive Translation

If the cursive component of the ETCH is given, the student has to translate a printed sentence and recopy it in cursive.

Composition

The student must compose a sentence and then write it. The occupational therapist should document how much support, such as suggestions for topics, is needed to be able to generate a sentence. Documenting how much time the student spends formulating his or her thoughts also is helpful. The time needed to formulate the thought should be compared to the amount of time needed to actually write the sentence. This helps the team determine if the problem lies with the writing process or with the mechanics of handwriting.

Legibility

Handwriting samples should be examined for the following problems that can affect legibility (Amundson, 1995; Cermak, 1991; Tseng & Cermak, 1991):
- Incorrect letter formation,
- Poor alignment of letters on the baseline or within the given writing area,
- Irregular spacing between letters or words,
- Inadequate letter ascenders and descenders,

- Uneven sizes of lowercase letters,
- Inconsistent height of letters,
- Incorrect use of capital letters,
- Use of mixed letter types (cursive and print, uppercase and lowercase),
- Slant (uphill or downhill) of the letters when writing in cursive,
- Reversals (letters written backward), and
- Inability to sustain the legibility of writing.

Handwriting Speed and Endurance

Amundson (1995) went on to indicate that handwriting speed and endurance can be affected by many factors. No exact data exists on specific writing speeds for letters per minute at each grade level. Endurance is observed during the actual writing task. Students who write poorly may have difficulty sustaining legibility as the length of their assignments increases.

When endurance is poor and writing speed is slow, a student does not have the same opportunity to practice letter formation as other students do. The occupational therapist and the teacher must work together to determine if the student's written productivity is adequate for the time constraints and volume of work involved.

Ergonomic Factors

Ergonomic factors such as posture; pencil grasp; and upper extremity control, including stability and mobility, also need to be observed and documented. To do this, the occupational therapist should document his or her observations of the following:

- Is the student able to maintain his or her head and trunk in an upright position while writing?
- Are the chair and desk heights appropriate for the height of the student?
- Does the student have adequate stability of the upper extremity to allow distal mobility of the hand for writing?
- Is the student's pencil grasp affecting his or her ability to write?

Visual–Motor Integration Scores

The VMI frequently is administered as part of the handwriting evaluation process, especially for those students with suspected or known cognitive deficits. Studies have shown a correlation between scores on this test and tests that measure intelligence, such as the Wechsler Intelligence Scale for Children–Revised (WISC–R; Beery, 1997). The standardized score on the VMI does appear to correlate with the full-scale IQ scores on the WISC–R.

For example, if a student's full-scale IQ is 75 and VMI score is 77, this should be taken into consideration when sharing evaluation information with the team. What this shows is that the student's visual–motor abilities are at the same developmental level as his or her cognitive abilities. This is important for the occupational therapist to understand when determining intervention strategies and expectations. The therapist also must be aware of the student's cognitive ability whenever the VMI is given in isolation. A below-average test score on the VMI should not be interpreted as a deficit if it is commensurate with the student's overall ability on his or her IQ test.

Interpreting Evaluation Results

Once background and evaluation information has been obtained, the occupational therapist needs to identify and consider the effect the performance components have on a student's ability to write. Information obtained from the Handwriting Teacher Questionnaire also should be considered because it affects the student's ability to write. Each student needs to be assessed individually.

Discriminating Between Letters and Numbers

A student's ability to identify and discriminate between letters and numbers needs to be determined. If the student does not know the letters that he or she is expected to write or copy, then this is equivalent to asking English-speaking adults to write in Chinese. Adults would not be able to write the symbols without a model, although they probably could copy them fairly accurately. The reproduced characters, however, would have no meaning to the writers. The same is true for students who cannot identify letters and numbers.

Reading and Comprehension Levels

A student's reading and comprehension levels must be considered because they affect how and if a child is able to read what he or she writes. If a student in fourth grade is reading at a first-grade level, then he or she should not be expected to generate ideas at a fourth-grade level. If his or her writing ability also is at a first-grade level, then his or her writing abilities are developmentally at the same level as his or her reading abilities. In this case, modifications could be considered, such as the use of software to generate ideas that an adult writes and the student copies.

Word Spacing

Another item to consider in relation to a student's ability to read is his or her ability to determine the spaces between words. If he or she has difficulty copying words, many times it is because he or she does not read the grouped letters as words. Often, as the reading ability improves, so does proper spacing and grouping between letters and words. It is therefore important to consider a student's reading ability when there are spacing issues instead of assuming that it is a visual–perceptual problem.

Spelling Ability

A student's ability to spell affects his or her ability to read his or her writing. When a teacher has concerns about the student's handwriting legibility, it is important to consider his or her ability to spell.

Content

The student's ability to read what he or she writes is affected not only by the legibility of his or her handwriting but also by the content of what he or she is asked to write.

Reading Cursive

If a student is expected to write in cursive but is having great difficulty, then it is important to know if the student can read cursive. More specifically, this applies to a student with a known cognitive deficit whose parents want him or her to learn cursive with his or her classmates. Students unable to read cursive will have difficulty writing in cursive and will not grasp the meaning of what they have written.

Other Factors

In addition to the factors just discussed, others must be considered, including the overall effect of a child's cognitive ability in relation to handwriting expectations. Do not expect a student with cognitive delays to be able to write at the same level, in terms of content, sizing, and spelling, as his or her peers. Students who rush through their work and fail to make corrections properly often have legibility issues. Frequently, these students do not take the time to go back and proofread their work before handing it in. When students rush, they do not form the letters as accurately as when they write more slowly. It is important to consider the speed of the writing when evaluating legibility.

A student's attitude toward handwriting and motivation to do his or her best work affects handwriting ease, comprehension, and legibility. When a student openly resists handwriting, it is very difficult to try to incorporate intervention strategies. Students must be motivated to work and respond to praise to be able to change the quality of their handwriting.

Support Options

If there are handwriting concerns that require support through either intervention or modifications, then it is important for the occupational therapist and the team to consider appropriate options based on a student's grade level and curriculum expectations. For example, if there are existing handwriting concerns with a special education student who is entering first grade, then the team needs to acknowledge that he or she will be exposed to formal handwriting as a part of the first-grade curriculum. The team needs to discuss whether additional intervention is needed, or if monitoring and remediation are sufficient.

Handwriting Interventions

As shown, the ability to produce written work can be affected by many factors. The mechanics of handwriting is just one factor. These include the ability to form letters and place them on the line with correct spacing so that the text is readable. All of this needs to happen efficiently, or it will interfere with the writing process. This process involves the selecting and organizing of words to convey a specific message. The message needs to be grammatically correct, that is, organized in such a way that the reader is able to follow the train of thought from the beginning to the end. The handwriting mechanics cannot interfere with the writing process, and they need to be considered separately from the writing process (Swinth & Anson, 1998).

It also is important to distinguish between difficulty with mechanics and difficulty with the writing process. This must be done to determine if the support of an occupational therapist is needed. The team must

determine if the speed of written output is being affected by problems with the writing process or if the writing process is being affected by problems with the mechanics of letter formation.

Handwriting problems can interfere with the writing process in terms of planning and generating ideas. If it is determined that a problem is related to the mechanics of handwriting, intervention can be provided. Such intervention can include remediation of specific letters, modifications (e.g., pencil grasps), and adaptive equipment (e.g., adapted paper, slanted surfaces).

A variety of approaches to handwriting intervention have been documented. Amundson (2001) described five theoretical frames of reference to intervention: neurodevelopmental, acquisitional (teaching–learning), sensory integrative (sensory–motor), biomechanical, and behavioral.

As a member of the educational team, the occupational therapist can provide a variety of resources based on these professional frames of reference. The techniques, strategies, and interventions from the identified theoretical approaches can be combined to create a program personalized to each student's needs. A comprehensive and challenging, yet motivational, intervention program can be developed and implemented to address specific handwriting needs (Amundson, 2001).

Neuromuscular Reference

The neuromuscular approach addresses postural control and stability, muscle tone, and the proximal joint stability needed for distal function. Preparation activities that target postural and upper extremity control are important components of a handwriting intervention program to develop the trunk control needed to provide the shoulder with the stability needed for hand function and writing. Development of wrist stability, in-hand manipulation, and a balanced interaction of intrinsic and extrinsic muscles also are necessary for the efficient and fluid movement required for handwriting. Specific intervention strategies that address these areas can be found in Chapter 5.

Acquisitional Reference

The acquisitional approach uses specific handwriting intervention programs based on the needs of the student. Graham and Miller (1980) described the conditions fundamental to making such a program successful and effective. They recommend that handwriting instruction be taught directly, implemented daily in short lessons, individualized to a student's specific needs, modified based on performance data, and applied in a meaningful context appropriate for the student.

Theories of motor learning categorize handwriting as a motor skill. There are three phases to learning a new motor skill: cognitive, associative, and autonomous (Fitts & Posner, 1967). First, the child develops a cognitive strategy for performing the necessary movements. Visual control and hand movement feedback are essential during this phase.

Next, in the associative phase, the child continues to adjust and refine the fundamental skills he or she has learned. The need for visual feedback declines as proprioceptive feedback becomes more important. In this phase, students need continued practice, instructional guidance, and self-monitoring strategies, such as doing worksheets with instruction on formation and checking his or her work.

In the final phase, the student is able to perform handwriting automatically with minimal conscious attention. At this autonomous level, the student is able to attend to other, higher level components of handwriting, including formulating thoughts and answering questions.

Intervention strategies for problems with spacing, alignment, sizing, and pencil grasp, as well as modifications and adaptive equipment, can be found through a variety of resources. One of these, *TRICS for Written Communication* (Amundson, 1998), provides a resource for educators, occupational therapists, and parents to improve students' written communication. The program incorporates strategies and techniques for improving written production in the classroom. This helps students be successful and functional writers as soon as possible. These techniques and strategies are listed on individual instructional pages that can be photocopied and used with individual students.

Fine Motor Dysfunction: Therapeutic Strategies in the Classroom, developed by Levine (1991), is a compilation of therapeutic suggestions, activities, and adaptations that address specific handwriting concerns. These can be photocopied and used with individual students. Other handwriting intervention programs that use the acquisitional approach are listed later in this chapter.

Sensory Integration

The sensory integration approach uses a variety of sensory experiences to encourage a student's nervous system to integrate information at the subcortical level so that effective and efficient motor output (e.g., legible handwriting) are produced. It encourages use of the multisensory format, including a variety of sensory input, mediums, and instructional materials. For example, a foam tray filled with modeling clay can be used to practice letter formation, providing the child with additional tactile and proprioceptive input as he or she forms letters, numbers, or words using a dowel rod or pencil. The tactile and proprioceptive input provides feedback to the child to assist in developing the muscle memory needed to form the letters. This approach takes issue with traditional approaches to handwriting intervention that require a student to sit at a desk performing tedious paper-and-pencil tasks, as this approach does not provide the same degree of sensory feedback needed to reinforce proper letter formation.

A multisensory approach allows the occupational therapist to use a variety of writing tools (e.g., markers, glitter crayons, grease markers); vertical, horizontal, or angled writing surfaces; and writing activities, including having students practice forming shapes or letters using trays filled with clay or a sealed plastic bag filled with finger paint or colored hair gel.

Students also are encouraged to self-talk, using the appropriate terminology needed to form the letters. For example, when writing the lowercase letter *a*, the student could say "around and straight line down."

Biomechanical Approach

The biomechanical approach addresses the ergonomic factors associated with handwriting dysfunction. Such factors include the need for a properly fitted desk, the use of adapted pencil grips, and the proper positioning of the writing paper to permit fluid writing.

Amundson and Weil (1996) and Amundson (2001) have indicated that team members may consider modifying a student's pencil grasp if he or she is holding the pencil so tightly that he or she repeatedly has to "shake out" the writing hand to relieve fatigue or if the pressure he or she exerts causes him or her to break the pencil lead. The student's grip also may need to be modified if the student holds the pencil tightly with her or her thumb wrapped around the pencil, closing the web space, which limits his or her ability to grade finger and thumb movements while manipulating the pencil.

Benbow (1990) noted that, once grasp patterns are established, they are difficult to change. She recommended not attempting to change a student's grasp pattern once he or she begins second grade. Thus, intervention should be done sooner rather than later, as correcting improper grips is difficult after age 7.

Behavioral Frame of Reference

An occupational therapist can use the behavioral frame of reference to establish a reinforcing environment. To maintain a student's motivation, the therapist needs to provide varied and new activities. Encouragement and reinforcement must be applied to assist the student in reaching realistic, attainable goals. Allowing the student such choices and control are empowering and motivational and promote success.

The occupational therapist also can enhance a student's social competence as well as his or her writing ability by having him or her participate in a handwriting intervention group that writes letters to other students (pen pals). When children are involved in a special activity or are a part of a special group, their enthusiasm and interest increase (Amundson, 2001).

Handwriting Intervention Studies

Peterson and Nelson (2003) examined whether or not occupational therapy intervention improved academic output (D'Nealian printing) in at-risk, economically disadvantaged first-graders. An occupational framework, including biomechanical, sensory integration, and acquisitional strategies were used for intervention.

The Minnesota Handwriting Assessment (MHT) was used, pretest and posttest, to evaluate legibility, letter and word spacing, line, placement, and letter size and form as well as speed. Students in the intervention group received occupational therapy intervention twice a week for 30 minutes for 10 weeks; the control group received only academic instruction without any individualized programming. The personalized sessions usually began with sensory integration activities.

The student then engaged in occupational forms (situations) to promote motor planning, motor memory, and self-monitoring performance. Strategies to promote proper letter and word spacing and proper letter size and alignment also were incorporated. A pictorial self-monitoring checklist was used to teach and reinforce these concepts. During the last 5 minutes of each session, students practiced D'Nealian printing. Posttest scores indicated a substantially greater increase in the scores of the MHT in the test group than the increase in scores of the control group.

A study conducted by Case-Smith (2002) investigated the effects of school-based occupational therapy services on handwriting. The work of students between ages 7 and 10 years who had identified poor handwriting legibility and who received direct occupational therapy services was compared to the work of students who did not receive occupational therapy services and yet still had handwriting problems. Handwriting legibility, speed, and associated performance components were examined.

Testing was done at the beginning of the school year and at the close of the school year. These tests evaluated visual–motor and visual–perception skills, in-hand manipulation, and handwriting legibility and speed. The intervention group received direct occupational therapy during the school year that incorporated a student's visual–motor skills in addition to handwriting practice.

As reported by the treating therapists, intervention strategies were provided from a variety of occupational frameworks. Individualized interventions were developed to address each student's specific handwriting needs. Visual–motor activities were implemented with a variety of handwriting interventions, including writing on the chalkboard or other vertical surface for strength and stability. Sensory integration techniques were used when children demonstrated specific problems, such as motor planning.

The treating occupational therapists were the primary professionals addressing the handwriting goals on each student's individual education plan (IEP). Collaboration was provided through communication with the students' teachers. Data was not collected regarding teacher support or carryover of intervention strategies into the classroom. Results indicated that the intervention group made significant gains in handwriting legibility, with an average improvement of 14.2 percent total legibility. The handwriting legibility of those students not receiving services remained unchanged over the course of the school year. In addition, students in the intervention group showed significant increases in in-hand manipulation and position-in-space scores.

In both of the studies described, the direct handwriting intervention provided integrated theoretical perspectives. The occupational frameworks included biomechanical, sensory–motor, and acquisitional principles applied from an occupational perspective.

Feder, Majnemer, and Synnes (2000), in surveying Canadian occupational therapists and reviewing the literature, found that the use of multiple theoretical frameworks is typical for occupational therapy intervention for handwriting. Combined with the results of the studies previously discussed, this information implies that integrating intervention strategies from a variety of occupational frameworks is appropriate when providing handwriting intervention. The role of the occupational therapist is to collaboratively develop and synthesize situations (occupational forms) that are meaningful and purposeful so that the student is able to engage in occupational performances (Peterson & Nelson, 2003).

An Intervention Option— The Sensible Pencil

The necessity of prewriting skills as a foundation for handwriting already has been discussed. Some children identified with a disability in the area of mental retardation or with other disabilities that may include mental retardation, such as multiple disabilities or autism, might never achieve all prewriting components, yet expectations are that the child will be exposed to handwriting as a part of his or her curriculum. The occupational therapist, as a member of the team, can assist other team members with intervention options to address this area.

Since 2000, the authors of this text successfully have used the Sensible Pencil handwriting intervention program (Becht, 1985) with students with autism, Down syndrome, and various degrees of mental retardation. It is an individualized, direct-instruction program that teaches how to print numbers and lowercase and uppercase letters. Prewriting strokes are taught prior to the introduction of letters, and verbal cues are paired with the formation of individual lines. Once mastered, the prewriting strokes are incorporated into the formation of letters. For example, a vertical line (down) is taught first, then a horizontal line (over) is taught. Finally, the two lines are combined using the terminology down, lift, and over to create a plus ("+" for prewriting strokes; "t" for letter formation).

The Sensible Pencil was developed by a special education teacher to teach children with special learning needs the skills necessary to write. Becht considered several important factors, such as prewriting ability, consistency, task analysis, progress or product, and review and mastery. These and other factors were incorporated into the program.

Prewriting

All manuscript letters and numbers are formed from 11 basic lines, or strokes. The Sensible Pencil allows students to learn to write these strokes in small, obtainable steps. Minimal verbal cues are provided to reinforce the formation of the line. Because minimal

verbiage is used when forming the strokes, the program is beneficial for those students who have difficulty processing verbal information, especially children with autism.

Because students often need to be able to write their names before they may have mastery of writing, Sensible Pencil terminology often is used to teach students how to write their names before being exposed to the individual letters.

Consistency

Instruction in the Sensible Pencil is consistent throughout the program. This creates fewer opportunities for confusion if different individuals work with the same student and makes the program easy to incorporate into the student's daily routine, increasing the potential for daily exposure.

The writing language, directions, and models used when teaching the lines, shapes, numbers, and letters are straightforward and easy to understand. All of the basic prewriting lines are introduced before they are used in letters. Only one type of line, shape, letter, or number is presented at a time and is worked on until mastered. Lowercase letters are introduced after prewriting strokes and shapes are learned.

Task Analysis

Skills previously taught in one-step instruction in other programs are taught in multiple steps. With the Sensible Pencil, these steps follow a logical progression from the simplest (vertical line) to the most difficult (diagonal line). This progression is both systematic and developmental. Therefore, the student is presented with numerous early positive experiences that provide a solid foundation for the writing process.

Specific strokes and letters must be mastered before students can move on, which means that they are not expected to learn all 52 uppercase and lowercase letters at once. In fact, letters are grouped by similarity in formation and are formed using a continuous stroke except for f, i, j, k, t, x, and y.

Process or Product

The Sensible Pencil focuses on how the student learns, not just on what the student learns. Each new task begins at a very basic level and progresses to increased difficulty. Worksheets supplement instruction, beginning with simple lines and progressing to print letters and numbers. These can be photocopied so that there is no need for additional workbooks or time spent creating worksheets and can be sent home for homework so that the parents are aware of their child's performance.

Review and Mastery

In the Sensible Pencil, one skill is learned before another skill is introduced. Each new word or skill presented is based on skills mastered in previous lessons. After a specific task is learned, it is incorporated permanently into the program. This continual review promotes skill retention.

Mastery tests assess each student's success, progress, and readiness to learn the next new task. Like the worksheets, these tests can be photocopied. They do ask that a child be able to write given letters when dictated within a designated area; however, teachers and the occupational therapist can modify these by allowing the student to copy the letters rather than writing them from dictation or modifying the paper that is used so that a larger space is provided.

Assistive Technology

Amundson (2001) indicated that some children with significant cognitive impairment may best meet their written communication needs through the use of assistive technology. Students who continue to have difficulty with letter formation and spacing may benefit from exposure to typing and keyboarding.

Students who need so much adult support when handwriting are unable to work independently to complete a task. Whereas these students often can generate a sentence verbally, it is difficult for them to remember it long enough to write it down on paper. Their difficulties with spelling, forming letters, and aligning and spacing letters and words affect their attempts to put their thoughts on paper. Adult support often is needed to compensate. Over time, students become dependent on adult support and expect it each time they attempt to perform a handwriting task, often looking to the adult for support before attempting to try something by themselves.

Rather than expecting students to generate and write a sentence independently, we have success having a student verbally generate a sentence that is scribed by an adult. The student then copies the sentence written by the adult using printing or keyboarding, depending on his or her ability. An example of an objective that addresses this is the section of this chapter on IEP goals.

For students who can manage the computer functions needed to use word processing, success also has been found by having them type words from their reading program into the computer one word at a time. The expectations are that a student will be able to use the keyboard to copy a single word displayed on a flip chart, hit the ENTER key two times to create a space, flip the chart to the next page, and begin the process again.

This approach works because the student has limited information (letters or words) on the page; there is minimal information to distract him or her or to copy. He or she is not required to attend to the task for a long period of time, and it requires minimal computer skills. Because of the repitition of the steps and limited demands required for this task, some students are able to perform it independently and require only an occasional verbal prompt from across the room.

For the student who has not been able to learn how to write his or her name after extended periods of exposure and practice, a name stamp may give a student a way to identify his or her work. Name stamps can be custom ordered online or from a local office supply store. Stamps come in font sizes that are big enough so that the name can be easily read.

Some students may have difficulty with stamps that are self-inking. If they do not understand the function of the stamp, they tend to continually press it down, creating multiple images. If a student is going to try to use a name stamp, an objective to have him or her stamp his or her name in a defined area may need to be developed.

Role of Occupational Therapy in Handwriting Intervention

If the educational team, including the parents and the occupational therapist, determine that handwriting intervention is necessary for a student to benefit from his or her educational program, the occupational therapist is usually involved in some aspect of the program. The therapist's role should be based on the student's needs as determined by the educational team.

Depending on the setting, the team may determine that the occupational therapist is responsible for providing direct intervention and also is primarily responsible for implementing the handwriting objectives on the student's IEP. This frequently is seen when handwriting is not systematically taught or when there is not a specific curriculum used within a particular district. The therapist is very qualified to assume this role, and research has indicated that students benefit from daily exposure to handwriting instruction (Graham & Weintaub, 1996; Vreeland, 1998).

If the team determines that the occupational therapist will provide direct intervention, then it is critical that he or she collaborate with the appropriate staff to ensure that handwriting intervention is provided at other times in addition to that provided by the therapist. Such collaboration may include

- Sharing techniques and terminology being used during therapy;
- Sharing any specific intervention programs that also can be used by the teacher for a specific student;
- Sharing any adaptations and modifications used during intervention (e.g., specific type of paper, highlighting baseline);
- Sharing copies of worksheets used to practice letter formation; and
- Developing homework packets. If homework packets are developed, it is important that the therapist instruct the parents so that the student can benefit from the practice, as someone needs to sit with the student to ensure that the letters are being formed as intended by the directions.

To help the occupational therapist develop a process for handwriting intervention, the following questions are presented. These should help the therapist evaluate any interventions currently being provided to determine if they are the most effective way of providing services, based on the information presented in this chapter.

- If an occupational therapy evaluation indicates deficits in handwriting, who determines if there is a need for occupational therapy services—the team or the occupational therapist?
- If occupational therapy services are needed, how is the type of intervention (e.g., direct, collaboration) determined?
- Is the type of service chosen dependent on the student's grade level, current exposure to handwriting within the classroom or resource room, or both? For example, if a first-grade student has handwriting concerns, will he or she receive handwriting instruction as a part of his or her daily curriculum and then be provided with support for areas of concern?

- Will the occupational therapist be functioning in a collaborative role because the general education or special education teacher already is providing the handwriting intervention needed?
- Is the occupational therapist the only person providing direct handwriting instruction for individual special education students?
- Does the occupational therapist use a specific handwriting intervention program?
- If yes, is any other team member using the same program with the student during the week? Is any other team member providing handwriting intervention during the week using a different approach than that of the occupational therapist?
- Are there specific handwriting objectives on the student's IEP? Are they written specifically enough so that data can easily be collected?
- If yes, does the general education or special education teacher provide any support for the handwriting objectives?

Other Handwriting Intervention Programs

Amundson (2001) included the following intervention programs for both print and cursive writing.

Callirobics

This program by Liora Laufer sets paper-and-pencil exercises to children's songs in preparation for both print and cursive writing (www.callirobics.com). The exercises consist of simple, repetitive writing patterns (straight and curved lines) set to music. The music component also benefits individuals who learn better auditorily than visually and encourages the development of the rhythm and flow needed for letter formation. The program can be implemented either individually or with groups, using the cassette tapes that accompany the student workbooks. Additional information can be obtained by calling 800-769-2891.

Handwriting Without Tears

This comprehensive set of manuals by Janet Z. Olsen, OTR, addresses general handwriting remediation in *Handwriting Without Tears,* print instruction in *Printing Power* and *My Printing Book,* and cursive writing in *Cursive Handwriting.* Visual and verbal cues accompany the lessons, and word and sentence writing are encouraged throughout each level of the program. Developmentally based, it is appropriate for students of all abilities. Multisensory teaching aids and methods can be used as part of the learning process. Lowercase letter formation is based on a continuous stroke concept. Letters are grouped by similarity in formation, which teaches students how to form most letters with only one stroke, instead of following the ball-and-stick approach. Specialized paper is used to decrease visual stimulation. Additional information can be obtained by calling 301-263-2700.

Loops and Other Groups: A Kinesthetic System

This system by Mary Benbow, MS, OTR, was developed to enable students to learn the formations of all lowercase cursive letters in 6 weeks. The alphabet is separated into four groups of letters that share common movement patterns. Students visualize and verbalize these patterns to experience the "feel" of the letter. The program provides a systematic approach for letter analysis and efficient motor and memory cues to simplify the learning of functional handwriting. The lead-in stroke for each letter is included as the letter is taught so that all letters begin on the writing line. The overall approach reduces the need for visual feedback, replacing it with ongoing kinesthetic feedback to increase handwriting efficiency. Additional information can be obtained from Therapy SkillBuilders at 800-872-1726.

Facilitating Functional Written Communication

Amundson and Weil (1996) have indicated that, when students are unable to improve their handwriting through remediation, compensatory strategies need to be considered. The occupational therapist may need to give a student with poor handwriting an alternative method for functional written communication. Such alternative methods can include the use of computers, augmentative communication systems in which responses are dictated into a tape recorder, and peer buddies who can assist with written assignments. The educational team must determine which approach is most functional for each student.

Keyboarding

Rubin and Henderson (1982) have stated that, when students struggle with the process of writing, their ability to express their knowledge can be compromised. Those who continue to display poor handwriting often are given lower grades on the content of their work when compared to students with good handwriting (Briggs, 1980).

At this point, the team needs to discuss alternative methods for producing written materials. MacArthur (1988) identified the benefits of using computers to help remediate and compensate for handwriting difficulties for students with learning disabilities. Keyboarding provides students with a more effective and efficient method to convey what they have learned. It is an appropriate accommodation and adaptation that allows students to be successful in the area of written communication without the skill of handwriting.

For the purpose of this section, use of keyboarding includes use of word prediction software. Portable word processing devices also are discussed.

Keyboarding as a technological support for students with disabilities is an intervention strategy recognized by IDEA. Assistive technology encompasses both devices and services. As defined, it includes "any item, device, or system used to increase, maintain, or improve functional capabilities of individuals with disabilities" (Swinth & Anson, 1998). Assistive technology services include any service that directly assists a child with a disability in the selection and acquisition of an assistive technology device. Correlating therapies, training, and technical assistance for individuals with disabilities are other assistive technology services provided under the law (Swinth & Anson, 1998).

Many public school systems have mandated keyboarding (i.e., word processing using a computer keyboard) instruction in elementary schools because of its benefits to students with difficulties writing (Balajthy, 1998). Keyboarding addresses the mechanics of the writing process. It also produces a neat product with correctly formed, spaced, and aligned letters and words that is readable by others (and not just by the teacher who has become accustomed to reading a student's handwriting and can decipher his or her work).

An additional benefit to keyboarding is that it assists students with other areas of the writing process, such as grammar, punctuation, and spelling. It allows ease of editing without recopying the work, reducing motor demands and improving the content quality and quantity of written work. For all of these reasons, students will find keyboarding to be a valuable life skill as they progress through their school careers.

Keyboarding Studies

Dunn and Reay (1989) found that students whose typing speeds equaled or exceeded their handwriting speeds displayed increased competence in the content of their writing when using word processing rather than handwriting. Cochran-Smith, Paris, and Kahn (1991) conducted a study that compared keyboarding to handwriting and found that students' composition skills increased with the use of word processing because they tended to write more and had more error-free text.

Rogers and Case-Smith (2002) conducted a study that examined the relationship between handwriting and keyboarding in sixth-grade students who had received standard keyboarding instruction. Before this training, the participants displayed the ability to write an average of 9.3 words per minute. After 30 sessions, they averaged 14.9 words per minute while keyboarding. Seventy percent of the students produced more text with keyboarding than with handwriting. Fifteen of the 20 slowest writers were able to type more letters per minute than they were able to write per minute. The study showed that students who have difficulty writing may become proficient in the use of keyboarding. Doing so simplifies their text production, which allows them to concentrate on the content of their compositions.

Another study (More, Deitz, Billingsley, & Coggins, 2003) investigated the effectiveness of occupational therapy intervention that focused on teaching children with learning disabilities and handwriting difficulties to use word processing. It was determined that intervention involving word processing and word prediction did improve the legibility and spelling of written assignments for some children with learning disabilities and handwriting difficulties.

Preminger, Weiss, and Weintraub (2004) attempted to determine if there was a correlation between handwriting speed and accuracy and keyboarding speed and accuracy. They also attempted to ascertain if handwriting and keyboarding share common underlying components. Handwriting requires the formation of specific letters and spatial organization abilities not required when keyboarding. Keyboarding requires the memorization of associations between locations (keys). Students must be able to position their fingers on the keys and press the appropriate keys. The researchers found that handwriting accuracy and keyboarding accuracy might entail different skills. Following keyboarding instruction, a significant correlation was found between handwriting and keyboarding speed but not accuracy in these tasks. This suggests that keyboarding may be a potential alternative strategy for students with handwriting difficulties.

Keyboarding and Word Processing Requirements

Some school districts require keyboarding as a part of the standard curriculum; however, it frequently is not introduced until middle school. Students having difficulty with handwriting need keyboarding skills before this time. It is important that students be exposed to keyboarding as soon as the need is identified. This must be done to facilitate efficiency, as students can usually write faster than they can keyboard if they have had no previous exposure to the latter. MacArthur (1988) stated that, for keyboarding to be efficient, students need to be able to type at the same rate (i.e., words per minute) that they are able to write. Freeman (1954) reported that the average adult writes approximately 26 words (or 130 letters) per minute but that a proficient typist can reach 100 words or more per minute.

To be proficient in word processing, the student must be able to create new documents and files, open and close these documents and files, save information, format text, edit content, space between words and lines, indent for new paragraphs, and manage the mouse (Cochran-Smith et al., 1991). These components are important to consider when working with children who have cognitive deficits.

Keyboarding for the Next Generation

Cochran-Smith and colleagues (1991) have indicated that students who will be using word processing as an alternative for written communication must learn keyboarding before using it for writing. In addition, they need to be given opportunities to practice on a regular basis, and they must receive feedback in small increments so that they can process and incorporate it into their routines. According to Swinth and Anson (1998), research indicates that, for students to become proficient enough to use the computer to complete classroom assignments, they must be able to keyboard (generate text) efficiently. Occupational therapists play a critical role when working with students with disabilities in this area. They need to ensure that students have the motor control and the cognitive and visual–motor skills to access the keyboard. If there are limitations in these areas, then adaptations to the teaching method may be required in addition to equipment and software modifications.

Before beginning a typing tutor program, a paper copy of the QWERTY keyboard can be used with students to help learn the locations of the letters. The letters can be color-coded to reflect right-hand use or left-hand use. Students can practice using the paper keyboard by touching the appropriate letters to spell out words on their spelling lists.

When a student is ready to begin using a typing tutor program at school, the parents are encouraged to use the same program at home. This provides consistency and additional practice opportunities. Most typing tutor programs have motivational games that the child can play to get additional practice. In addition, the programs track individual data to show progress, which also can be a motivator.

Keyboarding and Cognitive Impairments

When working with students with cognitive deficits, additional modifications often are needed. Many times, they are unable to utilize the home row (ASDF JKL) concept for finger placement but nonetheless are successful using the "hunt and peck" approach. They still should be encouraged to use the appropriate hand or fingers for those letters on the right side and left side of the keyboard. Otherwise, they will tend to use only one or two fingers on the preferred hand for all the letters, which decreases efficiency. They also should be encouraged to use their thumb for the space bar.

A larger font size and a contrast color can be used to decrease the amount of text on the screen. This makes it easier for students to read. Sometimes they may have difficulty finding the correct key when copying text from a paper because the keyboard letters are in uppercase but the text being copied includes lowercase letters.

Depending on what students are being asked to copy, such as personal information like their names, stick-on letters can be put on the keyboard in contrasting colors that include lowercase letters. Students can match the the stick-on letters to the word they are copying. For example, if a student is practicing copying her name—Angela—make stick-on letters that represent an uppercase *A* and lowercase *n-g-e-l-a*. This will make it easier for her to find the letters in her name on the keyboard.

Students with moderate cognitive delays, who are unable to copy individual words on paper without adult support, can use the keyboard to work more independently. Individual sight words are placed on a small flipchart next to the computer and in the same orientation as the screen. As discussed earlier, the student is taught to copy the word onto the computer, hit the ENTER key two times to provide spacing, flip to a new page, and begin the process again. Minimizing the motor component needed, eliminating the need to handwrite the word, and providing a designated area while presenting only one word at a time is a very effective formula for increasing a student's ability to work independently.

Word Prediction Software

A study by More and colleagues (2003) found that use of word processing and word prediction software improved the quality of written expression for 75% of the students with learning disabilities. The students practiced keyboarding, using a typing tutor program, four times a week. They also were taught to use the word prediction software *Co-Writer*. Word prediction programs facilitate more effective written communication.

As the first letter of a word is typed, a list of possible words appears. After each typed letter, the list is revised, until the intended word is predicted. The software uses rules of grammar and word frequency to predict the words that are listed when the student types in letters (More et al., 2003). These programs provide spelling support and improve understanding of grammar rules and punctuation. They also can increase typing speed by decreasing the number of keystrokes needed. As the predicted words are selected, the software automatically provides spaces after punctuation marks and capitalizes the beginning word of each sentence (Don Johnston, 2004).

Portable Word Processing Devices

Portable word processing devices can be used for simple word processing, such as taking notes, taking spelling tests, and completing worksheets that require short answers. As with any technology, these devices are con-

stantly being upgraded to provide more options. The following are a sample of portable word processing devices used in schools. Other types are available, however, so therapists are encouraged to seek additional information if those listed do not appear to meet a student's needs.

AlphaSmart. This small, lightweight, portable word processor can be used for note taking and simple word processing. It has a QWERTY keyboard and a small screen that displays four lines of text (4-line 40-character LCD display). It is battery powered for 700+ hours of use, has the ability to store up to 8 files (approximately 100 pages of single-spaced text), and spell checks. When connected via cable to a USB port, the device can function as a full-feature keyboard. It can print directly through the printer port or via Infared. The *AlphaSmart 3000* costs approximately $200 (for additional information, call 1-888-274-0680).

The Writer. The Writer is similar to the AlphaSmart and provides similar functions. In addition, it offers self-editing checklists to assist students with written composition. It has built-in keyboarding instruction software that allows students to work on keyboarding skills and tracks data on each student's progress. It costs approximately the same as the AlphaSmart (for additional information, call 1-800-797-7121).

Handwriting and Keyboarding IEP Objectives

Present Levels of Performance

When reporting information in the present levels of performance section on the IEP document, specifically describe what the student is currently able to do as it relates to the goals and objectives in the IEP. It is important to be specific in this section so that the objectives are less global and reflect specific areas of need. For example, "Sam can write all lowercase letters, except g, j, p, q, and y, when given a model so that they are readable." The objective should focus on the letters that cannot be formed: "Sam will write tail letters (g, j, p, q, and y) so that the tail of the letter descends below the baseline (80% for each letter)."

List the letters and numbers that the student can form, and indicate the support needed to write them. If there previously was an objective that was too advanced for a student ("Sam will compose a three-sentence paragraph using correct letter formation"), describe instead what the student can do ("Sam can generate three sentences verbally but is unable to write them on paper in complete words that are spelled correctly. If the sentences are dictated by Sam and scribed by an adult, he can copy them, at times having difficulty with the spacing between words and placement on the baseline"). Presenting the information this way describes what the student can do and provides information that can be used to generate specific objectives. The objective becomes, "When verbally generating a sentence that is copied by an adult, Sam will be able to copy the sentence correctly so that the words are on the baseline (75% of all words)."

Goals and Objectives

Please review the information in Chapter 2 for help writing goals and objectives. Objectives are written very specifically to be able to show progress.

For example, write "the name will be written with correct letter formation 80% of the time" rather than "80% of each letter." The former implies that *all* letters in the name have to be formed correctly 8 out of every 10 times the name is written.

The requirement for correct letter formation also should be avoided (when possible) when writing specific objectives. Students can have legible handwriting even though they may form some letters incorrectly, such as

starting letters at the bottom rather than from the top. Terminology such as "so that it is readable by two" is used rather than "so it is legible," because "readable by two" can be measured. While correct formation needs to be stressed early on, many students are able to form legible letters without using correct formation. Expecting correct letter formation and trying to collect data on each letter is unrealistic.

Prewriting Shapes

For prewriting objectives, the occupational therapist needs to describe the shapes that the student already can draw in the present levels of performance section of the IEP. Then the focus can be on the shapes with which the student continues to have difficulty, for example, "Alex is currently able to copy 4 out of 9 prewriting shapes. These shapes include copying a vertical line and a horizontal line, a circle, and a cross. Alex is unable to copy a square, right or left diagonal lines, an X, or a triangle."

1. For those students able to learn how to form the prewriting shapes, the following objective could be written: "Student will copy the 9 prewriting shapes needed for letter formation 80% for each shape." The occupational therapist also could add "within a designated area," if this is difficult for the student. For younger students, the therapist could write the following objective: "The student is expected to master the shapes in a developmental sequence as defined by the VMI" as

2. "Student will trace, imitate, or copy a vertical line, a horizontal line, and a circle. Criteria: 80% mastery of each shape."

3. "On mastery of (list shapes) _____, _____, _____, student will imitate, trace, copy (list shapes) _____, _____, _____. Criteria: 80% mastery for each shape."

Broken down in this way, the occupational therapist and teacher do not have to work on every prewriting shape at the same time. Breaking down an objective this way allows the therapist to observe the student's ability and provides ongoing data to determine if an adapted program (e.g., Sensible Pencil) is needed versus just using the VMI shape sequence.

If a student is using the Sensible Pencil curriculum, then objectives should be written to reflect the order in which Sensible Pencil shapes are introduced in that program. The shapes listed in each mastery test need to be listed when the objective is written. If the occupational therapist thinks that the student will master all of the prewriting shapes within the prewriting unit test, then the goal should be written to reflect that the student will copy all shapes within the Sensible Pencil's unit test.

When writing criteria for Sensible Pencil prewriting objectives, the occupational therapist should monitor the length of time that it is taking the student to form the given shapes and also remain within the designated boundaries as defined by the program. If, after an extended period of time, the student displays the ability to form the shapes but continues to have difficulty remaining in the boundary, the therapist has the discretion to modify the criteria for mastery (e.g., instead of writing "per mastery level as defined by program," criteria instead could state "per mastery level for formation as defined in the program"). So, the revised objectives may read like the following:

4. "Student will copy vertical line (down), horizontal line (over), and cross as defined within Mastery Test 1 of Sensible Pencil. Criteria: Mastery level as defined by program."
5. "Student will copy cross, circle, and vertical line (up) as defined within Mastery Test 2 of Sensible Pencil. Criteria: Mastery level as defined by program."
6. "Student will copy vertical line (down), horizontal line (over), cross, circle, verti-

cal line (up), horizontal line (back), and square as defined within the 'unit test of prewriting lines and shapes' of Sensible Pencil. Criteria: Mastery level as defined by the program."

Numbers

When writing number formation objectives, the occupational therapist needs to indicate in the present level of performance the numbers that the student is able to form consistently and legibly and note the type of support or prompting needed to write them, if applicable. Objectives can then reflect the numbers that the student continues to have difficulty forming.

7. "Student will imitate or copy [*list numbers of difficulty*] so that they are readable. Criteria: 80% mastery for each number." If using the Sensible Pencil program, write number objectives the same way as the letter objectives.
8. "Student will write numbers 0–9 so that they meet criteria as defined within the numbers unit test of the Sensible Pencil handwriting program. Criteria: Per mastery level as identified by the program" or "Per mastery level for formation as defined by the program."

Handwriting

Even if students are just being exposed to letters through the general education curriculum or through an adaptive program, often they work on writing their first and last names in combination with learning how to write all of the letters of the alphabet.

9. "Student will trace, copy, or write his first and last name using left-to-right progression and proper letter formation. Criteria: Uses L to R progression 95% of the time and proper letter formation 80% for each letter."

When writing letter formation objectives, the occupational therapist needs to be sure to indicate the letters that the student is able to form consistently and legibly in the present level of performance section of the IEP. The type of support or prompting needed (e.g., tracing, copying) to write these letters should be noted, if applicable. Objectives reflect the letters that the student continues to have difficulty forming. These objectives should be used for a student who has been exposed to all of the uppercase and lowercase letters within the curriculum.

10. "Student will imitate, copy, or write letters [*letters of difficulty*] of the uppercase and lowercase alphabet so that they are legible. Criteria: 80% for each letter." When using a program like Sensible Pencil or Handwriting Without Tears, write the objectives so that letters are introduced as mastery tests (Sensible Pencil) or as families. This allows the occupational therapist and the teacher to set realistic goals for the number of letters that a student is expected to master within a year instead of expecting mastery of all 52 uppercase and lowercase letters. The therapist must be sure to list the letters within the objectives so that the teacher and parent know what letters currently are being worked on.

11. "Student will write lowercase letters [*list letters*] so that they meet the criteria as defined in Mastery Test [*insert mastery test #*] of the Sensible Pencil handwriting program. Criteria: Per mastery level as identified by the program (see example below)."
    – Alex will write lowercase letters (a, o, l, t, i) so that they meet the criteria as defined in Mastery Test 3 of the Sensible Pencil handwriting program.
    – The following is the remainder of the mastery tests with the corresponding letters for the Sensible Pencil program: Mastery Test 4: r, h, n, m, c, e, s; Mastery Test 5: q, f, d, u, j, and g; Mastery

Test 6: p, b, v, w; Mastery Test 7: k, x, y, and z; Insert Capitals Mastery Test.

12. For Handwriting Without Tears, objectives may be written as, "Student will write letters within the 'Frog Jump Capitals' (F, E, D, P, B, R, N, and M), and the 'Starting Corner Capitals' (H, K, and L) so that they are readable. Criteria: 80% for each letter."

Depending on the setting, some kindergarten students are expected to write letters from top to bottom with left-to-right right progression, print uppercase and lowercase letters, correctly space letters, and leave spaces between words when writing. Occupational therapists need to find out what curriculum is being used in the classroom and if the district is using a specific curriculum. If a specific curriculum is being used, then the example objectives listed below are applicable. If students are only being exposed to letters within kindergarten and are not expected to master them, then the therapist should not be working on formal handwriting instruction for all uppercase and lowercase letters but can instead focus on letters in a student's first and last names.

For the student who did not receive formal handwriting instruction in kindergarten but will be receiving it as a part of the formal first-grade handwriting curriculum, objectives also can be written to reflect letters that the student is expected to learn during the first and second semester of the school year. In this way, the occupational therapist is not responsible for working on letters that have not yet been introduced. List the letters that the student is expected to learn during each semester in the Needs column on the IEP. Include a generalized statement in the present levels of performance that explains that formal handwriting instruction is occurring.

13. "When given a model, student will copy the letters of the alphabet that are introduced within the first semester of school

so that they are readable. Criteria: 80% for each letter introduced."

14. "On mastery of the uppercase and lowercase letters learned during the first semester, student will copy letters that are introduced during the second semester. Criteria: 80% for each letter introduced." If a student will receive formal handwriting instruction in kindergarten but not in first grade, then the therapist needs to determine which letters of the uppercase and lowercase alphabet the student continues to have difficulty forming. For this situation, reference Objective 10 for an example.

Objectives of Copying

For a student who has difficulty copying information, the following are ideas for writing objectives for this area. The occupational therapist needs to identify the student's area of concern (e.g., spelling words correctly, copying all of the words, spacing words correctly) and write the objectives that reflect these specific difficulties. The next two objectives also are applicable to those students who have difficulty composing a sentence independently. These students may need to give their responses orally, have an adult scribe the sentences, and then have the students copy the information.

15. "Student will copy a sentence from the chalkboard, paper, or book so that all words are present spelled correctly with proper spacing between the words so that they are readable. Criteria: 80% of attempts so that all words are present and spelled correctly with proper spacing between the words so that they are readable." (This objective is written with many components—only the components that the student is having difficulty with should be picked and included in the objective.)

16. "When copying a self-generated sentence (that is scribed by an adult) to the paper,

the student will accurately copy all words in the sentence so that it is readable. Criteria: all words accurately copied 80% of opportunities."

Objectives for Spacing, Size, and Alignment

If the student is having difficulty spacing letters and words (e.g., student runs words together as one long word or breaks words incorrectly), sizing letters (e.g., student writes lowercase *a* using the entire space within lined paper), or aligning specific letters (e.g., letters with tails or tall letters), then specific objectives can be written regarding these issues.

17. "When writing a sentence, student will provide space between words so that they are readable. Criteria: 80% of the time."
18. "Student will write letters remaining within area appropriate for the size for the letter case. Criteria: 80% of the letters."
19. "Student will write letters so that they fit within the designated space provided. Criteria: 80% of the letters."
20. "Student will place letters on the baseline of _____ grade paper or notebook paper. Criteria _____% of letters written on the line."
21. "Student will write tail letters (g, j, p, q, y) so that the tail of the letters descends below the baseline. Criteria: 80% for each letter."
22. "Student will write tall letters (b, d, f, h, k, l, t) so that they fit within the defined area. Criteria: 80% for each letter."
23. "When correcting work, student will completely erase mistakes before writing over the same area so that the correction is legible. Criteria: 80% of erasures."

Cursive Objectives

For cursive, objectives can be written the same way as previously discussed objectives. If cursive is just being introduced and the occupational therapist is assisting in instruction, the objectives can be written the same as Objectives 13 and 14. If a specific handwriting program (e.g., Handwriting Without Tears or Loops and Hoops) is being used, then objectives can be written in the same way as Objective 12.

If a student has received formal instruction in cursive handwriting and continues to have difficulty with formation of specific letters, then objectives can be written the same way as Objective 10. Objectives 24 and 25 specifically deal with writing a cursive signature. Also, Objective 26 is an example of what can be written to address those students having difficulty with connections and bridges between letters.

24. "Student will write letters in his first and last names in cursive in isolation so that they are legible. (Be sure to list the letters that are in entire name within the objective.) Criteria: 80% for each letter."

25. "Student will write his first and last names in cursive with proper bridges and connections so that they are readable. Criteria: 80% of the total number of connections."

26. "Student will write words in cursive using proper bridges and connections. Criteria: 80% of total number of connections."

Keyboarding Skills

For students who are learning to isolate their fingers to the home row of keys, working on this row in isolation or working on it with all other keys on the keyboard can be accomplished by using a typing tutor program. Students who display difficulty isolating their fingers or who are unable to use the home row can use the index fingers on both hands to access both the left side and right side of the keyboard.

27. "Student will use the appropriate hand (left or right) on those keys located on the same side of the keyboard when a divider is placed in the center of the keyboard. Criteria: Uses appropriate finger to press keys on left side or right side 80% of attempts."

28. "Student will move progressively through the lessons in [specific typing tutor program, e.g., Type to Learn] to increase keyboard awareness. Criteria: 80% mastery for each lesson over 5 consecutive sessions." When writing an objective to improve typing speed, it is important for the therapist to collect baseline information of the student's current typing speed, or letters per minute.

29. "When typing, student will increase letters typed per minute _____% from baseline. Criteria: _____% from baseline over 3 different opportunities." The student also needs to be able to perform basic functions required to access and use programs on the computer. An objective can be written that includes the functions that the student is unable to perform.

30. "Student will independently (with no prompts or assistance once initial directive is given) complete a variety of computer functions, such as using a mouse; turning on the computer; accessing the correct software program; saving information; closing out of a program; shutting down the computer; and using specific keys or functions within word processing programs, including space bar, return, delete, shift, spell check, using cursors to move to different lines or areas on the screen, and numbering items for a list."

For students completing assignments on the computer, the goal needs to specify whether they will be composing information as they type (e.g., typing spelling tests or paragraphs) or if they will be copying information from a written model. Objectives 15 and 16 in the handwriting section can be used as models for creating copying objectives. For composition objectives, be sure to specify what a student needs to complete when typing.

31. "Student will type a self-generated sentence using proper capitalization, punctuation, spelling, and spacing between words. Criteria: 80% for each item listed." (This objective is written with many components—pick only the components that the student is having difficulty with and include them in the objective.)

References

Alston, J. (1985). The handwriting of seven- to nine-year-olds. *British Journal of Special Education, 12,* 68–72.

Alston, J., & Taylor, J. (Eds.). (1987). *Handwriting: Theory, research, and practice.* London: Croom Helm.

Amundson, S. J. (1992). Handwriting: Evaluation and intervention in school setting. In J. Case-Smith & C. Pehoski (Eds.), *Development of hand skills in the child* (pp. 63–78). Rockville, MD: American Occupational Therapy Association.

Amundson, S. J. (1995). *Evaluation Tool of Children's Handwriting.* Homer, AK: OT Kids.

Amundson, S. J. (1998). *TRICS for written communication: Techniques for rebuilding and improving children's school skills.* Homer, AK: OT Kids.

Amundson, S. (2001). Prewriting and handwriting skills. In J. Case-Smith, (Ed.), *Occupational therapy for children* (pp. 524–541). St. Louis, MO: Mosby.

Amundson, S. J., & Weil, M. (1996). Prewriting and handwriting skills. In J. Case-Smith, A. S. Allen, & P. N. Pratt (Eds.), *Occupational therapy for children* (pp. 524–541). St. Louis, MO: Mosby.

Anderson, P. L. (1983). *Denver Handwriting Analysis.* Novato, CA: Academic Therapy.

Balajthy, E. (1988). Keyboarding, language arts, and the elementary school child. *Computing Teacher, 15*(5), 40–43.

Becht, L. (1985). *The sensible pencil: A handwriting program.* Birmingham, AL: EBSCO Curriculum Materials.

Beery, K. E. (1982). *The Developmental Test of Visual–Motor Integration.* Cleveland, OH: Modern Curriculum Press.

Beery, K. E. (1989). *The Developmental Test of Visual–Motor Integration* (3rd ed.). Cleveland, OH: Modern Curriculum Press.

Beery, K. E. (1997). *The Developmental Test of Visual–Motor Integration. Administration scoring and teaching manual.* Parsippany, NJ: Modern Curriculum Press.

Benbow, M. (1990). *Loops and other groups.* Tucson, AZ: Therapy SkillBuilders.

Benbow, M. (1995). Principles and practices of teaching handwriting. In A. Henderson & C. Pehoski (Eds.), *Hand function in the child: Foundations for remediation* (pp. 255–281). St. Louis, MO: Mosby.

Briggs, D. (1980). A study of the influence of handwriting upon grades using examination scripts. *Educational Review, 32,* 185–193.

Case-Smith, J. (2002). Effectiveness of school-based occupational therapy on handwriting. *American Journal of Occupational Therapy, 56,* 17–25.

Cermak, S. (1991). Somatosensory dyspraxia. In A. Fisher, E. A. Murray, & A. C. Bundy (Eds.), *Sensory integration: Theory and practice* (pp. 138–170), Philadelphia: F. A. Davis.

Cochran-Smith, M., Paris, C., & Kahn, J. (1991). *Learning to write differently: Beginning writers and word processing.* Norwood, NJ: Ablex.

Cornhill, H., & Case-Smith, J. (1996). Factors that relate to good and poor handwriting. *American Journal of Occupational Therapy, 50,* 732–739.

Dennis, J., & Swinth, Y. (2001). Pencil grasp and children's handwriting legibility during different–length writing tasks. *American Journal of Occupational Therapy, 55,* 175–183.

Don Johnston. (2004). Co:Writer. *The Don Johnston Catalog,* pp. 40–41.

Dunn, B., & Reay, D. (1989). Word processing and the keyboard: Comparative effects of transcription on achievement. *Journal of Educational Research, 84,* 237–245.

Exner, C. E. (1992). In-hand manipulation skills. In J. Case-Smith & C. Pehoski (Eds.), *Development of hand skills in the child* (pp. 35–45). Rockville, MD: American Occupational Therapy Association.

Feder, K., Majnemer, A., & Synne, A. (2000). Handwriting: Current trends in occupational therapy practice. *Canadian Journal of Occupational Therapy, 67,* 197–204.

Fitts, P., & Posner, M. (1967). *Human performance.* Belmont, CA: Brooks/Cole.

Freeman, F. (1954). Teaching handwriting. *What Research Says to Teachers, 4,* 1–33.

Gladstone, K. (2002). *Illegibility: Can America write?* Retrieved May 9, 2004, from http://www.global2000.net/handwritingrepair/Kate HwR.html.

Glass, A. L., & Holyoak, K. J. (1986). *Cognition* (2nd ed.). Reading, MA: Addison-Wesley.

Graham, S. (1992). Issues in handwriting instruction. *Focus on Exceptional Children, 25,* 1–4.

Graham, S., & Miller, L. (1980). Handwriting researcher practice: A unified approach. *Focus on Exceptional Children,* 13, 1–16.

Graham, S., & Weintraub, N. (1996). A review of handwriting research: Progress and prospects from 1980 to 1994. *Educational Psychology Review, 8,* 7–87.

Groff, P. J. (1961). New speeds of handwriting. *Elementary English, 38,* 564–565.

Hammerschmidt, S., & Sudsawad, P. (2004). Teachers survey on problems with handwriting: Referral, evaluation and outcomes. *American Journal of Occupational Therapy, 58,* 185–192.

Koziatek, S., & Powell, N. (2003). Pencil grip, legibility, and speed of fourth-graders' writing in cursive. *American Journal of Occupational Therapy, 57,* 284–288.

Larsen, S. C., & Hammill, D. D. (1989). *Test of Legible Handwriting.* Austin, TX: Pro-Ed.

Levine, K. J. (1991). *Fine motor dysfunction: Therapeutic strategies in the classroom.* Tucson, AZ: Therapy SkillBuilders.

Levine, M. (1985). *Pediatric Examination of Educational Readings at Middle Childhood (Peeramid).* Cambridge, MA: Educators Publishing Service.

Lidz, C. S. (1987). *Dynamic assessment.* New York: Guilford Press.

MacArthur, C. A. (1988). The impact of computers on the writing process. *Exceptional Children, 54,* 536–542.

Maeland, A. (1992). Handwriting and perceptual–motor skills in clumsy, dysgraphic, and "normal" children. *Perceptual and Motor Skills, 75,* 1207–1217.

McHale, K., & Cermak, S. (1992). Fine motor activities in elementary school: Preliminary findings and provisional implications for children with fine motor problems. *American Journal of Occupational Therapy, 46,* 898–903.

More, D., Deitz, J., Billingsley F., & Coggins, T. (2003). Facilitating written work using computer word processing and word prediction. *American Journal of Occupational Therapy, 57,* 139–151.

Oliver, C. E. (1990). A sensorimotor program for improving writing readiness skills in elementary-age children. *American Journal of Occupational Therapy, 44,* 111–124.

Peterson, C., & Nelson, D. (2003). Effect of an occupational intervention on printing in children with economic disadvantages. *American Journal of Occupational Therapy, 57,* 152–160.

Phelps, J., & Stempel, L. (1987). *The Children's Handwriting Evaluation Scale for Manuscript Writing.* Dallas: Texas Scottish Rite Hospital for Crippled Children.

Phelps, J., Stempel, L., & Speck, G. (1984). *The Children's Handwriting Evaluation Scale: A new diagnostic tool.* Dallas: Texas Scottish Rite Hospital for Crippled Children.

Preminger, P., Weiss, P., & Weintraub, N. (2004). Predicting occupational performance: Handwriting versus keyboarding. *American Journal of Occupational Therapy, 58,* 193–201.

Reisman, J. (1991). Poor handwriting: Who is referred? *American Journal of Occupational Therapy, 45,* 849–852.

Reisman, J. (1999). *Minnesota Handwriting Assessment.* San Antonio, TX: Therapy SkillBuilders.

Rogers, J., & Case-Smith, J. (2002). Relationship between handwriting and keyboarding performance of sixth-grade students. *American Journal of Occupational Therapy, 56,* 34–39.

Rubin, N., & Henderson, S. E. (1982). Two sides of the same coin: Variations in teaching methods and failure to learn to write. *Special Education: Forward Trends, 9*(4), 17–24.

Schneck, C. M. (1991). Comparison of pencil-grip patterns in first graders with good and poor writing skills. *American Journal of Occupational Therapy, 45,* 701–706.

Schneck, C. M., & Henderson, A. (1990). Descriptive analysis of the developmental progression of grip position for pencil and crayon control in nondysfunctional children. *American Journal of Occupational Therapy, 44,* 893–900.

Sovik, N. (1975). *Developmental cybernetics of handwriting and graphic behavior.* Oslo: Universitetsforlaget.

Swinth, Y., & Anson, D. (1998). Alternatives to handwriting: Keyboarding and text—Generation techniques for schools. In J. Case-Smith (Ed.), *Occupational therapy: Making a difference in school system practice* (p. 1–43). Rockville, MD: American Occupational Therapy Association.

Tseng, M. H. (1998). Development of pencil grip position in preschool children. *Occupational Therapy Journal of Research, 18,* 207–224.

Tseng, M. H., & Cermak, S. (1991). The evaluation

of handwriting in children. *Sensory Integration Quarterly, 19*(4), 2–12.

Tseng, M. H., & Cermak, S. A. (1993). The influence of ergonomic factors and perceptual–motor abilities on handwriting performance. *American Journal of Occupational Therapy, 47,* 919–926.

Tseng, M. H., & Murray, E. (1994). Differences in perceptual–motor measures in children with good and poor handwriting. *Occupational Therapy Journal of Research, 14,* 19–36.

Vreeland, E. (1998). *Handwriting: Not just in the hands.* Springfield, NH: Maxanna Learning Systems.

Weil, M., & Amundson, S. J. (1994). Relationship between visual motor and handwriting skills of children in kindergarten. *American Journal of Occupational Therapy, 48,* 982–988.

Ziviani, J., & Elkins, J. (1984). An evaluation of handwriting performance. *Educational Review, 36,* 249–261.

Appendix 6.1.
Handwriting Teacher Questionnaire

Student _____   Age _____

Date of Birth _____   Therapist _____

Teacher _____   Person Completing Form _____

School _____   Date _____

Special Education Classification _____   Does Student Have ADHD? (circle)   Yes   No

I. Background Information

1. Is the student able to print? Yes____ No ____

    Cursive? Yes ___ No ____

2. What is the primary method used for handwriting?

    Print ____ Cursive____

2a. (If grade appropriate) Has the child been taught cursive? Yes ___ No ____

2b. By whom? (please check)

    General education teacher ____

    Special education teacher ____

3. Is the student expected to use cursive during school day? Yes ___ No ____

    If Yes, for what assignments? _____

4. What curriculum is used for handwriting (e.g., Zaner Bloser)?

    Print ____ Cursive ____

5. Do teachers follow the curriculum identified in Item 4 specifically? Yes ___ No ____

    If no, what curriculum is used? _____

6. Do students have individual handwriting workbooks? Yes ___ No ____

    If not, what materials are used for instruction (e.g., teacher-prepared worksheets)? _____

II. Assessment Input

Can the student:

7. Copy the prewriting shapes needed for letter formation? Yes ___ No ____

8. Match and verbally identify alphabet letters and numbers in random order?

	Matching	Verbally Identify
Print uppercase:	Yes ___ No ___	Yes ___ No ___
Print lowercase:	Yes ___ No ___	Yes ___ No ___
Cursive uppercase:	Yes ___ No ___	Yes ___ No ___
Cursive lowercase	Yes ___ No ___	Yes ___ No ___

    Numbers up to: _____

9. Select own name in print when given different choices? Yes ___ No ____

10. Write first or last (circle which or both) name legibly?

    Print: Yes ___ No ____

    Cursive: Yes ___ No ____

11. Copy letters in uppercase and lowercase and numbers?

    In print? Yes ___ No ____

    In cursive? Yes ___ No ____

    Numbers (1–10)? Yes ___ No ____

12. Write uppercase and lowercase letters and numbers without a model?

    In print? Yes ___ No ____

    In cursive? Yes ___ No ____

    Numbers (1–10)? Yes ___ No ____

13. Accurately copy from the board or from a book to paper? Yes ___ No ____

(continued)

14. Write letters and numbers remaining within a designated space, such as lined paper? Yes ___ No ___

15. Write letters and numbers on the baseline of grade-appropriate paper? Yes ___ No ___

16. Organize written work on the page? Yes ___ No ___

17. Align vertical columns when writing (e.g., math problems? Yes ___ No ___

18. What is the student's reading ability?

    Grade-level equivalent: ___

    Comprehension level: ___

Comments:

_____

_____

_____

19. Read what written? Yes ___ No ___

20. Read cursive (if appropriate)? Yes ___ No ___

21a. Does the student have difficulty formulating and organizing thoughts? Yes ___ No ___

21b. Is the student able to compose a sentence and write it down with proper spelling? Yes ___ No ___

21c. Is it easier for the student to verbalize thoughts than to write them? Yes ___ No ___

Comments:

_____

_____

_____

22. Are the student's writing abilities commensurate with reading abilities? Yes ___ No ___

23. Is there a difference in the amount of time it takes the student to write when composing a sentence vs. when copying a sentence? Yes ___ No _____

Comments:

_____

_____

_____

24a. Does the student write quickly? Yes ___ No ___

24b. Does this affect the quality of the student's work? Yes ___ No ___

Comments:

_____

_____

_____

25. Rank the student's writing legibility compared to other students in the classroom (report as percentage): ___

III. Technology

26. Has the student been formally exposed to a typing tutor program that emphasizes keyboard awareness? Yes ___ No ___

    By whom? _____

27. What method does the student use for typing—hunt and peck or home row using both hands?

    _____

28a. Does the student have access to and the opportunity to use the computer at school to complete assignments? Yes ___ No ___

28b. Does the student have an opportunity to use a computer at home to complete assignments? Yes ___ No ___

29. What is the student's level of proficiency with using the computer (e.g., able to turn computer on and off, access programs, use keyboard to type; also list if adult assistance is needed to access the computer)? _____

    _____

30. Can the student enter or copy written information from paper or chalkboard into the computer accurately and efficiently? Yes ___ No ___

Comments:

_____

_____

_____

(continued)

IV. Areas of Concern

31. Describe the specific handwriting concerns: _____

   _____

   _____

   _____

   _____

32. How do these concerns affect the student's ability to benefit from the available educational programming (e.g., student cannot read assignment notepad, student gets answers marked wrong due to teacher's inability to read handwriting)? _____

   _____

   _____

   _____

   _____

33. In your professional opinion, what do you think is causing the handwriting problems? For example, student cannot visualize letters, does not know alphabet from memory, cannot spell words, writes too fast, or does not proofread completed work.

   _____

   _____

   _____

34. When does the student perform best? When does the student's performance break down (e.g., when copying information, when rushing, when information is dictated)? _____

   _____

   _____

   _____

35. What strategies currently are being tried within the classroom to assist in improving the student's handwriting?_____

   _____

   _____

   _____

36. Are there goals on the student's current IEP that address handwriting issues? Yes ___ No ___

37. What is the student's level of independence in completing handwriting tasks? _____

   _____

   _____

   _____

   _____

Created by Lynne Pape, MEd, OTR/L, and Kelly Ryba, OTR/L

Providing Occupational Therapy Services to Preschool Children

7

School-based occupational therapists frequently work with children ranging in age from 3 to 5 years who have been identified as *preschoolers with a disability*. This global term accounts for children at varying levels of functioning. The services provided may differ depending on the children's overall developmental levels and individualized needs.

Over the past 30 years, federal and state legislation has advocated rights and services not only for school-age children but also for toddlers and preschoolers. As a result of Part B, P.L. 94-142 of the Education of the Handicapped Act (EHA) that was originally passed in 1975, school districts are required to provide special education services to school-age children with special needs (Dunn et al., 1989). This includes access to related services if it is determined that a child would benefit from them.

In 1986, the EHA was amended through P.L. 99-457. This amendment mandated that school districts provide special education services to children between ages 3 and 5 years, whereas previously it had been optional for school districts to provide such services. The law's passage opened up many new opportunities for occupational therapists and occupational therapy assistants to become involved with and provide intervention for preschoolers in a school setting.

In 1990, the EHA was further amended and, ultimately, renamed the Individuals With Disabilities Education Act, or IDEA (Gartland, 2001). Reauthorizations and amendments were made to this act in 1997 and 1999. The act continues to support access to services for preschool-age children.

This chapter includes information on how a child qualifies as a "preschooler with a disability." The numerous roles of occupational therapists within a preschool classroom are examined, and different service delivery models are explored. In addition, assessments and evaluation procedures that can be used when evaluating preschool children are described, and considerations to remember when providing interventions are discussed.

Preschool Children: Varying Levels of Performance and Disability

Occupational therapists become involved with preschool-age children through the evaluation and intervention process. These children may present a variety of disabilities, including

- Deficits in fine motor skills development;
- Deficits in motor planning abilities;
- Mild to severe physical impairments, such as in cerebral palsy and spina bifida;
- Cognitive deficits, such as mental retardation;
- Autism spectrum disorder; and
- Global developmental delays in communication, gross motor skills, fine motor skills, daily living skills, and other areas.

Federal law does not have a separate definition for what constitutes a "preschooler with a disability." Preschoolers between ages 3 and 9 years fall under the global definition for a child with a disability. A "child with a disability" is defined as being between the ages 3 and 9 years who is experiencing delays as defined by the state and as measured by appropriate diagnostic instruments and procedures in one or more of the following areas: physical development, cognitive development, communication, social and emotional behavior, and adaptive behavior.

The federal government's definitions may be vague, but they provide guidelines as to what specific developmental areas the educational team must assess to determine if a disability is present. For example, the State of Ohio defines a preschool child with a disability as a child between ages of 3 and 6 years (a student must be 3 years old and remains eligible for services as long as his or her birthday falls after the cutoff date for entering kindergarten) who displays a disability as demonstrated by a documented deficit in one or more areas of development, which has an adverse effect on normal development and functioning (Ohio Department of Education, 2002). Educational teams are required to obtain evaluation data using a variety of methods, including structured interviews and observations. This information is combined with data from norm-referenced assessments and criterion-based or curriculum-based assessments. The areas that must be assessed include background information, such as developmental, family, medical, and education histories; adaptive behavior; cognitive ability; communication skills; hearing; vision; and pre-academic, sensory–motor, and social–emotional, or behavioral functioning. All of this is done to confirm that a disability is present that has an adverse effect on the child's normal development and functioning. The child has to score more than 2 standard deviations below the mean in one developmental area assessed or 1.5 standard deviations below the mean in two areas to qualify as a preschooler with a disability.

Location of Preschool Services

Preschool services are offered in a variety of locations depending on a child's individualized needs and the school district's framework for providing services to children. Some school districts have integrated preschool programs located within the district, either within a school building or at an off-site location. These classrooms usually consist of a designated number of children with special needs and children who are accessing the standard curriculum.

Other school districts are part of an education consortium, in which they may contract with an outside agency, such as the Head Start program or an educational services center, to provide preschool services to the children within their district. These classrooms may consist of children from numerous school districts located within the same county. An individual school district would be responsible for providing the related service providers to these facilities if the facilities do not have them on staff.

Children also may be seen for itinerant services. Itinerant service involves the occupational therapist or teacher going to a private preschool program and working with the child within that environment. This type of service is commonly used with children demonstrating delays in one or two areas, including fine motor development, social skills, and communication skills, but whose needs can be met within a private preschool program with other children who are part of a standard curriculum. An itinerant program is less restrictive than an integrated preschool. Providing such services also allows therapists to enter the community and affect preschool programs outside of a local school district. Finally, services may be provided within the child's home if the child is too medically fragile to attend an outside program

Cross-Categorical Environment of the Preschool

As discussed previously, preschool children with disabilities can present a wide range of functioning and ability levels. They do not have to be formally diagnosed to qualify for services. They also do not have to fit into one of the labeled areas of qualification (e.g., *learning disabled, autism, mental retardation*) required when qualifying for school-age services. A preschool classroom may include children with a wide range of motor abilities and cognitive levels, children who are nonverbal or who have limited communication skills, children with sensory–motor needs, and children with emotional and behavioral issues.

Due to the variation in the children's ability levels, educational teams, including occupational therapists, often have to be very dynamic when evaluating and determining appropriate goals, objectives, and services for children to meet each child's individualized needs. Such needs may include determining what assessments are appropriate to administer to the child to obtain the most accurate and reflective data. The team also needs to define the child's underlying strengths and weaknesses so that they can be addressed in the individualized education program (IEP). After these areas are assessed, the team must determine the type of environment and programming that would be most appropriate to help the child meet the individualized needs defined by the educational team members, including his parents.

Teachers also are presented with numerous challenges when planning lessons and activities to meet the needs of the children developing at varying levels. Differentiating instruction ensures that aspects of the activities conducted are meaningful to all of the children in the classroom and allow every child to be an active participant. Occupational therapists can assist teachers with this process by providing information on which activities are appropriate to meet students' varying developmental levels, providing suggestions on how to adapt equipment and materials for better access by the students, providing information on how to present tasks to optimize access, and assisting with organization of the classroom for optimum accessibility by all of the students.

Roles of the Occupational Therapist in a Preschool Setting

Occupational therapists working within a preschool environment assume numerous roles, including being a vital part of the screening process for children. Therapists may be involved in the team's initial screening of a child to determine if he or she should undergo a multifactored evaluation. This includes using developmentally based observation checklists designed by the district or therapist or more formal screening tools that look at the child's skills in multiple areas (see Appendix 7.1 for an example of a functional preschool checklist). If the team decides that there are enough concerns to warrant a multifactored evaluation, the occupational therapist may be included if concerns exist in the motor (both fine motor and sensorimotor) and self-help areas.

As related service providers and educational team members, occupational therapists may be involved in a child's initial evaluation to help determine if he or she qualifies for special education. Therapists may also become involved once a child is receiving special education services. During the evaluation process, therapists may incorporate a variety of methods, including standardized norm-referenced or criterion-referenced assessments, observation, and interviews, to obtain baseline information on a child's present level of functioning. Therapists also provide direct intervention to assist children with the development of or remediation of a skill within the classroom setting or in an individualized setting outside of the classroom.

Occupational therapists provide consultation and collaboration services to a child's preschool teacher, private therapist, and family. This includes assisting with the development of the IEP; determining what is needed to implement the goals and objectives, including materials, adapted equipment, instructional teaching methods, and services; and providing ongoing support to classroom staff and family members to problem solve in the areas of concern and to monitor the child's progress toward mastery of the identified skill areas.

Occupational therapists may be called on to evaluate and provide intervention for a variety of areas related to the preschooler's ability to independently manage the expectations of the school day. Possible areas include

- *Dressing skills*—Being able to put on and take off a coat, boots, gloves or mittens, hat, and art smock; being able to pull pants up or down during toileting; and managing clothing fasteners (e.g., engaging zipper on coat).
- *Fine motor skills*—Being able to appropriately use toys using a variety of grasps, developing a functional pencil grip, using both hands together to complete bilateral tasks, being able to cross midline, and being able to use classroom tools (e.g., scissors, pencils, paintbrushes, glue sticks).
- *Visual–motor skills*—Being able to draw prewriting shapes needed for letter formation, writing letters in name, cutting skills, and correctly using toys (e.g., stringing beads, replicating block designs, doing mazes and puzzles, matching, and beginning patterning).
- *Self-help skills*—Toileting; hand washing; managing belongings (e.g., coat, book bag,

take home folder); putting away toys at cleanup time; passing out napkins, cups, and food items at snack time; and independent feeding during snack time (e.g., managing drinking from a regular cup, finger feeding, using utensils).
- *Sensorimotor abilities*—Being able to process sensory information, including tactile, proprioceptive, vestibular, auditory, oral, and visual input in the classroom setting.

Evaluation Process

Methods used by school districts to conduct both initial and subsequent evaluations vary. A few of these methods are described below.

Play-Based Assessments/ Arena-Style Assessments

Some school districts conduct play-based assessments or arena-style assessments in which the parent brings the child to the preschool, where the team members (which may include the school psychologist, speech therapist, physical or occupational therapist, and special education teacher) conduct their evaluation. The child is initially observed playing within the preschool classroom. The special education teacher sets out specific toys or activities that the team would like to observe the child engage in, including fine motor toys (e.g., puzzles, art supplies, pegboards); dramatic play materials (e.g., those found in the housekeeping or dress up area); building blocks or LEGOs™; materials in the sensory table (e.g., shaving cream, sand, packing material); and gross motor activities on a climber in the classroom, in a separate gross motor room, or on the playground at the school.

The team can informally observe a few children at the same time. This provides the team with an opportunity to observe how the children interact with others. The children can engage in parallel or interactive play for a period of time.

After observing the child or multiple children play within the classroom, individual standardized assessments may be administered either in the classroom or in a separate location to obtain standardized scores reflective of the child's abilities. The benefit of conducting an assessment this way is that all of the team members observe the child's performance at the same time. A negative is that all of the testing is conducted in one day. If the child is having a bad day, the testing data may not reflect the child's actual abilities. If the child is unresponsive or refuses to participate in any part of the evaluation, the team should reschedule for a different day to see if the child's behavior improves during a second session. A second negative is that related service providers' schedules frequently do not allow for the time each week to devote to play-based assessments. This is particularly true for those therapists who travel between school buildings or districts.

Individual Assessments Conducted by Team Members

Some school districts have the school psychologist initially conduct an observation and screening of the child (either at home or at a building within the school district) and gather information from the child's parents to determine if a multifactored evaluation is needed. Based on this observation and screening, the psychologist determines which team members need to be involved in the initial evaluation process. For example, it may not be appropriate to have the occupational therapist assess a child whose primary area of concern is the area of communication (i.e., there are no fine motor or self-help concerns). On the other hand, if a child is entering the program and the primary concern is motor (e.g., a child with cerebral palsy or Down syndrome) or sensorimotor issues (e.g., a child

with autism), an occupational therapist may be needed to provide input. Each team member then conducts his or her part of the assessment at different times. The team collaborates on the child's results at an evaluation team meeting and determines if the child qualifies for special education services. If the child does qualify, the team defines the child's individualized needs.

The benefit to conducting an assessment using this format is that each team member observes and evaluates the child on a different day and can report on and compare the child's abilities and behaviors from multiple sessions. The negative to this type of assessment is that the team may disagree on the child's needs, as each team member is doing his or her own assessment of the child at different times and, possibly, locations. Team members also may not have time to collaborate regarding the child's performance prior to having the evaluation team meeting with the parent to share the results.

Assessments Conducted Once a Child Has Qualified for Special Education Services

An occupational therapist may be called on to evaluate a child after he or she has already qualified for special education and is receiving services. This type of referral often happens when a child initially demonstrates no discrepancies in motor and adaptive behavior but over time makes no progress in these areas. For example, a teacher may provide opportunities each week for a 5-year-old child to use a variety of writing utensils to practice drawing the prewriting shapes and letters in preparation for kindergarten. Even with repeated exposure in the classroom, the child continues to demonstrate a fisted grasp when holding writing utensils. The teacher has the child try a variety of pencil grippers and multiple types of utensils, including paintbrushes, crayons, markers, and Laddie pencils to complete the drawing activities, and the child has been encouraged to imitate and trace prewriting shapes and letters. Even after these interventions have been attempted, the child remains unable to accurately imitate or trace the basic prewriting shapes or letters. The teacher has requested a referral for an occupational therapy evaluation due to continued concerns regarding the child's immature pencil grip and possible visual–motor concerns.

It also is common to receive a referral as part of a child's transition from preschool to school-age services when moving to kindergarten. This referral may be initiated to obtain baseline information regarding the child's fine motor and self-help skills if the teacher suspects that the child's skills are not commensurate with other children his or her age, to provide the child's parents and upcoming teachers with suggestions and recommendations on how to assist the student with completing certain skills, or to determine if the child would benefit from direct intervention or consultation services prior to attending kindergarten or when transitioning to kindergarten the following school year.

Considerations When Conducting Assessments

For either type of assessment (the initial multifactored evaluation or evaluation once a student is already receiving services), the occupational therapist should use a combination of approaches to gain information on the child's current level of functioning. Completing an occupational profile through interviews with the child's parents and teacher provides background information about the child's developmental history and identifies overall strengths and current areas of concern. When evaluating the child's performance, the therapist can use a variety of approaches, including interviewing the parents and teacher, observing the child in his or her natural environments (e.g., school, home), and

completing standardized norm-referenced or criterion-referenced assessments. When conducting an assessment as a part of a child's initial multifactored evaluation to qualify for special education services, the psychologist may request that a formal assessment with standardized scores be administered. This helps qualify the child for special education services if standardized scores are needed to document fine motor, sensory–motor, or self-care deficits.

When completing an evaluation after the child has already qualified for special education services, the occupational therapist may not need to administer a standardized assessment. The therapist can use a combination of observation and interview to determine the child's current level of functioning and whether the child's skills are below average for his or her age and developmental level. The therapist can use standardized assessment tools to supplement the observations and interview data, depending on the child and situation. It is important for the therapist and the entire team to review other team members' evaluation and assessment data to gain an understanding of how the child is functioning across developmental domains. This will help the team determine what type of services the child will need to support his or her individual needs within the preschool environment.

Methods of Evaluating Occupational Performance

Parent/Teacher Interview

It is important to incorporate interviewing the child's teacher and parents during the evaluation process. For those children who are being evaluated at age 3 years and have had no prior school experience, interviewing the child's parents provides vital information about the child, including when he or she reached developmental milestones, and gives the occupational therapist a sense of the child's current abilities in fine and gross motor skills, beginning self-care skills, independence with feeding, and sensory processing abilities. Interviewing the parents also lets the therapist know whether the child has had exposure to certain activities. This is important in the evaluation process, as standardized assessments sometimes assess a child's ability to complete certain skills at a very young age.

For example, the Peabody Developmental Motor Skills (Folio & Fewell, 2000) evaluates a child's ability to snip paper with scissors at ages 25–26 months, but parents frequently have not allowed their children to use scissors at this age. Results from the assessment, therefore, may need to be skewed if the child is assessed on a skill to which he or she has had no exposure. Similarly, sometimes the child has not been required to complete certain self-help skills because an adult has always completed it for him or her. When interviewed, the parent may say, "I don't know if he can zip his coat because I always zip it for him." If the child has not been exposed to certain tasks, it may not be that the child is physically unable to complete the task but that the child has not been required to complete it at home.

If a child has received previous early intervention services through a county or state-run agency (e.g., Head Start, Board of Mental Retardation and Developmental Disabilities), it may be beneficial for the occupational therapist to collaborate with the child's teacher or other therapists to gain information on his or her abilities within the classroom setting and determine what skills have been focused on during earlier intervention services. Talking to the child's teacher provides the therapist with knowledge of the teacher's current concerns (e.g., behavior, ability to participate in fine motor activities in the classroom, self-help skills) and helps determine what tasks the child was having difficulty with and how

this interferes in the classroom. It also helps the team understand what activities and parts of the day the child is most and least successful participating in and completing.

The authors of this book have developed a Preschool Functional Educational Checklist (see Appendix 7.1) to be used as a guide during the interview and observation process with the child's teacher or parents. This checklist examines numerous skills required of children during their school day, including

- Gross motor skills
- Fine motor skills (including hand skills and tool use)
- Visual–motor skills
- Behavior and attention abilities
- Self-help skills
- Sensory processing abilities.

The Preschool Functional Educational Checklist assists therapists in structuring an interview with the child's parents or teacher to gain information about the child's current abilities and to help identify which of these areas need to be evaluated more directly.

Observation

Observing a Child at Home. When a child is initially assessed as a 3-year-old, the occupational therapist frequently goes to the child's home to complete the assessment. This provides a great opportunity to observe the child in his or her natural environment. While completing the observation, it is important to

- Gain an understanding of what toys the child prefers to play with regularly. The parents may be able to provide information on toys that the child tends to avoid. The therapist should determine if there is a pattern to the toys the child gravitates to or avoids (e.g., child avoids toys such as stringing beads, puzzles, or art projects that require fine motor skills).
- Determine if the child is able to play with toys purposefully and for their intended use. Does he or she engage in self-stimulatory

behaviors when watching the toys (e.g., flapping when a battery-operated train goes around on the track) or engage in repetitive play with toys (e.g., lining up cars and trains in a row or continuously spinning wheels on a car and watching it) instead of interacting with the toys appropriately? Does he or she appear to know the function of the toys? Is the child creative in play, or does he or she play with the toys in familiar and repetitive ways (e.g., rolling a car back and forth repeatedly instead of driving the car over a hill and under a bridge and through a tunnel)?

• Observe whether the child has the fine motor skills necessary to play and interact with toys (e.g., three-finger grasp, isolated index finger to poke, ability to use both hands together to play with bilateral toys, ability to cross midline to reach for or play with a toy). Does the child have toys that require him or her to use fine motor skills? Are the toys available to the child developmentally appropriate? Does the child have access to a variety of toys, or is the environment not stimulating?

• Observe the child's interactions with his or her parents and siblings, and observe reactions to playing and interacting with a stranger (e.g., the therapist). Is the child clingy, or does he or she easily separate from the parents? Does he or she appear to understand and follow directions? What occurs when he or she is told "no" or does not get his or her way? Does he or she attempt to control situations or other people's behavior? What happens if there is a change in his or her normal routine? What happens if someone takes a toy away or plays with the toy differently from how the child wants to play with it? All of these behaviors are important to observe, as the child needs to interact with a variety of people and toys in the preschool classroom, follow a classroom schedule, and complete teacher-directed tasks that are often not on his or her own terms.

• Observe the child eating a meal or snack to observe the child's ability to finger feed, use utensils, and drink from a regular cup or straw.

• Determine whether the child is able to independently maneuver around the home environment. Can he or she manage the stairs in the home? Is he or she able to transition in and out of a chair and up and down from the floor, and does he or she have adequate mobility to move throughout the environment by scooting, crawling, rolling, or walking? Was he or she observed to bump into items or people when moving from place to place? Does he or she use any adaptive equipment to walk (e.g., cane, walker, gait trainer)?

• Observe the child's attention to task. Does he or she need frequent reminders from the therapist to remain focused? Does he or she quickly abandon toys and move to the next task? Is he or she able to follow 1–2-step directions given by parents or the therapist during the administration of an assessment or when playing with toys?

• Determine if the child is able to tolerate a variety of sensory inputs, including tactile, proprioceptive, vestibular, oral, and auditory. Does the child react negatively to touch sensations? Does he or she avoid engaging in activities that involve interacting with tactile-related materials (e.g., finger paint, finger feeding, sand box). Does he or she overreact when his or her hands get dirty? Does the child crave deep pressure input or engage in activities such as crashing into others or objects or leaning heavily into people? Does he or she tolerate having his or her feet off the floor and playing on playground equipment, including the slide and swings? Does he or she cover his or her ears or become easily upset when the environment is loud? Does the child mouth objects, tolerate eating a variety of food textures, and tolerate having his or her teeth brushed?

Observing a Child in the Classroom. For a child who is already enrolled in a preschool program, it is important to conduct an observation within the classroom to see how he or she manages the classroom routine and to determine his or her ability to complete the required tasks within this setting. When conducting an observation in the classroom, it is important to

- Observe the child's ability to manage the daily classroom routine, including transitioning between activities (e.g., circle time, bathroom breaks, snack time, free play) and managing personal belongings (e.g., coat, take home folder, book bag, snow boots, art projects). Does the child overly rely on adult cueing and assistance, or is he or she able to do activities independently?
- Observe the child's overall behavior within the classroom.
  - Is the child able to interact with other peers and adults in an appropriate manner?
  - Does the child demand constant attention?
  - Does the child attempt to control play situations with others?
  - Is the child observed to have outbursts, such as temper tantrums, in response to situations such as transitions, being disciplined, not getting his or her way, a change in routine, or having to comply to a teacher-directed activity?
- Examine the child's overall ability to attend to classroom tasks.
  - How long, on average, is the child able to remain seated and attentive to a group activity such as circle time, reading a story, or a group art activity?
  - If off task, what is the child observed to do (e.g., become fidgety in the chair seat or on the floor, abandon the activity,

begin talking out or interrupting the teacher, fidget with objects in hands, reach out to others)?
  - Is the child able to be redirected to the task, or does he or she have to be removed from the situation to avoid distracting the other children?
  - Are there current intervention strategies in place to assist the child with attention issues (e.g., frequent redirection by the teacher, sitting the child near the teacher, incorporating movement breaks into the school day)?
- View the child's overall sensory processing skills.
  - Is the child able to tolerate interacting with a variety of materials (e.g., play dough, finger paint, items in the sensory table)?
  - Is the child able to tolerate being in line with other children and sitting near others?
  - Will the child eat a variety of foods during snack time?
  - Is the child observed to mouth objects and seek oral input?
  - Does the child seek deep pressure proprioceptive input by climbing, running into things, or banging into objects or other children?
  - Is the child observed to engage in self-stimulatory or self-abusive behaviors?
  - Will the child tolerate vestibular input, including playing on the playground equipment and engaging in gross motor activities (e.g., dancing; playing ring around the rosie; or using equipment such as a tricycle, scooter, or swing)?
  - Does the child cover his or her ears when there is music playing, children singing, a teacher talking, or an announcement being made over the intercom?

The child's tactile, proprioceptive, vestibular, visual, oral, and auditory sensory processing skills can be observed throughout the school day. If the teacher has observed that the child is having difficulty tolerating a particular type of input (e.g., tactile input), the teacher should plan activities that are tactile based so that the occupational therapist can observe the child's interactions with the materials and reaction to the activities.

The occupational therapist should observe whether the child is able to manage the daily living tasks that are required of him or her during the school day, including managing a coat, book bag, and take home folder; managing clothing when using the restroom; toileting; washing his or her hands; pouring a drink from a pitcher at snack time; and passing out napkins or snack items to peers. The therapist should also note whether the child is able to participate in and complete required fine motor tasks. This includes interacting with toys; picking up and releasing objects; using two hands together to complete bilateral tasks; and using tools during art time, including scissors and writing utensils. Can the child complete multistep fine motor tasks that are commonly completed within a preschool classroom? Tasks include completing a color, cut, and paste project in which the child has to remember the steps in the correct order to finish the activity.

If the child is unable to complete any of these activities, the therapist should note the reason for the child's lack of ability.

Standardized Assessment Tools Used in Schools

Richardson (2001) described two main types of standardized assessment tools used by occupational therapists within a school setting: criterion-referenced assessments and norm-referenced assessments. Assessments used by pediatric occupational therapists are norm-referenced, criterion-referenced, or both.

Norm-Referenced Assessments. This type of assessment develops "norms" (or average scores) through administering the assess-

ment to the "normative sample," which comprises a large group (usually hundreds) of typically developing children from various ethnic and socioeconomic backgrounds and geographic locations to ensure that the sample is representative of the population in the United States at that point in time.

When an occupational therapist performs a norm-referenced assessment, the score is compared to the standard scores established by the tool to determine the child's level of functioning. This type of assessment provides standard scores and percentiles to provide this comparison. Norm-referenced assessments usually include more general test items that at times have no functional application within a school setting. It is up to the therapist to interpret the child's low score on certain assessment items based on how it relates to and affects his or her ability to perform functional activities in the classroom setting.

These assessments have standardized protocols and must be administered using the specific procedures outlined by the assessment. Some norm-referenced assessments are the Bruininks–Oseretsky Test of Motor Proficiency (Bruininks, 1978), the Peabody Developmental Motor Scales (Folio & Fewell, 2000), and the Pediatric Evaluation of Disability Inventory (Haley, Coster, Ludlow, Haltiwanger, & Andrellos, 1992).

Criterion-Referenced Assessments. This type of assessment is designed to provide information on a child's performance of specific tasks. The child's performance is compared to a particular criterion established for each test item through administering the assessment to a large group of children. Test items on criterion-referenced assessments are usually more specific than those on norm-referenced assessments, meaning that a child has to meet the specific criterion established by the assessment to receive credit for the specific skill. The test results indicate the particular skills that the child could and could not complete and may be used as a baseline when planning for intervention. For example, in the Peabody Developmental Motor Scales (Folio & Fewell, 2000), which is both criterion-referenced and norm-referenced, the authors devised specific criteria for each test item. Based on the child's performance, the child receives a score of 2 (mastered the skill), 1 (skill is emerging), or 0 (unable to complete the skill). The therapist can review the child's results to see what skills the child received 1s and 0s in to plan the intervention.

Criterion-referenced assessments may or may not have standardized protocols for administration, depending on the assessment used. This type of assessment does not yield standard or mean scores to compare to peers. Examples of criterion-referenced assessments include the Pediatric Evaluation of Disability Inventory (Haley et al., 1992) and the Peabody Developmental Motor Scales (Folio & Fewell, 2000).

Norm-Referenced and Criterion-Referenced Assessments. Some assessments are both norm-referenced and criterion-referenced. This means that the test provides statistical analysis as in norm-referenced assessments but includes skills that are both developmental and functional that can be used as a basis for intervention planning as seen in criterion-referenced assessments. Examples of assessments that are both criterion-referenced and norm-referenced include the Peabody Developmental Motor Scales (Folio & Fewell, 2000) and the Pediatric Evaluation of Disability Inventory (Haley et al., 1992).

Standardized Assessment Tools Commonly Used for Preschoolers

The following are common assessment tools used by occupational therapists to evaluate preschool-age children's fine motor, self-care skills, and sensory–motor abilities.

Fine Motor and Self-Care Assessments.
Batelle Developmental Inventory. (See Newborg, Stock, Wnek, Guidubaldi, & Suinicki, 1998)

- Has a daily living skills section and a motor skills section.
- Daily living skills section examines the child's ability to complete self-care tasks in four domains: dressing, grooming, toileting, and eating.
- Motor skills section examines the child's fine motor, gross motor, and perceptual motor skills.
- Can be used for children from birth to age 8 years.
- Obtains information through parent/teacher interview, observation, and direct assessment.
- Provides evaluator with a standard score, percentile, and age equivalent for the child's skills in relation to same-age peers.
- Can be used with children of varying developmental and cognitive levels.

Brigance Diagnostic Inventory of Early Development. (See Brigance, 1978)

- Examines a child's performance of fine motor and self-care tasks.
- Fine motor assessments include general eye/finger/hand manipulation skills, block tower building, prehandwriting (including pencil grasp, drawing, name writing, and tracing/copying of upper- and lowercase letters), drawing of forms (copying prewriting shapes), and cutting.
- Self-care assessments include feeding/eating skills, dressing skills, managing fasteners, toileting, bathing, and grooming.
- Can be used for children from birth to age 7 years.
- Obtains information through parent/teacher interview, observation, and direct assessment.
- Provides developmental age ranges for individual test items to indicate at which level a child is functioning.

- Baseline information obtained from the assessment can be used to indicate present levels of performance and measure progress when readministered.
- Can be used with children of varying developmental and cognitive levels.

Pediatric Evaluation of Disability Inventory. (See Haley et al., 1992)

- Comprehensive clinical instrument that examines key functional capabilities and performance in self-care, mobility, and social function using two subscales—functional skills (197 items) and caregiver assistance (20 items).
- Can be used with children ranging in age from 6 months to 7 ½ years of age.
- Obtains information through parent/ teacher interview, observation, and direct assessment.
- Both norm-referenced and criterion-referenced, providing normative standard scores and scaled scores based on the standardization sample of children without disabilities.
- Can be used with all children but is particularly appropriate for lower functioning children to evaluate the level of independence and amount of caregiver assistance needed to complete tasks.

Beery Developmental Test of Visual–Motor Integration. (4th ed., rev.; see Beery, 1997)

- Commonly used and well-recognized assessment that measures a child's visual–motor skills.
- Requires the child to copy a variety of shapes and geometric designs to help identify if the child is having visual–motor deficits in nine basic prewriting strokes needed for letter formation, including vertical and horizontal lines, circles, crosses, right and left diagonal lines, squares, Xs, and triangles.
- Provides developmental age equivalents for skill levels of copying individual shapes and designs.

- Has a short format for children ages 3 to 7 years and a long format for children of all ages.
- Has standardized supplemental tests that measure a child's visual perception and motor coordination that may be administered after the assessment if it is suspected that the child has deficits in these areas.
- Helpful when looking at objectives for a child who remains unable to form all of the prewriting strokes needed for letter formation (taking into account developmental age norms for acquisition of the prewriting strokes).

Bruininks–Oseretsky Test of Motor Proficiency. (See Bruininks, 1978)

- Assesses motor functioning in children age 4 ½ to 14 ½ years.
- Includes a complete battery and a short form.
- Complete battery comprises 8 subtests with a total of 46 test items, providing individual measures of fine motor and gross motor skills and a comprehensive index of the child's overall motor proficiency. The subtests on the assessment include
  - Running speed and agility
  - Balance
  - Bilateral coordination
  - Strength
  - Upper-limb coordination
  - Response speed
  - Visual–motor control
  - Upper-limb speed and dexterity.
- Short form comprises 14 test items and can be used a screening tool of general motor proficiency.
- Norm-referenced and provides standard scores for individual subtests and standard scores, percentiles, and stanines for each of the composite scores; age equivalents for each of the 8 subtests also are provided.
- Complete battery takes 45–60 minutes to administer, and the short form takes 15–20 minutes to administer.

Peabody Developmental Motor Scales–2nd Edition. (2nd ed., see Folio & Fewell, 2000)

- New version released in 2000.
- Norm-referenced and criterion-referenced assessment tool designed to assess motor skills in children ranging in age from birth to 6 years.
- Composed of six subtests:
  - *Reflexes:* Measures the child's ability to automatically react to environmental events
  - *Stationary:* Measures the child's ability to sustain control of his or her body within the center of gravity and retain equilibrium
  - *Locomotion:* Measures the child's ability to transport his or her body from one base of support to another
  - *Object manipulation:* Measures the child's ability to throw, catch, and kick balls
  - *Grasping:* Measures the child's ability to use his or her hands and fingers
  - *Visual–motor integration:* Measures the child's ability to integrate and use visual–perceptual skills to perform complex eye–hand coordination tasks.
- Takes 45–60 minutes to administer.
- Often therapists administer only the grasping and visual–motor integration subtests.
- Results can be used to estimate child's motor competence relative to his or her peers.
- Provides standard scores; scaled scores; percentiles; and fine motor, gross motor, and total motor quotient scores.
- Authors also have written a motor activities program consisting of 104 activities designed to developmentally target the skills tested within the six subtests on the Peabody.

Miller Assessment for Preschoolers. (See Miller, 1988)

- Consists of 27 test items arranged into 5 performance indices (foundations, coordi-nation, verbal, nonverbal, and complex tasks) that assess a child's developmental status across different content domains (e.g., behavioral, motor, cognitive).
- Each performance index falls into one of three types of developmental abilities:
  1. *Sensory and motor abilities:* Consists of items found in the foundations index and the coordination index. Items in the foundations index examine the child's basic motor skills and awareness of sensations, including the child's sense of position and movement, sense of touch, development of basic components of movement, and sensory integration and neurodevelopment. Items in the coordination index assess the child's sensory and motor abilities simultaneously, including complex gross motor, fine motor, and oral motor tasks.
  2. *Cognitive abilities:* Consists of items found in the verbal index and nonverbal index. The verbal index examines the child's memory, sequencing, comprehension, association, and expression in a verbal context. The nonverbal index measures the child's memory, sequencing, visualization, and performance of mental manipulations not requiring spoken language.
  3. *Combined abilities:* Consists of items found in the complex tasks index, which measures the child's sensorimotor abilities in conjunction with his or her cognitive abilities.
- Takes 25–35 minutes to administer.
- Provides normed scores expressed as percentiles for the child's total score and for each performance index.
- Provides a "Behavior During Testing Checklist" to note atypical or abnormal behavior while administering the assessment; is used as supplemental information. If abnormal behaviors are present during the administration of the assessment, the

Miller Assessment for Preschoolers total score may not indicate the child's true sensory, motor, or cognitive capabilities secondary to his or her behavior.

Sensory Assessments.

Sensory Profile. Developed by Winnie Dunn in 1999, this instrument is organized as a questionnaire for the child's caregiver to complete. The assessment measures the child's sensory processing abilities and determines the effect of sensory processing his or her daily functional performance; it is recommended to be used with children ages 5 to 10 years. The assessment also offers an infant/toddler version (used for children from birth to age 36 months). This assessment can be used on children with varying disabilities, including learning disability, mental retardation, speech impairment, autism, Asperger's syndrome, visual or hearing impairment, cerebral palsy, traumatic brain injury, and multiple disabilities.

The questionnaire comprises 125 items grouped into three major areas: sensory processing, sensory modulation, and emotional and behavioral responses. The sensory processing area assesses auditory, visual, vestibular, multisensory, and oral sensory processing abilities. The modulation area looks at endurance and tone, body position and movement, activity levels, and modulation of sensory input (including visual input) that affects the child's emotional responses. In the behavioral and emotional response area, the caregiver reports on the child's activity level, attention, and behavioral and emotional responses to activities and situations.

The caregiver defines if the behaviors are exhibited always, frequently, occasionally, seldom, or never. Each response corresponds to a graduated point system. The points are totaled to determine the overall raw score for each section. The totaled raw scores from each section are interpreted and grouped into

one of three categories (typical performance, probable difference, definite difference) to determine where the child's performance is compared to that of typically developing peers. In addition to providing information on the child's performance in each of the sections, the assessment groups test items into factors, including sensory seeking, emotionally reactive, low endurance/tone, oral sensory sensitivity, inattention/distractibility, poor registration, sensory sensitivity, sedentary, and fine motor/perceptual factors.

The factor summaries assist in revealing patterns related to the child's response to types of stimuli within the environment. The scores are classified into three groups based on the performance of the child in relation to typically developing children:

- *Typical performance:* Child scores at or above 1.00 standard deviation below the mean.
- *Probable difference:* Child scores fall between 1.00 to 2.00 standard deviations below the mean.
- *Definite difference:* Child's scores fall below 2.00 standard deviations below the mean.

Dunn developed a theoretical model for sensory processing that can be used in the interpretation and reporting process. The child's scores are organized into a behavioral response continuum that includes four quadrants: poor registration, sensation seeking, sensitivity to stimuli, and sensation avoiding. Organizing the scores in this way assists in targeting specific intervention strategies to coincide with the child's profile.

Sensory Integration Inventory–Revised, For Individuals With Developmental Disabilities. Developed by Judith Reisman and Barbara Hanschu in 1992 and revised in 2001 to be used as a screening tool to determine if a child would benefit from further assessment in the area of sensory processing and if he or she would benefit from therapy targeting deficits in that area, this inventory can be completed by a child's caregiver or staff (e.g., occupational therapist, teacher) familiar with the child. The inventory assists in determining if a child's behaviors are a result of a sensory processing issue.

The inventory is organized into four sections: vestibular processing, tactile processing, proprioceptive processing, and general reactions to sensory input. Items within the sections are checked to report whether the child is exhibiting the behaviors listed. The "yes" responses are placed on the inventory rating form. Trends or patterns can be identified in the four major categories of dysfunction defined by the inventory: sensory modulation, sensory defensiveness, sensory registration, or sensory integration. Treatment can be developed to address the specific areas of difficulty the child is exhibiting as defined by the inventory.

DeGangi–Berk Test of Sensory Integration. This screening tool was developed by Ronald A. Berk and Georgia A. DeGangi in 1983 to provide an overall measure of sensory integration functioning for preschool children ages 3 to 5 years. The test comprises 36 items providing information about the child's overall sensory integrative functioning. The items are organized into three subdomains: postural control, bilateral motor integration, and reflex integration.

The DeGangi–Berk Test is a criterion-referenced assessment, designed to be used for children suspected to have delays in their sensory, motor, or perceptual skills or for children suspected of having learning problems. The test was designed to measure a child's abilities related to postural control, bilateral motor integration, and reflex integration. The test can be administered in about one-half hour. Results help determine whether a child is functioning in the normal range of performance, is at risk for a sensory integrative dysfunction, or has definite deficits in sensory integrative functioning.

Temperament and Atypical Behavior Scale. This assessment, developed in 1999 by John T. Neisworth, Stephen J. Bagnato, John Salvia, and Frances M. Hunt, is norm-referenced and provides a measure of dysfunctional behavior in children between ages 11 and 71 months. The intended purpose is to assist in identifying children who are "at risk" or who are developing atypically in the areas of temperament and self-regulation. The assessment tool comprises 55 test items arranged in a checklist format. The items are arranged into four subtests: detached, hypersensitive/active, underreactive, and dysregulated.

The respondent (usually the child's parent or caregiver) records whether the child is exhibiting the stated behaviors listed and whether help is needed with managing the child's behavior in the stated areas. The raw scores for each of the four subtests are totaled, and standard scores and percentiles can be derived for the child's score in each area. The raw scores for all four subtests are then totaled to determine the overall temperament and regulatory index, which has a standard score of 100 with a standard deviation of 15. Because the items on the TABS are written in specific behavioral terms, they easily can be targeted for intervention on child's IEP in the area of behavior.

Reporting Results of Assessments

After administering and completing the standardized assessment and conducting interviews and observations, the occupational therapist needs to write up the child's results. Performing standardized assessments provides the educational team with information on how the child performs certain skills when compared to peers. When reporting results of these assessments, it is important to try to relate the information obtained to how it affects or may affect the child's ability to function in the preschool classroom.

Items on norm-referenced or criterion-referenced assessments often are isolated skills, but they do not provide insight on how the child's inability to complete this skill will affect him or her functionally in the classroom. For example, what is the functional impact if the child is unable to isolate touching each finger to his or her thumb as measured on the Peabody Developmental Motor Scales (Folio & Fewell, 2000)? The therapist needs to determine if the child understood the directions required to complete the task, whether the child's motor abilities are affecting his or her ability to complete the task, if he or she does not understand the language used in the verbal directions given, or whether he or she is displaying difficulty imitating the motor act after being provided with a demonstration by the therapist.

The occupational therapist needs to evaluate how the child's inability to complete a skill would affect educational performance in the classroom. For example, Bobby is unable to bring each of his fingers individually to his thumb, which may affect his ability to separate the two sides of his hands when completing fine motor tasks, resulting in him using his hand as a whole unit when picking up items from the table, using a gross grasp when holding a utensil, or placing all of his fingers into the holes of scissors.

Although standardized test results should be reported within evaluation write-ups (including standard scores, percentages, and standard deviations), they should not be used as the sole basis of qualification for occupational therapy services. When a child undergoes a multifactored evaluation to determine qualification for special education, a low standard score or standard deviation below the mean may assist in qualifying the child for special education programming, but this does not necessarily mean that the child qualifies for occupational therapy services. A child may score below the mean but remain functional at home or in the classroom. The child currently may be able to manage at home and in the classroom even through he or she was unable to do the very specific fine motor or self-care test items on the assessment tool. In this case, the child may still qualify for special education services in the motor or adaptive area, but the special education teacher, rather than an occupational therapist, may be able to meet the child's IEP needs. However, the child may qualify for occupational therapy as he or she gets older and the demands of the classroom become increasingly difficult.

The occupational therapist and educational team must take into account all of the assessment information, including observation, interview, and the results of standardized assessment, to determine the child's needs, annual goals, short-term objectives, and types of services needed to benefit from educational programming. The therapist should never comment on what type of service is needed to support the child's deficits within the evaluation write-up. Determination of whether the child would qualify for special education services and benefit from occupational therapy services in a school setting should be made by the entire educational team after all information regarding the child's overall developmental level of functioning is reported.

The Role of Occupational Therapists in Program Planning

After the evaluation process is completed and the education team determines that the child is eligible for special education services, the next step is for the team to develop and write the child's IEP. This includes determining appropriate goals and objectives for the child to focus on and what services will be needed to support his or her goals and objectives.

It is important for occupational therapists to collaborate with all team members in determining appropriate goals and objectives and prioritizing areas to focus on at the present time. For example, it is not recommended that goals and objectives be written for using a tripod grasp and forming prewriting shapes for an incoming 3-year-old child if the focus in the classroom is not on completing prewriting tasks requiring the child to use a writing utensil. If teachers have both morning and afternoon classes, they frequently try to gear the morning class toward younger children and the afternoon class toward older children. The focus of the 3-year-old class is to assist children in learning the structure and routine of the classroom, promote interaction between peers, develop play skills, and participate in teacher-directed activities. Fine motor tasks and manipulatives are incorporated into free play so that children can gain exposure. For this age group, objectives regarding releasing objects, using two hands together to complete bilateral tasks, completing a 1- or 2-step fine motor task, managing personal belongings, and using a three-finger or pincer grasp to pick up objects may be more appropriate areas to focus on.

In the classrooms with older children, structured times are usually set aside for completing art activities that require the children to complete multistep color, cut, and paste tasks; write their names on paper; and draw shapes in preparation for kindergarten. At this time, it would be more appropriate for the IEP to focus on the child's pencil grasp, prewriting and writing skills, and cutting skills.

The results of the evaluation reported by the occupational therapist need to be compared to the child's overall level of functioning to determine the priority areas to address in the child's IEP. The prioritized items need to be developed into goals and objectives as part of the child's IEP. The team will decide whether the goals and objectives developed need to be supported by the occupational

therapist. The child may need to initially get adjusted to the structure of a school day and obtain exposure to a variety of materials as presented by the teacher to further develop his or her skills before being considered for related services like occupational therapy. On the other hand, the team may also determine that the child and teacher would benefit from occupational therapy consultation and collaboration to provide ideas for the identified areas and monitor the child's progress. Finally, the team may decide that the child would benefit from direct occupational therapy as a related service to the child's IEP to work on the prioritized areas.

It is important that occupational therapists proactively educate team members about the varying roles that an occupational therapist can perform and when the different types of service delivery models (e.g., consultation and collaboration vs. direct service) would be appropriate and effective. Often when children with disabilities display deficits in fine motor, sensory, or self-care areas enter a school-based program it is assumed that they will receive direct occupational therapy services. These children may receive services privately in the community or have received services in an early intervention program. The educational team needs to follow the IEP process as intended, including identifying the child's educational needs, establishing goals and objectives, and determining what services are needed. Determination of the type of service that is needed (whether consultative or direct) should be based on the needs of the student within the context of the classroom and not solely on whether the student receives private therapy services, scores a certain way on an assessment, or has a specific diagnosis.

School-based occupational therapists need to educate team members (including teachers and parents) about the types of service delivery models and describe the pros and cons of each. For example, teachers and parents often are hesitant to have the student receive only consultation services and not direct services because they fear the student will not see the occupational therapist weekly. The therapist needs to describe the benefit of frequent consultation services and the impact it can have on a child's performance. By using consultation, the child can participate in the classroom in activities designed by the occupational therapist on a daily basis that support the child's areas of need. Staff can be trained to implement these activities. At times, this can be a more effective service than having the occupational therapist meet with the student in isolation once a week for a direct therapy session.

If the team determines that the type of service provided by the occupational therapist is not effective for the child, the IEP team can reconvene and revise the services as needed. Many studies have been conducted regarding the effectiveness of a consultative model with preschool children versus a direct service model. These studies will be described in depth below.

According to Case-Smith and Berry (1998), the level of occupational therapy services should be modified throughout the child's career. This may include decreasing direct service over time and increasing consultation and collaboration with the child's teachers and parents as the child makes gains or if it is determined that the child's needs can be addressed throughout the school day by the teacher with the support of the occupational therapist. Preschool children are exposed to a wide variety of fine motor and self-help activities as a part of their school day, and this exposure may be enough to assist the child in improving his or her skills. Occupational therapists can collaborate with teachers to help them develop activities and materials to work on identified skills and to aid in structuring the classroom

and school day to ensure that the activities are being naturally incorporated.

Service Delivery Models

Occupational therapists working in a preschool setting can provide an array of services to meet children's needs. This includes one-on-one direct intervention in the classroom, direct intervention with a small group of children within the classroom, one-on-one direct intervention using a pull-out method in an environment outside of the classroom, and consultation and collaboration with the child's teachers and family.

Providing Consultation Services to Preschool Children

Consultation is one way to deliver services within the preschool environment. Consultation services commonly occur between the occupational therapist and the child's teacher and parents but can occur between the therapist and any of the educational team members.

In consultation the therapist uses his or her knowledge to allow another person to successfully interact with the child or group of children in a way that promotes functional skills (Richardson & Schultz-Krohn, 2001). Consultation services may involve meeting with the child's teacher or parent who has identified a concern, observing the child in the classroom or at home when participating in the activity of concern, and providing recommendations to the teaching staff or parent on ways to work on the identified skills.

The occupational therapist should be involved in the IEP process by assisting the teacher in writing the child's goals and objectives. When the educational team decides that the child would benefit from consultation services, it should be identified on the child's IEP. The therapist may be attached to specific goals and objectives or may be identified strictly as a service within the services section on the IEP. The minimum amount of consultation that will be provided to the child should be identified within this section (e.g., "Occupational therapy consultation 30 minutes per month to support objectives 1a, 1b," or "Occupational therapy consultation services 15 minutes a month to support any concerns in sensory processing or fine motor skills").

The occupational therapist can affect the classroom as a whole and the child individually by providing consultative services. The therapist's responsibilities may include making recommendations for positioning the child or equipment for optimum performance by the child. For example, when completing art projects, the therapist might remind the teacher of the importance of having the child sit at a table that is of appropriate height in a chair that allows for his or her feet to be supported by the floor. The therapist may also provide recommendations on where activities should be positioned for the child either for optimum access or to challenge the child to work on a specific skill (e.g., crossing midline). For example, when working with a child with cerebral palsy who is seated in a wheelchair with a tray, the therapist may recommend that the switch or communication device be positioned slightly on the child's left side so that the child is forced to cross midline to activate the switch when using his or her right hand, a goal on the child's IEP.

The therapist also is responsible for making recommendations on how to modify the environment to meet child's individualized needs. For example, for a child with achondroplasia (small stature), the therapist would recommend lowering the child's coat hook for easier access, providing a bench for the child to stand on to access the sink and toilet in the classroom, and providing a foot rest under the table to support the child's feet when seated at the table to complete fine motor tasks.

The therapist also makes recommendations on how to modify an activity to meet the child's needs. This includes having the child use thicker paper while cutting for easier management when having to turn the paper. For a preschool child with a visual impairment, the occupational therapist may recommend that the teacher position the child's worksheets on a slant board, enlarge the child's worksheets for increased size, and copy the child's worksheets on yellow paper for greater contrast.

Occupational therapists can adapt equipment or order supplies for children to allow them to be as independent as possible in the classroom (e.g., making footrests or back supports out of phone books, ordering pencil grippers and Handiwriters [HandiThings, P.O. Box 41, New Melle, MO 63365; 636-398-4081] for older preschool children who have nonfunctional pencil grips and are working on prewriting skills, and ordering smaller scissors for children who have difficulty managing the larger Fiskar scissors).

Another responsibility is making recommendations for the arrangement of the classroom to support the child's needs. For example, a child with autism or attention issues may benefit from having a separate closed-off workstation in the classroom (made using dividers) for completing pre-academic or writing tasks. This would provide the child with a private, quieter environment where he or she can complete his or her work and then rejoin the rest of the class for group activities.

The occupational therapist should assist the teacher in designing materials for individual children. The therapist also may assist the teacher in designing child's picture schedules (using actual photographs or Boardmaker™ [Mayer-Johnson, Inc., P.O. Box 1579, Solana Beach, CA 92075; 800-588-4548; mayerj@mayer-johnson.com] pictures) and visual reinforcement systems that can be used with children in the classroom and when they travel to see related service providers (e.g., speech-language pathology, physical therapy). This ensures that all staff members are consistent in managing the child's behaviors, in supporting the child's communication, and in maintaining the child's routine. For example, the occupational therapist provides consultation services to a child with autism who is using a picture schedule in the classroom. The therapist has developed a sensory plan to be incorporated daily into the child's school day. The therapist recommends that the child be offered choices for the sensory activities by being shown pictures of the different activities and allowing the child to choose. The therapist may assist in collecting the pictures of the sensory activities, designing the choice board, and demonstrating to staff how to use it with the child.

Occupational therapists may consult with teaching staff and parents by providing in-service training relating to child development in fine motor, visual–motor, self-care, or sensory–motor development. This ensures that teachers and parents are setting realistic expectations for children (e.g., not expecting a 3-year-old to engage the zipper on his or her coat) and that developmentally appropriate activities are being incorporated into the child's day.

A study by Dreiling and Bundy (2003) attempted to determine if there was a difference in the amount of progress a preschool child made toward his or her goals and objectives when receiving direct occupational therapy services versus when receiving consultation services. The authors divided a group of children in half, with half of the 20 students in the study receiving consultation services from an occupational therapist and the other half receiving direct therapy services. They observed the children for one school year. The results indicated that a consultation model of service delivery was as effective in assisting a child in meeting educational goals as the direct intervention model.

The researchers also found that the child retained skills throughout the school week when the child received services through a consultative model. The study determined that consultation services took as much time, if not more, than direct intervention initially in the school year, but over the course of the school year the amount of consultation time decreased as programs became established and as staff became increasingly familiar with the strategies implemented to assist the child with his or her skill deficits.

Providing frequent consultation to teachers can be an effective way of providing services to preschool students. The therapist can observe the child engaging in certain selected tasks in the classroom, problem solve with the teacher regarding skills that the student is demonstrating difficulty with performing in the classroom, provide recommendations to the teacher on how to assist the child in further developing these skills, educate the teacher on what to observe when the child is completing the skills (e.g., position of the forearms next to the body when completing cutting tasks), and make recommendations for or provide adapted equipment (e.g., adapted scissors, pencil gripper, slant board) to enable the child to perform the skills more effectively. See Exhibit 7.1 for an example.

Providing Direct Intervention to Preschool Children

Direct service involves the occupational therapist or occupational therapy assistant working one-on-one or in a small group with the child to provide intervention on individual skills. The therapist works with the child to target the specific goals and objectives that are outlined on the IEP, designing preparation activities and intervention strategies. Direct services are provided when the team determines that the child would benefit from hands-on intervention and monitoring by the

Exhibit 7.1. Case Study

An occupational therapist consults monthly with a preschool teacher regarding a 5-year-old preschool student with fine motor deficits who currently has self-care objectives on his IEP. The child is able to take off his jacket but has difficulty putting on his jacket independently. He is able to pull the zipper up and down once engaged but is unable to engage the zipper. He also has difficulty hanging up his coat on a hook in the hallway. He remains unable to manage clothing fasteners that he commonly wears to school, including the snaps on his pants.

The therapist observes the child periodically in the classroom during a fine motor activity time and meets monthly with his special education teacher to discuss the effectiveness of recommended interventions and determine if progress has been made toward his goals and objectives. The therapist provided suggestions to focus on these skill deficits, including having the student use the "flip-over" method

to put on his coat, lowering his coat hook so that it is at eye level, placing his coat hook at the end of the row to limit distractions and provide him with additional space, and adding a zipper pull to the zipper on his coat to allow for a larger surface area for him to grasp when pulling the zipper up and down.

The therapist also met with the child's parent and teacher and recommended that the child have a "fine motor kit" available to him during the school day. The fine motor kit included activities that promoted the child using a three-finger grasp and increasing finger strength, including popping bubble wrap, opening/closing clothespins, and finding coins in Theraputty and placing them into a resistive container. The teacher agreed to have the child spend a few minutes each day with an educational assistant in the classroom completing fine motor tasks in the kit that targeted the development of specific hand skills and then have the child practice on one of the individualized

self-care goals on his IEP daily, including putting on his coat, engaging the zipper, and managing snaps on his pants.

The fine motor preparation activities and work tasks alternated throughout the week. The opportunities to practice the skills throughout the week provided the child with one-on-one attention that focused on his identified individualized needs. A list of the activity suggestions also was provided to the child's parents so that the skills could be reinforced at home. The occupational therapist was used as a consult to the parent, teacher, and teaching assistant to observe the child performing the tasks, to problem solve on skills he was having difficulty with, to determine why he was unable to complete the skills (e.g., poor in-hand manipulation skills, decreased hand strength, poor bilateral coordination), and to add activities to the fine motor kit and update materials throughout the year to account for the child's progress with the identified skills.

occupational therapist to focus on specific skill deficits (e.g., in-hand manipulation skills, pencil grasp, prewriting and other visual–motor skills, self-help skills).

Case-Smith and Berry (1998) conducted a study comparing the effectiveness of providing direct intervention to children in a small group versus a one-on-one direct instruction. The study found that the children made the same amount of progress whether the services were provided individually or within a small group. She reported that the advantage of working with children in a small group was that the therapist could target the child's social skills in addition to fine

motor skills during the group session and that the groups combined children with varying ability levels, providing the children with peer models to reference for assistance while completing the tasks.

Direct services may be provided in a variety of settings, including in the child's home, in a private preschool program in the community, in the child's classroom, or in a separate environment (e.g., a therapist's treatment room) at an integrated preschool program. There are pros and cons to providing preschool therapy services in the classroom or in a pull-out model, as described in Tables 7.1 and 7.2.

Table 7.1. Pros and Cons to Providing Direct Services in the Preschool Classroom

Pros	Cons
• Children are able to engage in the activities as they occur naturally throughout the school day (e.g., practicing dressing skills when taking off or putting on a coat, practicing pulling pants up and down when using the restroom).	• Children may not want to work with the therapist on certain skills because they do not want to miss what the other children are doing in the classroom.
• Children have the opportunity to observe their peers to see how they approach and complete tasks.	• For children with poor attention spans, it may be difficult to focus on very specific skills (e.g., prewriting, in-hand manipulation, clothing fasteners) when other children are nearby or when the environment is noisy or chaotic.
• The classroom teacher and assistants are able to observe the therapy, which assists in carryover of intervention strategies in the classroom.	• It may be more difficult for the therapist to collect data on specific goals and objectives. Because the therapist sees the children only for a certain period of time, it may be difficult to coordinate the children's goals and objectives into the treatment session.

Communicating With Teachers and Parents About Direct Service. If consultation time is not built into the IEP, the occupational therapist should attempt to communicate with the child's teacher and parents what is occurring within occupational therapy treatment sessions, what interventions or modifications assist the child in completing selected tasks, and what should be focused on or integrated into the child's day (both at home and school) to reinforce the skills. This may need to occur weekly or as needed when the therapist observes a change in the child's performance or observes a technique that is effective for the child.

Preschool teachers often create daily communication logs for parents to assist them in knowing what occurred at preschool

Table 7.2. Pros and Cons to Providing Direct Services to Preschool Children Using a Pull-Out Model

Pros	Cons
• Children are able to work one-on-one with the therapist on specific skills in a quiet environment.	• Children are pulled out of their natural environment and work on skills in a simulated setting.
• Children may be better able to focus their attention to the tasks without the distractions common in the classroom setting.	• Children are unable to observe how their peers would approach or complete the tasks.
• The therapist can design intervention strategies that target the children's individual goals and objectives so that numerical data can be collected to report the children's progress.	• Children may not want to leave their peers and may demonstrate difficulty transitioning out of the classroom to work with the therapist.
	• The teacher is unable to observe what is occurring in the treatment sessions, which could affect the carryover of the skills throughout the week in the classroom setting.

that day. This allows parents to talk to their children about the activities when they get home. The occupational therapist could ask the teacher to provide an area on the daily communication sheet for the therapist to fill in about what the child did in therapy that day and what the child should focus on during the upcoming week. This would allow for the teacher and parent to read the remarks and implement the suggestions in the classroom or at home.

Some parents have their own communication logs that they design for staff members who work with their child to complete. Using this form, the occupational therapist also can provide the parent with information on the preparation activities and intervention strategies that were conducted and the child's progress and performance. Suggested activities can be given for the parent and teacher to work on during the upcoming week.

Occupational therapists should encourage parents to reinforce skills with their child at home. A great way for therapists to check if parents are reinforcing skills at home is to assign homework. Each week the therapist provides one suggestion or activity (e.g., letter writing or prewriting, cutting, a fine motor activity, a self-help task) for the parent to complete with the child. The child then brings in the work sample the following week, or the parent provides written feedback in the daily communication notebook detailing how the child did and how much assistance was needed for him or her to complete the task. The therapist can then provide the parent with suggestions based on the feedback.

Another way to assist parents in reinforcing skills with their children is to write a monthly newsletter that can be sent home with children that focuses on different skills and provides sample activities and suggestions for parents to do with their children. Teachers often have their own Web pages within the school district's Web site. The oc-

cupational therapist could collaborate with the district's administration and technology coordinator to see if an occupational therapy Web page could be created to display these activities or if the therapist could incorporate information into the preschool teacher's Web page and then parents could be notified each month to check the site for that particular month's activity focus (e.g., October: Cutting, November: Facilitating a Three-Finger Grasp, December: Pre-writing Skills). A sample newsletter is provided in Exhibit 7.2.

Managing Considerations for Direct Service. When providing direct services to children in a preschool setting, occupational therapists should consider that scheduling preschoolers can be a difficult task, due to the structure of the school day. The shorter school day (usually 2 ½ hours) allows for a maximum of only 4 to 5 children to be seen directly (using a one-on-one format) during one school day. Therapists frequently have to schedule children around snack time, circle time, and music or physical education. If a child's IEP goals address feeding, the therapist should consider scheduling that child during snack time. If the child has a goal to manage his or her coat and book bag, then the therapist can see the child at the beginning or end of the school day to work on these skills as they occur naturally.

If the therapist provides direct intervention to numerous children in the same class, block scheduling of children may be an effective technique. Using this technique, the therapist spends a large portion or the entire school day in that classroom. This allows the therapist to be available to see the children during opening and closing routines, snack time, circle time, and centers (e.g., housekeeping center, art center) to work on needed skills. If the therapist provides intervention for children in multiple preschool classrooms, he or she may want to consider collaborating with the teachers to see if they can alternate

Exhibit 7.2. Sample Occupational Therapy Newsletter

Fun Activities to Work on Your Child's Cutting Skills

Preparation Activities

There are many preparation activities that you can do with your child at home that will work on the hand movements needed in order to cut. These include

- Having your child use tweezers or tongs to pick up small objects (e.g., small food items, cotton balls, fabric balls, candy).
- Having your child use a plant sprayer to water your houseplants. Pressing the trigger in and out mimics the movements used when cutting.
- Using tweezer scissors (typically used to pluck eyebrows, similar to scissors but with flattened tips at the end) to pick up items and place them in a designated area. Make sure that you present the items to the child in midline (the midsection of the child's body) in a horizontal plane (e.g., hold up an index card in your child's midline at the child's chest level so that he or she has to use a "thumbs-up" position (with child's thumb pointing toward the sky) to grasp and hold on to the card using the tweezer scissors). This can be made into a game by having the child match index cards based on colors, letters, or numbers. It assists the child with learning the open/close movements needed for cutting with scissors.
- Having your child practice cutting on a variety of materials, including play dough, straws, sandpaper, corrugated paper, and other paper with varying thickness (e.g., cardboard vs. copy paper). Once the child has demonstrated the ability to open and close the scissors to make continuous cuts in paper, increase the difficulty by having him or her follow a straight line, curved path, and then shapes requiring changes in direction, including a circle, square, or triangle.

What to Look for When Your Child Is Cutting

- Make sure that your child is seated in a chair that allows his or her feet to touch the ground. Ensure that the height of the table is appropriate for your child's height (the top of the table should be around the child's elbow level).
- When your child is cutting, his or her forearms should be at the side of his or her body, and he or she should stabilize the paper using a "thumbs-up" position. This will assist in turning the paper to cut around shapes requiring changes in direction. The hand your child uses to cut also should be in a "thumbs-up" position.
- Make sure that your child is looking at the paper when cutting. The eyes drive the hands, so if your child is not looking at the paper, it will be difficult for him or her to remain on the lines.

Happy cutting!
Sincerely,
Kelly Ryba, OTR/L

when activities will occur to support the related service providers' schedule. By ensuring that the children do not all have circle time or snack time at the same time, the teachers allow for all available time during the school day to be used for direct service. Therapists should also collaborate with other related service providers at the beginning of the school year to ensure that there will not be conflicts in scheduling for children that are seen by multiple related service (e.g., physical therapy, speech-language pathology, occupational therapy).

When seeing children in a small group, it may be beneficial to group children with similar goals and objectives to promote easier data collection. The small group can meet in the preschool classroom or in a separate setting (e.g., the therapy room). If a group of children have goals and objectives addressing cutting and prewriting skills, the therapist can design preparation activities and intervention activities or projects to address each child's goals and objectives. If the group includes children who are at different levels of performance, the projects can be graded to meet their ability levels, using a charting system to collect data on each child's goal and objectives. See Chapter 2 for details in collecting data and sample forms to use to chart activities, record numerical data, and document narrative information.

Another way to provide direct intervention to children is to combine a one-on-one with a small group approach. For example, the occupational therapist can collaborate with the preschool teacher in designing fun art activities that focus on the child's goals and objectives (e.g., cutting, prewriting, pencil grasp, bilateral hand skills). The therapist then divides the treatment session into two parts: assisting children in a small group as they complete the classroom art activity and pulling the children for the remaining half of the treatment session for one-on-one intervention to focus on specific skills. This allows the teacher to observe the types of cues, intervention strategies, and modifications the therapist uses with the child and allows for the therapist to address specific skills and gather specific data toward goal and objectives in a one-on-one setting.

This is an effective technique to use when the occupational therapist only has a few children in a preschool classroom. It is also effective when the therapist sees children on a consultative basis. The therapist and teacher can plan activities to focus on the child's IEP goals and objectives, and then the therapist would be a part of the activity to not only observe the children perform the activity but also to provide recommendations for carryover when completing similar activities the other days of the school week.

Combining Direct and Consultation Services

Often occupational therapists are asked by team members whether the child needs direct service or consultation. A good answer is, "Why not both?" Providing a combination not only allows for the therapist to work one-on-one or in a small group with the child but it also allows the therapist to collaborate with the teacher regarding what is observed during the direct therapy time and to make recommendations for what needs to be carried over in the classroom setting on a daily basis.

Depending on the child's needs, the therapist may initially see the child directly once a week and collaborate with the teacher once a month. Over time, the therapist may decrease the amount of direct service time each month and increase the amount of consultation time. Over time (e.g., as child transitions to a school-age program), the child may require only consultation services by the therapist. This is a great way for therapists to define their role more globally with parents and teachers from the beginning of the child's career and not be forced into a direct service model for the child's entire education. If the parents can see the effectiveness of a consultation model from the start of their child's education, they may not be as hesitant to shift from direct service when the team feels that consultation services would meet the child's needs.

Intervention Considerations for Areas Commonly Supported by Occupational Therapists

Children With Sensory Processing Problems

After determining that a child has deficits in sensory processing skills, the occupational therapist needs to determine how to provide intervention or accommodations to meet the child's individualized sensory needs. Meeting the preschool child's sensory needs can be done in a variety of ways, including developing an individualized sensory plan that targets the child's sensory needs that can be implemented daily, incorporating sensory-based activities into the classroom, and structuring the environment to support the child's sensory needs.

Implementing Individualized Sensory Plans. Developing an individualized sensory plan that includes activities that can be incorporated in the child's school day daily is typically the recommended approach when a child presents with sensory–motor issues that are interfering with his or her ability to participate in the school day. The teacher and occupational therapist should identify specific times during the day in which the child is displaying difficulty.

For example, the teacher reports that the child demonstrates difficulty engaging in art tasks due to not wanting to interact with tactile materials, including glue and finger paint, or not wanting to get his or her hands dirty when using markers. The therapist may suggest a few tactile preparation activities that provide deep pressure input to be conducted prior to the classroom art activity. This may include engaging the child in a lotion and towel rub that provides the child's hands with deep pressure desensitizing input prior to engaging in the activity (see Chapter 8 for more discussion of sensory integration activities). The teacher or assistant could have the child engage in this activity daily for a period of time (e.g., over a span of a few weeks) to determine if the child is better able to tolerate the materials used after the tactile preparation activity is conducted.

Another example would be designing strategies for a child demonstrating difficulty remaining seated and attending during circle time (averaging 10–15 minutes) each day. Depending on the child's individual needs, the occupational therapist may recommend that the child engage in a movement-based activity for 5 minutes prior to circle time (e.g., bouncing on a therapy ball, jumping on trampoline) or in a calming activity prior to circle time (e.g., steam roller, slow linear swinging, sitting in a rocking chair) for additional input

prior to having to remain seated. The therapist may also recommend that the child wear a weighted vest and sit on a Movin' Sit (Gymnic, Ledraplastic S.p.a., Via Brigata Re nr. 1, 33010 Osoppo (UD), Italy; www.gymnic.com) cushion during circle time, providing additional deep pressure input to help him or her with organizing himself or herself to improve concentration. Each of these activities may need to be introduced separately over time so that staff can determine which interventions work.

Incorporating Sensory–Motor Activities Into the School Day. The second method of meeting a student's sensory needs is having the staff incorporate sensory–motor-based activities conducted with all of the children into the school day. The occupational therapist may consult with the teacher to design activities that can be conducted in the classroom setting. Preschool children often rotate through stations or centers, and teachers may include a sensory center for the children to go to each day. At this center, the teacher can incorporate movement activities, including dancing; gross motor activities, including wheelbarrow walking or animal walking; Brain Gym activities; playing on a climber in the classroom; or playing at a sensory table filled with different tactile materials (e.g., rice, noodles, shaving cream). The teacher could incorporate movement activities throughout the school day, including crab crawling between centers, dancing or doing gross motor activities at circle time, and using vibrating toothbrushes to "wake up" the children's mouths prior to having snack. If a particular child has more severe sensory processing issues that require specific activities to be designed, then an individualized sensory plan would be needed.

Structuring the Child's Environment. Another method of supporting the child's sensory needs is through structuring the environment. This method is particularly successful for children with autism or behavior issues who display difficulty managing the daily classroom routine (e.g., transitioning, following teacher-directed tasks, initiating and completing work independently). For some children, structuring the environment provides support for their success throughout the day. For others, structuring the environment may need to be combined with the first or second method discussed to meet their sensory and behavioral needs. The following suggestions have been successful:

- *Having a consistent schedule:* Children usually benefit from having a routine schedule each day (e.g., enter classroom, circle time, centers, snack, story time, special, get ready to go home). This is particularly important for a child who has difficulty making transitions. This child desires a structured, predictable routine. Occupational therapists can help teachers better structure their school day to meet the needs of the children in their classroom. This may include setting up a classroom schedule, rotating centers for the children to rotate through, providing exposure to a variety of activities (so children do not pick the same 2 or 3 activities every day), or designing individual strategies for a particular student to assist with better understanding the daily routine.
- *Picture schedules:* For children who display difficulty managing transitions and following the daily classroom routine, individual picture schedules can be designed and used. This may include using object cues (for a child who is unable to understand photographs or picture representations), actual photographs of the child engaging in the activities, or picture representations of the activities like those found in the Boardmaker™ (Mayer-Johnson, Inc., P.O. Box 1579, Solana Beach, CA 92075; 800-588-4548; mayerj@mayer-johnson.com) program.

The individual picture icons or object cues can be arranged in the order they occur during the school day. Teachers attach the icons to a laminated file folder or binder with Velcro™ or to a wall in the classroom. Before each activity ends and a transition occurs, the teacher prompts the child to check the schedule. The child then can do a variety of things to indicate completion of one task and readiness for the next. To indicate he or she is finished with an activity, the child could turn that icon over and attach it to the Velcro™ strip, put that icon on the "finished folder," or put the icon into an envelope labeled "Finished." The picture schedule provides additional structure to the school day by preparing the child for the activities that will occur.

- *First–then board:* Using a first–then board with a child assists in structuring the day by defining what he or she has to complete first before moving on to the next activity. For example, if a child really loves to play in the block area but needs to complete the daily art activity (a nonpreferred activity), the teacher may state, "Connor, first you have to do the art activity, then you can play in the block area." This defines what Connor needs to do before he can engage in the preferred activity. This is a good strategy to use for children who always want to engage in the same activities every day. The child must first do one nonpreferred activity before engaging in the reinforcer. This also is an effective strategy for students who become overwhelmed by seeing the entire list of activities for the day, especially when seeing activities listed that the student does not enjoy.
- *Use of a timer:* Teachers often use timers when rotating through centers to ensure that each center lasts the same amount of time, allowing the children to rotate through all of the centers. Timers also can be used for individual children to assist in

defining how long they have to engage in an activity. The teacher and therapist need to determine if the child responds better to a visual timer or a timer that rings a bell. For example, the teacher may say, "Connor, you need to paint for 5 minutes. I will set the timer; when you hear it ring, you will be done."

- *Defining the child's personal space:* When the children are seated on the floor (e.g., during circle time or story time), some children have difficulty maintaining their personal space. These children lean into others, lie down, or scoot around on the floor, at times disrupting the other children. These children may benefit from having their space defined for them. The teacher can accomplish this by having children sit on individual carpet squares or Movin'sit cushions (Gymnic Line—The Way to Move, Ledraplastic S.p.a., Via Brigata Re nr.1, 33010 Osoppo (UD), Italy). This allows the children to know their boundaries and the teacher to prompt the children back to their designated spaces.

- *Use of social stories:* Speech therapists and teachers often develop social stories to help children deal with difficult situations (e.g., managing transitions, sharing toys, following directions, behaving appropriately with peers). Social stories also may help children prepare for new activities or transitions during the school day (e.g., for an assembly, class party, field trip, unexpected classroom task).

The occupational therapist, in collaboration with the preschool teacher and education team members, will have to determine the best method to use to meet the child's individualized sensory needs in the classroom setting.

Children With Fine Motor Deficits

Occupational therapists are frequently called on to provide consultation or direct service for children with fine motor difficulties. "Fine motor skills" is a very generalized term that is often used by teachers. Therapists need to conduct further analysis to determine the teacher's concerns about the child's fine motor skills and how they are affecting the child's ability to perform in the classroom. A child with deficits in fine motor skills may present difficulties with

- Picking up and manipulating objects
- Displaying developed palmar arches, having separation of the sides of the hands, and demonstrating beginning in-hand manipulation skills when interacting with objects or completing tasks
- Using both hands together to complete bilateral tasks
- Grasping a writing utensil and completing prewriting and writing tasks
- Positioning scissors correctly in fingers to cut out lines and shapes
- Managing fasteners on clothing, including engaging a zipper or snapping his or her pants.

Occupational therapists can be valuable resources when designing programs to target preschool children with fine motor difficulties, including providing information on the development of fine motor skills. Therapists can be instrumental in providing parents and teachers with what are realistic expectations for a child with fine motor deficits. Therapists can share with parents and teachers the developmental age norms for acquiring different skills and can provide insight as to what is affecting the child's ability to attain certain skills.

For example, a parent may report, "My child is unable to draw his prewriting shapes and therefore needs occupational therapy." After reviewing the child's work samples, the therapist may find that the child is able to complete the prewriting shapes that are developmentally appropriate for his age (e.g., the child just turned 4 years old and can copy a vertical line, horizontal line, circle, and cross but cannot yet draw a square or triangle, which is normally achieved at age 5. Because the parent does not know the age norms for drawing prewriting shapes, she would not know that her son was able to draw age-appropriate shapes. It also is important for therapists to observe the teacher's expectations of the children to ensure that teachers are not requiring them to perform tasks that are developmentally inappropriate and may lead to frustration (e.g., requiring a 3-year-old to write his or her first name).

In many classrooms, children are required to complete "must-do" tasks each day. This usually includes a manipulative task or art activity. Other classrooms have centers that the children rotate between that incorporate working on different skills (e.g., dramatic play center, block center, art center). Therapists can assist teachers in structuring tasks that can be completed during these times that focus on fine motor skills. This may include having children complete puzzles; string beads; use manipulatives or play dough activities that require tools; perform resistive manipulative tasks like pop beads and pop tubes; and work on prewriting, writing, and cutting tasks. Because the children would be divided into smaller groups, the teacher or classroom assistants can devote individual time to children.

Individual time is particularly important when working on prewriting and writing skills. Many times teachers set out name templates for children to trace over or practice copying their names. While the children are practicing tracing their name, no one is providing individualized instruction on how to form the letters, leading to the child drawing over the letters but not forming them using proper letter formation. The occupational therapist can suggest that this task be incorporated into a smaller group time, when the teacher or assistant can teach the actual formations. Once the children have demonstrat-

ed mastery of the formations, this skill could be reinforced daily by having them write their names independently on art projects or papers. It is important to ensure that all individuals working with the children (e.g., parent, teacher, assistant, occupational therapist) are introducing the letter formations the same way. It is important for therapists to check with teachers and educate parents to ensure that they are familiar with either the writing curriculum used by the school district or an adapted curriculum that, in the therapist's and teacher's professional opinions, would be most successful for the child to use.

As discussed in Chapter 5, the development of hand skills should be a fundamental part of a preschool program for children ages 3 to 5. During the preschool years, children are increasing their repertoire of fine motor function through learning to use their hands to interact with a variety of objects; refining their grasp and release skills; using their hands together to complete more refined tasks, including cutting, writing, and pulling apart or pushing together toys; and stabilizing objects with one hand while manipulating an object with the other hand. Children also further develop their in-hand manipulation skills, which affects their ability to interact with objects with increased refinement and their ability to complete self-care tasks (e.g., buttoning, zipping). Children are beginning to use tools to complete a variety of tasks including feeding (e.g., using utensils, pouring from a pitcher), prewriting (e.g., grasping a writing utensil), and cutting (e.g., positioning scissors correctly, opening and closing the scissors to cut paper). Case-Smith and Beery (1996) have discussed the numerous components that contribute to the child's development of hand function, including

- *Biomechanical components*—Range of motion, postural control, muscle tone
- *Somatosensory components*—Tactile and proprioceptive input

- *Visual–perceptual skills*—Position in space, figure ground, spatial relations, visual–motor integration, form constancy
- *Cognitive components*—Attention, interaction, planning/sequencing, problem solving, levels of play, learning
- *Neuromotor components*—Motor control, coordination/dexterity, strength, in-hand manipulation, bilateral coordination
- *Psychosocial components*—Motivation, interpersonal skills, self-concept, and coping skills.

Through observation and assessment, occupational therapists can be instrumental in observing and identifying the specific hand skill components with which children are having difficulty. (See Chapter 5 for information about the developmental age norms for acquiring hand skills and for detailed information related to the evaluation of hand skills.) In addition to identifying a child's hand skill deficits, the occupational therapist can recommend activities to incorporate into the school day to focus on specific skills and to discuss the proper positioning of activities or materials.

For example, the occupational therapist can recommend that the teacher attach pegboards to a wall in the classroom to provide a vertical surface for the child. This encourages children to use wrist extension when placing pegs into the pegboard versus using wrist flexion, which is commonly seen when inserting the pegs into a pegboard that is positioned on a flat surface. The therapist also may recommend presenting small snack items to children in a raised vertical position to support using a three-finger or pincer grasp to grasp the object and bring it to their mouth. When food items are left on the table, children may rake the items into their palms using all fingers as a unit instead of isolating the index finger against the thumb to pick them up.

In addition to providing recommendations about the positioning or presentation of items to support the development of a child's hand skills, occupational therapists also can develop activities and order equipment for activities that target specific hand skills in the classroom setting. This may include equipment that focuses on the development of a three-finger grasp. All of the equipment could be housed in separate bins that are labeled for the skills they target and brought out during centers or individual work time during the school day. Hand skills development may include

- Doing Theraputty activities
- Picking up coins and placing them in a piggy bank or resistive container
- Doing resistive pegboard activities or Geoboards
- Using wind-up toys and spinning tops for older children
- Popping bubbles on packing material
- Attaching clothespins to a surface (could match labeled clothespins to letters in name, numbers, colors)
- Using tweezers, test tube holders, or tongs to pick up objects (e.g., cotton balls, fabric balls, LEGOs™)
- Using eyedroppers to paint or to collect and release water
- Using squirt bottles to water flowers in the classroom or to erase the chalkboard
- Doing resistive activities using pop beads or pop tubes
- Screwing and unscrewing tiny nuts and bolts
- Playing commercial games like Lite-Brite™ and Connect Four.

Similar fine motor bins containing activities could be made for bilateral skills, prewriting skills, and preparation activities for cutting. Prior to having the children engage in an activity, the teacher could pull out the specific bins and conduct a preparation activity that focuses on that skill (e.g., have children use tweezer scissors or tongs to pick up objects and place them into a container as preparation for a cutting task). Many preparation activities can be incorporated naturally into the school day. Teachers may incorporate an activity for cutting during snack time by having the children use tongs to pick up their snack foods. Teachers can incorporate instruction on drawing prewriting shapes by having the children circle or draw a square or rectangle around their name to sign in at the beginning of day for attendance. Finding ways to incorporate fine motor and visual–motor or visual–perceptual activities naturally into the school day reinforces the skills on a daily basis.

Children With Autism and Cognitive Impairments

Many teachers who have children with autism spectrum disorder in their classrooms incorporate instruction techniques from the TEACCH curriculum (Treatment and Education of Autistic and Related Communication Handicapped Children; Lord & Schopler, 1994), a program founded in 1972 at the Department of Psychiatry at the University of North Carolina at Chapel Hill. The curriculum includes providing structured teaching to children. At the preschool level this involves having children learn individually or in small groups, with an emphasis placed on structuring the environment to increase the development of communication and social skills, fine and gross motor development, and self-help skills. Teachers organize the room so that specific tasks always occur in defined areas of the room. This structure allows children to predict what events will occur in each area and be prepared for those events to occur. The teacher could designate areas of the room for cognitive preacademic tasks and fine motor tasks, self-care, and play (to work on socialization skills and interactive play skills). The children have individual daily schedules posted at a convenient area in the classroom so that they are visible from all areas of the room.

Common activities incorporated into the children's individual workstations are called "bin tasks" or "shoe box tasks" (premade tasks can be ordered from www.shoeboxtasks.com). These tasks work on specific cognitive and fine motor abilities and become progressively more difficult (increasing the complexity of the task and the number of steps) over time as the child masters the beginning bin tasks. These tasks can be designed to meet each student's developmental level and individualized needs. Examples include picking up items and placing them into a container, sorting items by similarity, and completing multistep tasks such as placing pegs inside a film canister or putting a toothbrush in a toothbrush holder.

Using this type of program is very effective for children with autism or cognitive impairments and attention issues because

- It provides structure to the children's day and can be incorporated into their daily picture schedule
- It provides a defined beginning and end to an activity (e.g., complete two bin tasks and then you will be done)
- It provides a way for the children to complete tasks independently and
- It provides a graded program by increasing the level of difficulty and duration of completing work tasks over time.

[handwritten: Let them choose the boxes you want them to use.]

Occupational therapists can assist with this process by ordering or making the shoebox tasks. Therapists also can design other tasks or suggest activities that could be incorporated into the children's work system time that target fine motor, perceptual–motor, or self-help skills.

Occupational therapists can assist teachers when placing their classroom orders each school year by helping them determine what types of activities to focus on. Therapists can make recommendations for effective and fun fine motor activities that target various skills (including facilitating a pincer grasp, bilateral hand skill development, upper extremity and finger strength, and in-hand manipulation skills) and can recommend adapted equipment (including pencil grippers, Handiwriters, slant boards, and adapted scissors).

Children With Deficits in Self-Help Skills

Self-help tasks commonly expected of preschool children during the school day include putting on, taking off, and hanging a coat on a hook; assisting with managing clothing fasteners; zipping and unzipping a book bag; putting items in and taking items out of a book bag; toileting and hand washing; and finger feeding, using utensils, pouring liquid into a cup using a pitcher, and drinking from a regular cup. Therapists can educate all team members on what is developmentally appropriate for each child.

When identifying what tasks a child is having difficulty with, it is important that occupational therapists keep in mind developmental ages for the acquisition of certain skills to ensure realistic expectations for each child.

Managing Coat and Book Bag. Depending on the child's cognitive level and severity of the disability, 3- and 4-year-old children should be encouraged to assist with putting on and taking off their jackets and pulling the zipper up and down once it has been engaged by an adult. Zipper pulls attached to jackets often help children better grasp the zipper to pull it up and down. Children often are more successful using the "flip-over method" to put on their jackets, which allows a child to simply place his or her arms through the sleeves of the jacket and flip it over the head. Older preschool children (ages 5–6 years) may be encouraged to practice the traditional method of putting on their coats. Chapter 4 provides developmental age ranges for all clothing fasteners and can help therapists be realistic when writing goals and objectives.

Occupational therapists should ensure that a child's book bag is not too difficult to manage. Many types of book bags are available for children, ranging from an open bag without a fastener, a book bag with a zipper, or a suitcase-style bag on wheels. If the child is unable to open the zipper (even after a zipper pull is attached), the therapist may recommend that the parent buy a bag that is open and does not require the child to manage a fastener. The therapist also should ensure that the child's book bag is not too large or too heavy to carry.

Occupational therapists need to ensure that children have access to their hooks to hang up coats and book bags. Children who demonstrate difficulty hanging up their belongings may benefit from having their hooks positioned at the end of the row (where they do not have to stand in the middle of other children while completing the task). If a child's hook is too high, it should be lowered for easier access, or a bench should be provided for the child to stand on while completing the task. If a child has difficulty locating the hook, highlighting the hook using paint may assist in distinguishing the child's hook from others in the class.

If a child is easily distracted while completing this task as other children are completing it, he or she may benefit from being dismissed a few minutes early to begin putting on his or her coat at the end of the day or allowed to take off his or her coat a few minutes after class begins at the start of the day. This limits the distractions within the hallway or classroom so that the child can focus on the task.

Using a picture schedule also will assist a child with completing this daily routine. The picture cues can be aligned directly above the child's hook or cubby to reference. Over time, an adult can prompt the child to reference the picture icon schedule instead of having to provide more restrictive cueing.

Hand Washing/Toileting. A child may benefit from using a picture icon schedule to break down the steps required for hand-washing and toileting. The child can reference the pictures to complete the individual steps. (See Chapter 4 for intervention strategies for targeting effective hand washing.)

Through a consultative model, occupational therapists may be able to assist teachers and parents with helping the child gain more independence in toileting. There are usually established times during the school day in which the children use the restroom. The child would be encouraged to go at this specific time. In addition, children who are just beginning to work on toilet training may benefit from having toileting included in the schedule more frequently. The therapist should observe the toileting process to determine what step the child is having difficulty with (e.g., managing pulling clothing up and down, wiping, reaching the toilet to sit on or stand in front of) and then target intervention strategies for those individual steps.

Snack Time. During snack time, children are encouraged to spread out their napkins, take their snack items from a bowl, pour their own juice or water, feed themselves using their hands or utensils, and drink from a regular cup. This is an instrumental time for teachers and occupational therapists to work on a variety of skills.

If a child is having difficulty picking up food items using a three-finger grasp or continues to eat off of his or her palm or the side of his or her hand, an adult should position food items in a vertical plane in front of the child. The child also may be encouraged to wear a mitten that has been cut, allowing for only the thumb, index finger, and middle finger to be exposed. The therapist can try a variety of utensils and cups to determine which type the child has the greatest success using. For a child who is just learning to use a spoon or fork, raising the plate or bowl up off of the table will bring the bowl closer and decrease the distance he or she has to keep the food on the spoon. This also may assist in decreasing spilling. (See Chapter 4 for more specific techniques for working on feeding skills with children.)

Summary and Conclusion

Occupational therapists are involved in many aspects related to delivering services to preschool children with disabilities. This includes evaluating children who may qualify for special education services or who are already receiving special education services. Therapists should become familiar with the federal law and their individual state laws and regulations that define the standards for qualification as a preschooler with a disability.

When evaluating children, occupational therapists should incorporate a variety of techniques, including using standardized assessments, interviewing the child's parents and teachers, and observing the child at home or at school. The data collected from the assessment should be reviewed with the educational team and compared to the child's overall developmental level to determine if he or she would benefit from occupational therapy.

Therapists should not jump into providing direct service for all children; instead, the educational team should consider whether direct services are needed or whether the consultative or collaboration model of service would be a better option. Therapists need to keep the lines of communication open with the child's teachers and parents to ensure consistency and reinforcement of skills in all settings. Interventions can be designed to target specific skills and should be incorporated naturally into the child's daily curriculum.

References

Beery, K. E. (1997). *The Beery–Buktenica Developmental Test of Visual Motor Integration* (4th ed., rev.). Parsippany, NJ: Modern Curriculum Press.

Berk, R. A., & DeGangi, G. A. (1983). *DeGangi–Berk Test of Sensory Integration*. Los Angeles, CA: Western Psychological Services.

Brigance, A. H. (1978). *Diagnostic Inventory of Early Development*. North Billerica, MA: Curriculum Associates.

Bruininks, R. H. (1978). *The Bruininks–Oseretsky Test of Motor Proficiency*. Circle Pines, MN: American Guidance Service.

Case-Smith, J., & Berry, J. (1998). Preschool hand skills. In J. Case-Smith (Ed.), *Making a difference in school system practice* (pp. 1–41). Bethesda, MD: American Occupational Therapy Association.

Dreiling, D. S., & Bundy, A. C. (2003). Brief report: A comparison of consultative model and direct–indirect intervention with preschoolers. *American Journal of Occupational Therapy, 57,* 566–569.

Dunn, W. (1999). *Sensory Profile*. San Antonio, TX: Psychological Corporation.

Dunn, W., et al. (1989). *Guidelines for occupational therapy in early intervention and preschool services*. Rockville, MD: American Occupational Therapy Association.

Education for All Handicapped Children Act of 1975, P.L. 94-142, 20 U.S.C. §1401.

Education of the Handicapped Amendments of 1986, P.L. 94-457, 20 U.S.C. §1401.

Folio, M. R., & Fewell, R. R. (2000). *Peabody Developmental Motor Scales* (2nd ed.). Austin, TX: Pro-Ed.

Gartland, S. (2001). Occupational therapy in preschool and child care settings. In J. Case-Smith (Ed.), *Occupational therapy for children* (4th ed., pp. 731–755). St. Louis, MO: Mosby.

Haley, S. M., Coster, W. L., Ludlow, L. H., Haltiwanger, J. T., & Andrellos, P. J. (1992). *Pediatric Evaluation of Disability Inventory*. Boston: New England Medical Center Hospital & PEDI Research Group.

Individuals With Disabilities Education Act, P.L. 102-119, 20 U.S.C. §1401 (1991).

Lord, C., & Schopler, E. (1994). TEACCH services for preschool children. In S. L. Harris & J. S. Handleman (Eds.), *Preschool education programs for children with autism* (pp. 87–106). Austin, TX: Pro-Ed.

Miller, L. J. (1988). *Miller Assessment for Preschoolers*. San Antonio, TX: Psychological Corporation.

Neisworth, J. T., Bagnato, S. J., Salvia, J., & Hunt, F. M. (1999). *Temperament and Atypical Behavior Scale*. Baltimore, MD: Paul H. Brookes.

Newborg, J., Stock, J. R., Wnek, L., Guidubaldi, J., & Suinicki, A. (1988). *Batelle Developmental Inventory*. Chicago: Riverside.

Ohio Department of Education. (2002). *Operating standards for Ohio's schools serving children with disabilities*. Columbus: Author.

Reisman, J. E., & Hanschu, B. (1992). *Sensory Integration Inventory–Revised for individuals with developmental disabilities*. Hugo, MN: PDP Press.

Richardson, P. K. (2001). Use of standardized tests in pediatric practice. In J. Case-Smith (Ed.), *Occupational therapy for children* (4th ed., pp. 217–245). St. Louis, MO: Mosby.

Richardson, P. K., & Schultz-Krohn, W. (2001). Planning and implementing services. In J. Case-Smith (Ed.), *Occupational therapy for children* (4th ed., pp. 246–264). St. Louis, MO: Mosby.

Appendix 7.1.
Preschool Functional Educational Checklist

The intent of the Preschool Functional Educational Checklist is to help occupational therapists identify skills that a child currently possesses and to define areas of concern that may affect the child's ability to complete a variety of tasks in the preschool setting.

The checklist can be sent to the child's parents, classroom teacher (if a child received early intervention services or attended a private preschool), or special education teacher (for a child already in an integrated preschool program) to complete prior to the therapist observing and evaluating the child.

The checklist can be used by the therapist as a tool to interview the child's teacher or parents to help identify areas that may affect the child's ability to complete tasks at home or at school.

If the Preschool Functional Educational Checklist has already been filled out, the therapist still will need to meet with the person who completed it to review the responses and ask additional information. Based on those responses, the therapist should observe and evaluate the areas of concern that have been identified as affecting the child's ability to function in school.

Interpretation of Results

An interpretation section is included to help occupational therapists summarize and synthesize the information identified on the checklist by identifying the components that the child is lacking to perform specific tasks and to list strategies that can be used to remediate the skill deficits. This provides the therapist with information that can be used

when developing goals and objectives on a student's IEP.

After completing the observation and direct evaluation, the therapist should complete the interpretation section at the end of the checklist.

In Section I, the therapist should identify the specific areas of concern that appear to have the greatest impact on the child's ability to function in the school setting. If there are many areas, the therapist should attempt to prioritize those that seem to have the greatest impact. Input from classroom staff may be necessary to do this.

In Section II, the therapist should list the components that are preventing the child from completing the tasks identified in Section I to look for common components. If there appear to be other factors—such as lack of attention, inability to understand what was being asked, or refusal to perform the request or task—those factors also should be listed, especially if it appears that the child has the motor components to complete a task.

The intent of Section III is to encourage the therapist to identify specific intervention strategies (or preparation tasks) to address the components identified in Section II rather than having the child practice the task he or she was unable to complete. An example of this would be giving the child small pieces of food during snack time to get him or her to use a three-finger grasp. The intent would be to work on specific intervention strategies needed to develop the grasp. The therapist would follow up by giving him or her small pieces of food at the end of the session to see if the grasp has changed.

Preschool Functional Educational Checklist

Child _____

Date of Birth _____

Teacher _____

School   AM   PM _____

Age _____

Therapist _____

Person Completing Form _____

Date _____

I. Areas of Concern

___ Fine Motor   ___ Gross Motor

___ Self-Care   ___ Sensory–Motor

II. Areas of Qualification (Check the specific areas in which the child initially qualified as a preschooler with a disability)

___ Adaptive Behavior   ___ Cognitive Ability

___ Communication   ___ Gross/Fine Motor

___ Hearing Ability   ___ Pre-academic Skills

___ Social/Emotional/   ___ Vision Ability
Behavioral

III. Specific Concerns (Please complete sections in specific areas of concern)

A. Hand Use/Fine Motor

Yes   No   Does the child:

___ ___ 1. Does the child use a preferred hand? Which one? _____

___ ___ 2a. Is the child able to isolate the index finger to point?

___ ___ 2b. Is the child able to push down and activate a toy using the index finger?

___ ___ 3a. When an object is placed in the child's hand, will the child grasp the object?

___ ___ 3b. When an object is presented, does child pick it up and hold it?

4. When the child picks up small objects, which of the following grasps are observed? (Please check)

___ Raking grasp (uses all fingers to rake objects into palm)

___ 3-finger grasp (grasp object with thumb and 1st and 2nd fingers)

___ 2-finger grasp (grasp object with thumb and index finger)

___ ___ 5. Is the child able to release an object into a designated area?

6. What is the smallest item the child is able to release (e.g., stuffed animal, block, cereal)? _____

___ ___ 7. Is the child able to bring his or her hands together to play with an object or to clap?

___ ___ 8. When holding an object, will the child transfer it to the opposite hand?

___ ___ 9. Does the child use one hand to hold or stabilize an object while performing a task with the other hand (e.g., stirring, stringing beads, playing musical instruments, putting notebook into book bag, holding paper while cutting or writing)?

Tool Use

Yes   No

___ ___ 1. Does the child use a fisted grasp when holding a writing utensil?

___ ___ 2. Does the child use a 3-finger grasp (grasp with thumb and pad of index finger with utensil resting against side of middle finger)?

___ ___ 3. Does the child position scissors correctly in fingers?

B. Visual–Motor

Yes   No

___ ___ 1. Does the child visually attend to objects during interaction (e.g., cutting, prewriting tasks)?

(continued)

___ ___ 2. Can the child complete a 3-shape form board?

3. Is the child able to copy the shapes listed below as commensurate with the child's ages as stated on the Test of Visual–Motor Integration (Beery, 1997)?

Shape	Chronological Age
___ ___ Vertical line	2–10
___ ___ Horizontal line	3–0
___ ___ Circle	3–0
___ ___ Cross	4–1
___ ___ Right diagonal line (/)	4–4
___ ___ Square	4–6
___ ___ Left diagonal line (\)	4–7
___ ___ X	4–11
___ ___ Triangle	5–3

4. When coloring: (Please include work sample)

___ The child makes random marks on the paper.

___ The child attempts to remain in defined area.

___ The child fills approximately ____ amount of the shape/area.

___ ___ 5a. Has printing students' name been introduced in the classroom?

___ ___ 5b. Can the child independently trace the letters in his or her first name?

___ ___ 5c. Can the child independently print his or her name when given a model?

___ ___ 5d. Can the child independently print his or her name without a model?

___ ___ 6a. Can the child snip paper with scissors?

___ ___ 6b. Can the child cut a piece of 8 ½" x 11" paper in half?

___ ___ 6c. Can the child cut on a straight line?

___ ___ 6d. Can the child cut out a circle?

___ ___ 6e. Can the child cut out a square?

C. Self-Care/Adaptive Behavior

Yes   No

___ ___ 1. Is the child able to self-feed a variety of sizes of finger foods?

___ ___ 2. Is the child able to use a spoon to self-feed?

___ ___ 3. Can the child pour liquid from a pitcher without spilling?

___ ___ 4. Is the child able to drink from a regular cup without spilling?

___ ___ 5. Is the child able to place a cup on the table after drinking?

___ ___ 6. Is the child able to suck from a straw?

___ ___ 7. Is the child able to wash his or her hands? If "no," what steps can the child complete? _____

___ ___ 8. Is the child independent with toileting? If "no," what steps can the child complete?

_____

___ ___ 9. Is the child able to put on and take off a coat? What method is used for putting the coat on (e.g., traditional method or flip-over method)? _____

___ ___ 10. Is the child able to thread the zipper on a jacket and pull the zipper up and down?

___ ___ 11. Is the child able to put on and take off and open and close a book bag?

___ ___ 12. Is the child able to hang up a coat and book bag on a hook?

___ ___ 13. Can the child put shoes on the correct feet?

D. Gross Motor

Yes   No

___ ___ 1. Is the child able to sit and stand independently and unsupported?

___ ___ 2a. Can the child stand on one foot?

___ ___ 2b. Can the child jump up, clearing both feet off of the ground?

___ ___ 2c. Can the child hop on one foot?

(continued)

__ __ 3. Describe how the child walks up and down the stairs: _____
_____

__ __ 4. Is the child able to keep up with peers when (please check):

___ Walking down the hall in line?

___ Walking up and down stairs?

__ __ 5. Is the child able to run?

__ __ 6. Is the child able to get on and off a riding toy?

__ __ 7. Is the child able to pedal a tricycle?

__ __ 8a. Can the child get in and out of a small chair?

__ __ 8b. Can the child push a chair toward and from the table?

__ __ 9. Can the child get up from and down onto the floor?

__ __ 10. Can the child manage self on different terrains (e.g., grass, gravel, carpet, going up a hill)?

__ __ 11. Can the child navigate around and over objects on the floor?

__ __ 12. Can the child maintain balance when challenged?

__ __ 13. Does the child trip or fall easily?

__ __ 14. Can the child access playground equipment that is appropriate for his or her size?

E. Sensory–Motor

Yes No

Tactile

__ __ 1. Can the child tolerate others in his or her personal space (e.g., during circle time, in line, free play)?

__ __ 2. Can the child tolerate a variety of textures on his or her hands (e.g., glue, finger paint, shaving cream, sand)?

__ __ 3. Does the child appear irritated by certain clothing textures (e.g., does the child itch or push up his or her sleeves)?

__ __ 4. Does the child resist having his or her face or hands washed?

__ __ 5. Does the child have specific and/or limited food preferences?

Vestibular

__ __ 6. Does the child resist utilizing playground equipment? What type?_____
_____
_____

__ __ 7. Does the child appear fearful or cautious with movement (e.g., on steps, when climbing or walking)?

Proprioceptive

__ __ 8. Is the child clumsy or awkward?

__ __ 9. Does the child display self-abusive or self-stimulatory behaviors (e.g., hitting self, head banging)? Describe:_____
_____
_____

__ __ 10. Does the child bump into objects?

__ __ 11. Is the child a messy eater?

Auditory

__ __ 12. Does the child appear sensitive to sounds in the classroom (e.g., loud toys, other children talking, school bell, fire alarms)?

__ __ 13. What does the child do to demonstrate that he or she is sensitive to sounds (e.g., cover ears)? Describe:_____
_____
_____

F. Miscellaneous

Yes No

__ __ 1. Is the child able to follow 2–3-step directions?

__ __ 2. Does the child display a high level of activity?

__ __ 3. Is the child able to maintain the attention needed to complete a task?

(continued)

Interpretation Section (For therapist's use only):

1. Identify the specific areas of concern (e.g., child is unable to manage coat and book bag, child is unable to drink from a regular cup).

_____

_____

_____

_____

_____

_____

_____

2. What is interfering with the child's ability to complete the identified tasks (e.g., child does not demonstrate proper lip closure around the cup when drinking, child has difficulty coordinating using two hands together to complete bilateral tasks)?

_____

_____

_____

_____

_____

_____

_____

_____

3. What intervention strategies will be used to remediate the skill deficit(s)?

_____

_____

_____

_____

_____

_____

_____

_____

Created by Lynne Pape, MEd, OTR/L, and Kelly Ryba, OTR/L
Updated 5/04

Sensory-Based Issues: Identification, Evaluation, and Program Development

8

Sensory stimulation bombards students each day at school: loud noises on the bus, in the cafeteria, in the classroom, and during physical education class and visual input on classroom walls, worksheets, and textbooks. During this, children have to sustain their attention to lessons and tasks.

Students with typically developing sensory processing abilities are able to take in all of this information and filter out nonrelevant information to remain calm and organized to attend to and learn from lessons. To assist with remaining attentive and focused on tasks throughout the day, typically developing children may be observed to engage in behaviors such as chewing their fingernails, shaking their legs under the desk, fidgeting with objects, and taking a break to get a drink of water. Children with deficits in sensory processing skills have difficulty remaining focused on classwork or engaging in teacher-directed lessons and are observed to engage in more noticeable behaviors such as not being able to sit still, constantly fidgeting with objects in their hands or mouth, and having difficulty following directions to complete classroom tasks (especially directions including multiple steps) or following the class routine. These behaviors affect students' ability to learn and benefit from an education.

Children have two main occupations: school and play (Haack & Haldy, 1998). In regard to the occupation of school, a child's responsibilities start before entering the school building. He or she must complete numerous tasks in order to be ready to go to school each day, including bathing, brushing teeth, get-ting dressed, eating breakfast, packing a book bag, putting on a coat, and catching the bus or walking to school. At school, the child has to attend and participate in class lessons, follow directions and manage the classroom routine, work cooperatively with peers, complete all necessary academic assignments, manage self-help tasks (e.g., toileting, managing clothing fasteners and personal belongings), and participate appropriately in nonacademic extracurricular activities (e.g., clubs, sports).

Play occurs both at school and at home. At school, the child is expected to play cooperatively with peers during recess, physical education activities, and classroom games or activities. Outside of school, the child may be involved in extracurricular activities or engage in play with siblings or peers at home. Play involves working cooperatively with others, understanding the function of toys to allow for increased imagination and creativity, and being able to socially interact in an appropriate manner with other children of similar age groups. For a student with a deficit in sensory processing skills, the ability to effectively and successfully complete the responsibilities of his or her occupations (of school and play) may be affected.

This chapter provides an overview of the major sensory systems, describes observable characteristics of dysfunction in sensory processing skills, and discusses common sensory-based problems that are observed in a school setting. The chapter also reviews evaluation techniques (including both formal and informal assessments) for identifying sensory-based problems, service delivery options, and interventions and classroom modifications.

Overview of Sensory Integration Theory

Dr. A. Jean Ayres (1979) described *sensory integration* as "the organization of sensation for use" (p. 5). Sensations provide the body with a multitude of information about the environment. If the sensations flow in a well-organized manner and the brain is working effectively, it can use the sensory input to form perceptions and behaviors to learn from the experience. Effective sensory integration abilities lead to successful adaptive responses to environmental situations.

Ayres (1979) defined an *adaptive response* as a "purposeful, goal-directed response to a sensory experience" (p. 6). Adaptive responses include pedaling a bicycle, reaching for a toy, or throwing a ball toward a basketball hoop.

Sensory integration is viewed as a dynamic process. An individual does not simply gather and process information from one sensory system at a time; he or she gathers information from multiple sensory systems and integrates all of the input to respond in an organized manner. The sensory systems depend on each other and work together to produce an effective response, which is the basis for the sensory–motor–sensory feedback cycle. The body takes in sensory input, processes the input to produce a motor response, and provides sensory feedback to the body. Over time, if the process works correctly, the body builds on this feedback to produce quality adapted responses. If a breakdown occurs at any step in the cycle, the ability to produce adapted responses may be affected.

Three major postulates to the sensory integration theory originally were developed by Ayres (Fischer & Murray, 1991). These postulates provide an understanding of sensory integration and how to gear intervention for those with deficits:

1. Individuals take in sensory information from the environment and movement of the body, the central nervous system processes and integrates these sensory inputs, and individuals use the sensory information to organize their behavior.
2. Deficits in sensory integration results in deficits in conceptual and motor learning.
3. Providing sensory experiences within the context of a meaningful activity and the planning and production of an adaptive response results in enhanced sensory integration and, in turn, enhanced learning.

Fisher and Murray's discussion of the assumptions that underlie the postulates of sensory integration theory are described in Table 8.1.

According to Ayres (1979), children have an inner drive to seek out sensory input from the environment. Based on the feedback from this interaction, children are able to process a multitude of sensory input that allows them to respond appropriately and successfully to the situation. Over time, as children increase their exposure to different sensory experiences, they are able to build on basic experiences and function in more complex ways. Children may no longer have to think about and process every aspect of the experience because it is already a part of their memory. This allows them to build on their experiences and apply their foundational knowledge to novel and more complex tasks.

Ayres's research and sensory integration theory were based on children with learning disabilities without overt brain damage. The children had to demonstrate evidence of underlying deficits in the central processing of proprioceptive, vestibular, or tactile sensory inputs that were not attributed to peripheral or cortical central nervous system damage (Fisher & Murray, 1991). It was understood that children with damage to the central nervous system (e.g., cerebral palsy, mental retardation) may show coinciding deficits in processing sensory information (e.g., abnormalities in muscle tone, tolerating tactile

Table 8.1. Postulates for Sensory Integration Theory

Neural plasticity	The ability of the brain structures to be changed or modified over time as a result of ongoing sensory experiences (tactile, proprioceptive, and vestibular).
Sensory integration occurs as a developmental sequence	In normal development, the child is presented with increasingly complex behaviors, and as a result of the sensory–motor–sensory feedback loop, the child develops increasingly complex responses to the behaviors.
Nervous system hierarchy	The brain functions as an integrated whole but consists of systems that are hierarchically organized. "Higher level" functions (cortical structures) emerge and are dependent on "lower level" functions (subcortical structures).
Adaptive response/behavior	Purposeful and goal-directed movement allows an individual to successfully meet "just-right challenges" and learn something new. Adaptive behavior supports sensory integration, and thus the ability to produce adaptive responses is dependent on sensory integration. If any step of the process is incorrect, the child is unable to have an adaptive response.
Inner drive	Each person has an inner drive to develop sensory integration through participation in sensory activities in the environment.

Adapted from "Integration to sensory integration theory" by A. G. Fisher & E. A. Murray. In A. G. Fisher, E. A. Murray, & A. C. Bundy (Eds.), *Sensory integration: Theory and practice* (pp. 3–26), © 1991 by F. A. Davis. Adapted with permission.

input, proximal stability, equilibrium responses, and motor coordination), but these deficits may be a result of the damage to the brain rather than a deficit in integrating sensory input.

Sensorimotor intervention techniques often are used and may prove beneficial for both types of students. Fisher and Murray (1991) stated that, when implementing sensory treatment techniques, it is important to differentiate between a sensory integration treatment program, which may be implemented for students who have difficulty with sensory integration, "and a sensorimotor treatment program into which sensory integration treatment procedures have been incorporated," as would be the case when implementing sensory techniques for a student with cerebral palsy.

Sensory Integration in Child Development

In the first few years of a child's life, he or she is presented with a variety of experiences that allow him or her to move from being completely dependent on adults for basic needs to gaining control over his or her body and the environment. During this time, a child develops head, neck, and trunk stability; sits independently; and becomes mobile, beginning to crawl and walk and then maneuvering through the environment. The child gains the ability to sustain visual attention on and follow a moving object, reach for objects or toys using the hands, and refines hand skills to use tools. The child gains independence in self-care tasks (e.g., drinking from a cup, assisting with dressing and toileting), which affects overall self-esteem and sense of accomplishment.

All of the sensations that a child actively takes in over the first few years of life are organized in the nervous system to enable him or her to learn from the experience and about the environment. Ayres (1979) described the development of a child as follows:

- *Birth–6 months:* During the first 6 months of life, children move from predominantly reflexive movement to more purposeful active movement. Children's hands are no longer controlled by the grasping reflex, and, by age 6 months, they are able to use a pincer grasp to pick up objects and use their hands together to interact with toys. Children develop the ability to gain head and neck stability, which affects their ability to keep their eyes stable on an object or a person. By the sixth month, children can look at their hands as they play with toys, can visually track an object in different planes, and can follow a moving object. As children gain more extension throughout the body, they are able to maintain a prone extension position and begin to bear weight on extended forearms and hands in prone to play with toys. They begin to sit up independently without losing their balance. By age 6 months, children enjoy a variety of movement input (e.g., being rocked to sleep by a parent, rolling over).

- *6–12 months:* During this stage, children begin to develop bilateral control through crawling, creeping, and pulling to stand. Children refine their hand skills by using a pincer grasp to pick up and manipulate small objects, crossing midline to reach for or play with objects, and beginning to hold objects and tools within their hands to interact with toys (e.g., using a hammer to pound a ball into a hole). With movement comes exploration of the environment. Children now begin to understand the space around them and the relative distance between objects in the environment. Children also begin to search out toys in certain locations (e.g., a toy cabinet or basket).

- *1–2 years:* Children now can walk and are very interested in interacting and moving in the environment. At this point they begin to gain body awareness. They begin to talk and interact with people and are able to understand and follow directions given by an adult. They attempt to exert independence and do not always want to follow directions. They interact in increasingly complex ways with toys and become creative in their play with toys. Their tac-

tile discrimination skills are becoming refined, enabling them to purposefully interact with toys in a more sophisticated way.

- *3–7 years:* Children can plan for and sequence more complex gross motor movements that may require eye–hand coordination and balance (e.g., soccer, riding a bike). They are further developing their cognitive and language skills (both receptive and expressive) and can rely more on their auditory skills than visual skills to understand and complete tasks. They develop the ability to use tools in a refined way (e.g., using feeding utensils, writing utensils, scissors) to complete self-care (e.g., managing fasteners, opening containers) and fine motor tasks (e.g., writing, cutting, playing with toys).

During these formative years it is crucial that children be presented with opportunities to take in and actively participate in an environment that provides enriched sensory input. Children need to experience weight bearing through their arms to fully develop the palmar arches and to gain shoulder stability that will later affect tool use as it relates to writing. Children need to be given the opportunity to be mobile in the environment (through crawling or walking) to begin to develop balance, body awareness, and spatial relations skills. Movement input (including being rocked, going down a slide, jumping on a trampoline, or swinging on a swing) provide a child's body with a variety of tactile, proprioceptive, and vestibular input that further assist the child to develop the previously mentioned skills. Children who have been deprived of this vital sensory input (e.g., a child who has been neglected or abused, a child who spent a large amount of time in a crib) lacked receiving this variety of sensory input early in life. This may affect their ability to meet motor milestones, tolerate sensory input (especially tactile and vestibular input), and develop the early social emotional and cognitive skills that come with interacting with toys and other people.

Neurological Background

According to Ayres (1979), "over 80% of the nervous system is involved in processing or organizing sensory input" (p. 28). Neurons (nerve cells) comprise a cell body, dendrites (which receive messages), and an axon (which sends impulses from the cell body to dendrites of other nerve cells). Sensory and motor neurons connect the brain and spinal cord to the rest of the body. Sensory neurons contain specialized receptor cells that target each type of sensory stimuli. These receptors receive input from the body or from the environment and are able to sense the intensity, duration, and location of stimuli. They travel and connect to other neurons (either sensory or motor) in the body to produce a response, inhibitory or excitatory. Motor neurons receive input from sensory receptors and produce a specific motor response to the given input. These sensory and motor responses provide feedback to the brain and body.

The nervous system comprises many parts that have specific functions related to the processing and integrating of sensory stimulation. The spinal cord contains the nerve tracts that carry sensory information to the brain and then carry the motor output from the brain back down to the nerves, which transmits to the body's muscles and organs. A limited amount of sensory integration occurs at the spinal cord level, but the information does travel through this area. Some reflexes are generated at the spinal cord level, including the muscle stretch reflex and knee-jerk reflex (Murray-Slutsky & Paris, 2000).

The brain stem and midbrain area is vital to the sensory integration process. This level contains the reticular formation, pons, hypothalamus, and thalamus. The brain stem is considered the crossroads of the brain. Input from the left side of the body crosses to the right hemisphere, and information from the right side of the body is directed to the left hemisphere. This results in communication between the two sides of the brain to direct the movement responses.

The reticular formation is spread throughout the pons, hypothalamus, and thalamus (described below; Murray-Slutsky & Paris, 2000). Many types of sensory input converge in this area. The reticular formation acts as a "filter" to sensory input and is responsible for connecting every sensory system to motor neurons and other parts of the brain. It contributes in regulating arousal states (e.g., awake, asleep, alertness and attention levels). It also is involved in processing vestibular sensations involved in hearing, balance, and coordinating eye movements. Dysfunction of the reticular formation can affect a child's ability to regulate input, modulate arousal states, and regulate behavior.

The thalamus is termed the "relay station" of the brain. All sensory input (except olfactory input) passes through the thalamus and is sent to the sensory and motor areas in the cortex for further processing.

The pons connects the spinal cord and cerebral hemispheres to the cerebellum. Many types of fibers pass through the pons, which convey proprioceptive and vestibular input to the cerebellum. The pons also has ascending sensory fibers passing through on their way to the thalamus and descending motor tracts passing through from the cortex on their way to the spinal cord.

The primary role of the hypothalamus is the maintenance of homeostasis. It is involved in regulating the body's temperature, hunger and thirst needs, blood pressure and heart rate, and gastrointestinal functions.

The vestibular nuclei area processes information from the gravity and movement receptors located in the inner ear and uses the information to assist the body in keeping an upright posture and maintaining equilibrium and is important for processing information from all other senses, especially those from the joints and muscles (Ayres, 1979).

The cerebellum processes all types of sensation but is responsible for assisting in organizing gravity (vestibular) and movement sensations (proprioceptive) to ensure coordinated and accurate movements. The cerebellum plays a large role in motor planning (especially timing and sequencing of movements) and execution of movements. It also assists in coordinating the body's muscle tone and sense of balance.

The limbic system plays an important role in the formation of memories and emotions, control of visceral functions, and olfaction (Martin, 1996). It consists of structures located within the cerebral hemispheres, the main structures being the hippocampus and amygdala. The hippocampus works closely with the cerebral cortex through a loop system that sends information from the cortex to the hypothalamus and thalamus and then receives input back from these areas. It plays a role in learning, memory, cognition, motivation, and our emotions, such as regulating attention and arousal and aids in regulation of emotional tone. A disruption results in fluctuation of emotional tone, irritability, confusion, and disorganization (Murray-Slutsky & Paris, 2000). The amygdala plays a role in the body's emotions and in coordinating the body's response to stressful and threatening situations by controlling what the body responds to, how overt responses to stimuli are, and the internal responses of the body's organs (Martin, 1996).

The cerebral hemispheres is the highly specialized area of the brain, responsible for processing information from each body sense and receiving and processing information from other senses. The hemispheres contain association areas that are responsible for coordinating many types of sensory input to unify the brain as a whole (Ayres, 1979). Four major lobes to the cerebral hemispheres process different types of input and work together to integrate sensory input:

- *Occipital lobe:* Processes visual information. Visual information begins to be processed in this lobe and then is sent to the parietal and temporal lobes for further processing.
- *Parietal lobe:* Processes proprioceptive input regarding body movements and position in space and refined tactile information, including pain, temperature, vibration, and discriminative touch. Contains an area involved in motor planning, development of body awareness, and understanding of language.
- *Temporal lobe:* Processes auditory information; contributes to the interpretation and understanding of language; and contributes to memory abilities, cognitive skills, and regulation of emotions.
- *Frontal lobe:* Associated with motor behavior, speech production, higher level cognitive processing, and aspects of personality and emotions. Considered the "executive thinking" lobe for higher level thinking.

Major Sensory Systems

There are three major sensory systems: tactile, vestibular, and proprioceptive.

Tactile System

The tactile sensory system is the first sensory system to develop in utero (Royeen & Lane, 1991). The tactile receptors are located in the skin and detect light touch, pressure, vibration, movement, pain, and temperature. There are certain areas on the body that are more sensitive to touch input, including the palms of the hands, soles of the feet, stomach, and mouth. There are two components to the tactile

Table 8.2. Functions of the Tactile System

System	Protective	Discriminative
Responsible for	Provides body with survival response—"Fight, fright, or flight"	Provides brain with precise information about objects including size, shape, and texture
Receptors	Located on the skin surface and stimulated by light touch, pain, and temperature	Located deeper under the skin surface and stimulated by touch pressure
Sensation	Diffuse, general sensory input (e.g., arm is touched, and child is unable to isolate the location of the touch input)	Specific, discrete sensory input (e.g., arm is touched, and child is able to localize the input)
Processing	Considered to be more primal; processing occurs at brain stem level	Considered to be more sophisticated; processing occurs at cortex level
Function	Provides a general awareness about the environment	Assists with tactile discrimination, gives meaning to touch sensations, assists with stereognosis

system: protective and discriminative. Table 8.2 provides an explanation of both components.

When dysfunction occurs in the tactile system, it can take place in either the protective or discriminative component. Dysfunction in the protective component may range from not being able to perceive pain or touch to being overly sensitive to touch. This is termed *tactile defensiveness*. When dysfunction occurs in the discriminative component, the child demonstrates difficulty assigning meaning to tactile experiences. Input remains general and vague instead of specific. This results in the child displaying difficulty identifying objects and properties of objects through their sense of touch alone. The child must rely on other senses to assist in this process. Table 8.3 provides a comparison of

dysfunctions in the protective and discriminative components.

Tactile defensiveness. Ayres (1979) described a child with tactile defensiveness as "having a tendency to react negatively and emotionally to touch sensations that other people would hardly feel or would not find harmful" (p. 107). The child lacks the ability to inhibit tactile sensations and thus is overly focused on the input. Incoming tactile sensations are not modulated correctly, resulting in the tactile input being viewed as aversive. In a child with tactile defensiveness, there is too much protective activity and not enough discriminatory activity occurring. Instead of the child finding out what the sensations mean, the child immediately reacts with a fight or flight response (Ayres, 1979). This

Table 8.3. Dysfunction of the Tactile System

Protective	Discriminative
Child has difficulty perceiving pain and temperature (hot vs. cold).	Child has difficulty with stereognosis.
Child is not able to localize the source of pain.	Child demonstrates poor tactile discrimination and has difficulty recognizing characteristics of objects.
Child exhibits tactile defensiveness.	Child demonstrates poor in-hand manipulation skills of objects.

results in the child usually being easily distracted, emotionally unbalanced, and at times hyperactive.

The child does not like to engage in everyday sensations that others find enjoyable, which may include playing in the sandbox or in the grass in the backyard, finger painting, or bathing. The child is averse to light touch input and touch initiated by others. Even though the child is bothered by certain touch input, he or she may crave deep-pressure input, including rough-and-tumble play or hugs from a parent and may actually seek out this type of input as a way of receiving tactile sensations.

Tactile defensiveness can

- Impact an infant's overall development, including not wanting to lie in a prone position on the floor and not wanting to place weight on his or her arms or through the hands, and can affect the development of walking if the child is averse to placing his or her feet on a variety of surfaces and textures.
- Impact the child's ability to engage in and tolerate self-care activities, including getting his or her hair cut or brushed, nails trimmed, or teeth brushed.
- Impact a child's ability to tolerate certain food textures; he or she may refuse certain foods (e.g., foods with lumps like yogurt or mashed potatoes) or spit out foods while eating.
- Impact a child's functioning in the school setting, including tolerating sitting or standing near peers (e.g., on the floor during circle or carpet time, when interacting in a group, standing in line, or sitting next to other students in the lunchroom or classroom).
- Impact a child's ability to interact with a variety of tactile-related materials (e.g., paints, glue) that may be used in classroom or art activities; over time, this also can af-

fect the child's tool use, due to not wanting to hold objects, and he or she may be observed to hold objects only with the tips of his or her fingers.

- Impact a child's ability to build interpersonal relationships with caregivers and others; the child is overly focused on the possibility of being touched and is unable to interact with and tolerate having people and objects in his or her personal space.

Poor tactile discrimination. *Tactile discrimination* is the ability to understand attributes of tactile sensations. This includes determining if the input is light touch or deep-pressure; pinpointing the location of where the body was touched; and understanding the properties of objects, including their size, shape, temperature, and texture. The discriminative sense develops over time as the body begins inhibiting the protective system. Even though both protective and discriminative systems perform different functions, they continue to work together throughout life to remain balanced (Ayres, 1979). The discriminative sense allows the child to learn about objects and the environment through the sense of touch. Dysfunction in the discriminative system can result in

- Difficulty interacting with toys effectively. The child may not be able to control the force of his or her movements as he or she interacts with toys, resulting in either using too little or too much force and pressure when activating a toy. This is the result of dysfunction of the sensory system, not due to a motor dysfunction.
- Difficulty localizing where touch input has occurred on the body.
- Difficulty registering pain and localizing where the painful experience is occurring on the body.
- Difficulty defining the properties of the objects through touch alone, resulting in the child relying on the sense of vision.

- Weak in-hand manipulation skills due to receiving poor feedback in the hands. This results in the child displaying difficulty with completing complex tasks, including managing clothing fasteners and tool use (e.g., writing tools, scissors).

Vestibular System

The vestibular system provides the body with information on the position of the head and body in relation to the ground. Receptors are located in the inner ear and respond to changes in head position and movement, including both acceleration and deceleration (Ayres, 1979). The receptors react to linear movement (e.g., up and down, side to side, back and forth) and rotary movement (e.g., moving in circles such as spinning on a platform swing). The vestibular sensations are processed both in the vestibular nuclei and cerebellum. They are then sent through the spinal cord and into the brain stem, where they combine the vestibular and proprioceptive input. Some of the sensations are then sent to the cerebral hemispheres, where they combine with proprioceptive and visual input. The functions of the vestibular system include

- Helping the body regulate balance and upright posture. It also helps the body make discrete automatic changes in posture or movement to remain stable, providing the body with postural and gravitational security.
- Coordinating movements so they are smooth, accurate, and properly timed.
- Providing information about the orientation of the body and movement of the body in space.
- Helping the body control eye movements, including maintaining a stable visual field and focus on objects, shifting eye gaze to track objects, and informing the brain of the surroundings, such as knowing

whether objects (e.g., the body) are moving in the environment, whether the surroundings are moving, or whether the body is on something that is moving (e.g., an escalator or elevator).
- Regulating muscle tone, especially the body's extensor tone.
- Assisting the body in being able to use both sides of the body in a coordinated manner (bilateral coordination).

The vestibular system is connected with and influences many other sensory systems and plays a vital role in the body. Dysfunction in the vestibular system can result in

- *Low muscle tone:* The child may lean or prop him- or herself up for additional support when seated at a desk, may sit with a rounded posture, and may become easily tired as a result of having to exert so much effort just to keep his or her body up.
- *Poor postural background movements and balance:* The child may fall frequently and be unable to automatically and quickly catch him- or herself. He or she may have a rigid posture and walk in a high guard position. The child may appear clumsy and not exhibit the correct timing and accuracy when interacting with objects.
- *Postural and gravitational insecurity:* The child may become upset by changes in body position or when he or she has to engage in movement activities. The child is fearful of having his or her feet off of the ground and prefers to have feet on the floor. He or she becomes distressed when forced to engage in movement activities, including using playground equipment (e.g., the slide or swings), riding on a roller coaster, or going up or down steps or curbs on the street.
- *Poor bilateral coordination:* The child is unable to use both hands to complete similar tasks (e.g., holding a box) or different tasks (e.g., holding paper with one hand while cutting using the other hand).

• *Poor eye movements:* The child may display difficulty tracking objects, especially across midline. He or she also may have difficulty shifting his or her gaze to copy information from the chalkboard to paper.

Proprioceptive System

Proprioception is the unconscious sense of body movement. Proprioceptive receptors are located in the muscles, muscle tendons, and joints and respond to movement and gravity. The proprioceptors respond to active movement that is initiated by the child. Minimal proprioceptive input is provided when the movement is passive (e.g., passively ranging a child's arms and legs; Blanche & Schaaf, 2001). The function of the proprioceptive system is to provide the body with information regarding where the body is in space (external map) and where body parts are in relation to one another (internal map). It assists the child in developing awareness about the body to form a body image and plays a role in assisting the body in maintaining postural control, motor coordination, and motor planning (see Chapter 5 for more information regarding motor planning). The proprioceptive system works very closely with the tactile and vestibular systems to perform the functions described above.

A child with dysfunction of the proprioceptive system may have difficulty with planning and coordinating movements. The child may exhibit low muscle tone; have difficulty grading movements (e.g., overshoots or undershoots movements) when playing with toys, causing the toys to break; and has difficulty performing gross motor movements. Another disorder associated with the proprioceptive system includes those children who seek a great deal of proprioceptive input to help remain modulated. These children often appear hyperactive. They run and seek out deep-pressure input in different and at times unsafe ways, including jumping off of objects

to crash into something, playing aggressively with siblings or peers (e.g., hitting, pushing, and biting), and engaging in self-stimulatory behaviors (e.g., banging his or her head, hitting himself or herself, and pinching or biting himself or herself; Blanche & Schaaf, 2001).

In addition to evaluating and providing interventions for students with sensory processing issues in the tactile, proprioceptive, and vestibular systems, occupational therapists also must remember to consider the visual, olfactory, and auditory systems when evaluating a student's area of need. Therapists can use the information obtained through the evaluation process to develop an intervention plan. Although intensive sensory integration treatment can be difficult to conduct in a school setting, numerous interventions and modifications can be implemented to help the child be successful throughout the school day.

Common Terms Used in Sensory Integration Literature

It is at times difficult to distinguish between the terms used in sensory integration literature, including processing, registration, modulation, regulation, integration, and defensiveness. The more commonly used terms are defined below.

Sensory processing: The ability to register sensory input. The brain gathers sensory input and filters out irrelevant input. The input is continually organized and interpreted to maintain an optimal state of arousal in the nervous system (Haack & Haldy, 1998).

Sensory registration: The brain's ability to detect and respond adequately to sensations coming in from the environment (Hanschu, 2003). Royeen and Lane (1991) described sensory registration as a continuum. A child can be overresponsive (leading to defensive behaviors) or underresponsive to sensory input. When a child is underresponsive to sensory input, he or she shows minimal or no response to sensory stimuli. If the student is over- or underresponsive to sensory input, he or she will be unable to properly modulate it. Intervention techniques commonly used for modulation disorders can be utilized with the student who has registration issues.

Sensory modulation: Can be described in physiological and behavior terms (Miller, Reisman, McIntosh, & Simon, 2001). Behaviorally, modulation refers to the child's ability to regulate and organize responses to sensations in a graded and adaptive manner to meet situational demands. Physiologically, modulation refers to the neural mechanisms that affect the body's ability to stimulate or inhibit sensations to act in accordance with the situational demands.

Sensory modulation disorders fall on a continuum from sensory dormancy (a complete lack of or limited response to sensory input) to sensory defensiveness (overresponding to sensory input). Behavioral symptoms of sensory modulation dysfunction include fluctuating responses to sensory stimuli (hyperresponsive or hyporesponsive); exhibiting sensory seeking and sensory avoiding behaviors; fluctuating emotional states (e.g., depression, anger, anxiety); and attention concerns, including hyperactivity, impulsivity, disorganization, and distractibility. All of these issues affect the child's ability to perform in work and play, interact socially, and complete activities of daily living (Miller et al., 2001).

Over time the child begins to habituate sensory input (Ayres, 1979). The child establishes a high threshold for a certain type of sensory input and becomes less responsive to that input, allowing the child to filter out familiar sensations so that attention can be focused on novel or more important sensory information. Children with autism and attention deficit disorders commonly meet the criteria for a sensory modulation disorder.

These children have difficulty maintaining their attention throughout varying times of the day, may be hyperactive or easily distracted, and may have fluctuating arousal and mood states.

Sensory regulation/self-regulation: A child's ability to maintain homeostasis, internally regulate information entering the brain and make the needed adjustments to maintain organization and control in the brain. Reeves (2001) defined *homeostasis* as "the maintenance of internal stability through automatic adjustments and coordination in the physiological systems and neural processes to regulate arousal to maintain order and balance" (p. 90). Sensory integration is reliant on receiving and modulating sensory input so that the child can regulate his or her behavior and emotions (Ayres, 1979). Sensory regulation and integration are interdependent and interrelated processes (Reeves, 2001).

Sensory defensiveness: Originally defined as an exaggerated, disorganized response to sensory input resulting from an imbalance between inhibition and excitation in the nervous system (Knickerbocker, 1980). Wilbarger and Wilbarger (1991) defined *sensory defensiveness* as a "tendency to react negatively or with alarm to sensory input that is generally considered harmless or nonirritating" (p. 3). Children with sensory defensiveness often appear hyperactive, are easily distracted, and are disorganized. They may develop learned patterns and habits around avoiding sensory situations or seek out sensations that they find comforting.

Defensiveness can occur along a continuum from mild to moderate to severe (Wilbarger & Wilbarger, 1991). Students who are mildly affected may be those who are often referred to as picky or choosy. Students affected moderately are affected in two or more aspects of their life. This may include the student's social skills, emotional state, ability to complete academics, or ability to be independent in self-help skills. A student who is severely affected by sensory defensiveness would be affected in all aspects of his or her life. Wilbarger and Wilbarger (1991) reported that often these students have other diagnostic labels that also affect their ability to complete certain functional tasks (e.g., multiple disabilities, severe developmental delays, autism). Sensory defensiveness can occur in many of the sensory systems, including visual, auditory, olfactory, vestibular, and tactile input. Sensory defensiveness also is considered a sensory modulation disorder.

When evaluating a student with sensory concerns, it is important to keep all of these considerations in mind (e.g., is it a sensory modulation, registration, or defensiveness issue?).

Evaluating a Student With Sensory Integration Concerns

> Evaluation of sensory integration provides information about the client's sensory processing and perception and how these impact on planning and function. Evaluation also includes analysis of sensory, motor, and cognitive demands of the activities, social and physical characteristics of the environment, and the effectiveness of the student's performance skills and patterns in those activities and environments. The results are interpreted in conjunction with information obtained through the occupational profile, and an intervention plan is developed. (Smith Roley, Clark, & Bissell, 2003)

Occupational therapists in a school setting may evaluate a student's sensory processing needs as part of an initial multifactored evaluation or reevaluation or may be called on to evaluate the sensory processing needs of students who have already qualified for special education services and have an in-

dividualized education program (IEP). A student's teacher may be the first professional to identify that he or she is having sensory issues. The teacher may express concerns to the educational team, which includes the occupational therapist and occupational therapy assistant, regarding how the student is easily off task and is impulsive in the classroom, has difficulty following the classroom routine or multistep directions, seems bothered by loud sounds like the fire drill or public announcement system, has difficulty standing next to others in line or when seated at circle time, or may be demonstrating aggressive behaviors.

It is important to use a variety of methods when evaluating a student's sensory processing needs. Methods include using a screening tool or standardized assessment, conducting a teacher and parent interview, and observing the student in a variety of settings within the school (especially in those settings with which the student is having the most difficulty). For example, if the student is displaying defensive behaviors to auditory input, he or she may demonstrate difficulty in music class on days when instruments are played, have difficulty eating lunch in the lunchroom, or display difficulty riding the bus to and from school. All of these areas of difficulty would need to be explored (through observation or interview) during the evaluation process.

Parent and Teacher Interview

It is always important to collect information from the student's teachers and parents when completing a sensory evaluation. Completing an occupational profile with data provided by the student (if possible) and the student's parents and teachers provides information regarding the student's history, the reason for the referral for the sensory assessment, the student's strengths and areas of concern, and the occupations that are meaningful to the student and also can help the therapist understand the desired outcomes of the family and student. This profile can be completed using an informal checklist and may be combined with data collected by completing a standardized assessment or inventory, examples of which are described below.

It is always important to clarify responses that are checked on the assessment tool to personalize the information. Receiving input from parents and teachers assists in determining if the student's behavior is different at school and at home. Students often can hold it together while at school but fall apart once they get home. For this type of student, providing recommendations and activity suggestions that the family could perform at home would be helpful. Another student may exhibit behavior such as refusing to do work, temper tantrums, noncompliance, putting his or her head down on the desk, and fidgeting more at school than at home. The student may be expected to complete tasks independently, work at tasks that remain difficult to complete or that are of low interest, and remain attentive throughout the lengthy school day. Obtaining this information in addition to specific areas of concern related to the student's behavior and specific sensory processing needs is an important part of the evaluation process.

Structured Evaluation Tools for Sensory Integration

Sensory screening tools, questionnaires, and assessments can be used as a guide in the evaluation process.

Sensory Profile. This instrument (Dunn, 1999) is organized in a questionnaire that the child's caregiver completes. The assessment measures the child's sensory processing abilities and determines the effect of sensory processing on the child's daily functional performance. The profile is recommended to be used with children ages 5–10 years. The assessment also offers an infant/toddler version (used for children from birth to 36 months) and an adolescent/adult version (used for individuals ages 11–65+ years). This assessment can be used with a wide range of students with varying disabilities including learning disabilities, mental retardation, speech impairments, autism, Asperger's syndrome, visual or hearing impairment, cerebral palsy, traumatic brain injury, and multiple disabilities.

The questionnaire consists of 125 items grouped into three major areas: sensory processing, sensory modulation, and emotional and behavioral responses. Items assessed in the sensory processing area include auditory, visual, vestibular, touch, multisensory, and oral sensory processing abilities. The modulation area examines endurance and tone, body position and movement, activity levels, and modulation of sensory input (including visual input) that affect the child's emotional responses. In the behavioral and emotional response area, the caregiver reports on the child's activity level, attention, and behavioral and emotional responses to activities and situations.

The caregiver defines if the child exhibits the behaviors always, frequently, occasionally, seldom, or never. Each response corresponds to a graduated point system. The points are totaled to determine the raw score for each section. The totaled raw scores from each section are interpreted and grouped into one of three categories (typical performance, probable difference, definite difference) to determine where the student's performance is compared to that of typically developing same-age peers. In addition to providing information on the child's performance in each section, the assessment groups test items into factors, including sensory seeking, emotionally reactive, low endurance/tone, oral sensory sensitivity, inattention/distractibility, poor registration, sensory sensitivity, sedentary, and fine motor/perceptual.

The purpose of the factor summaries is to assist in revealing patterns related to the child's response to various types of stimuli within the environment. The scores are classified into three groups based on the performance of the child in relation to typically developing children.

- *Typical performance:* Child's scores at or above 1.00 standard deviation below the mean.
- *Probable difference:* Child's scores fall between 1.00 to 2.00 standard deviations below the mean.
- *Definite difference:* Child's scores fall below 2.00 standard deviations below the mean.

Dunn (1991) developed a theoretical model for sensory processing that can be used in the interpretation and reporting process. The child's scores are organized into a behavioral response continuum that includes four quadrants: poor registration, sensation seeking, sensitivity to stimuli, and sensation avoiding. Organizing the scores in this way can assist in targeting specific intervention strategies that coincide with the child's profile.

Sensory Integration Inventory–Revised, For Individuals With Developmental Disabilities. This screening tool was developed by Judith Reisman and Barbara Hanschu and revised in 1992 and is meant to be used as a screening tool to determine if the student would benefit from further assessment and therapy targeting deficits in sensory processing. The inventory can be completed by a child's caregiver or staff (e.g., occupational therapist, teacher) that are very familiar with the student. It can assist in determining if a student's behaviors are a result of a sensory processing issue. The inventory is organized into four sections: vestibular processing, tac-tile processing, proprioceptive processing, and general reactions to sensory input.

Items within the sections are checked ("yes" or "no") to report whether the student is exhibiting the behaviors listed. The "yes" responses are then placed on the inventory rating form. Trends or patterns can be identified in the four major categories of dysfunction defined by the inventory: sensory modulation, sensory defensiveness, sensory registration, and sensory integration. Treatment activities then can be developed and focused to address the specific areas in which the student is exhibiting difficulty.

DeGangi–Berk Test of Sensory Integration. This tool (Berk & DeGangi, 1983) provides an overall measure of sensory integration functioning for preschool children ages 3–5 years. The test consists of 36 items providing information about the child's overall sensory integrative functioning. The test items are organized into three subdomains: postural control, bilateral motor integration, and reflex integration.

The DeGangi–Berk Test is a criterion-referenced assessment. It was designed for use with children who are suspected of having sensory, motor, or perceptual delays or for students suspected of having problems learning. The test can be administered in about 30 minutes. Test results can be interpreted to determine if the student is functioning in the normal range of performance, is at risk for a sensory integrative dysfunction, or has definite deficits in sensory integrative functioning.

Temperament and Atypical Behavior Scale. This assessment (Neisworth, Bagnato, Salvia, & Hunt, 1999) is norm-referenced and provides a measure of dysfunctional behavior in children between the ages of 11 and 71 months. The intended purpose is to assist in identifying children who are "at risk" or who are developing atypically in the areas of temperament and self-regulation. The assessment tool includes 55 items arranged in a checklist format. Items are arranged into four subtests: detached, hypersensitive/hyperactive, underreactive, and dysregulated.

The respondent (usually a parent or caregiver) records whether the child is exhibiting the behaviors listed and whether he or she needs help managing the child's behavior in those areas. The raw scores for each of the four subtests are totaled, and standard scores and percentiles can be derived for the child's score in each area. The raw scores for all four subtests are then totaled to determine the overall Temperament and Regulatory Index, which has a standard score of 100, with a standard deviation of 15. Because the items are written in specific behavioral terms, they easily can be targeted for intervention on the student's IEP in the area of behavior.

Sensory Integration and Praxis Tests. These tests are designed to be used with children between ages 4 and 8 years who exhibit mild to moderate learning, behavioral, or developmental disorders (Ayres & Marr, 1991). Seventeen individually administered tests require the student to perform various tasks: kinesthesia, finger identification, graphesthesia, localization of tactile stimuli, postrotary nystagmus, standing and walking balance, space visualization, figure-ground perception, manual form perception, motor accuracy, design copying, constructional praxis, postural praxis, praxis on verbal command, sequencing praxis, oral praxis, and bilateral motor coordination.

Test results are computer scored and provide information regarding the child's performance on each of the 17 tests. It also plots the student's overall pattern of socres compared to patterns that characterize the six diagnostic clusters: deficit in bilateral integration and sequencing, visuo- and somatodyspraxia, dyspraxia on verbal command,

generalized sensory integrative dysfunction, low-average sensory integration and praxis, and high-average sensory integration and praxis (Ayres & Marr, 1991). A therapist must receive specialized training to be able to administer this assessment. Due to the amount of time it takes to administer this assessment, the cost incurred to receive the training on administering the assessment, and the fact that the assessment is scored by a computer, plus the need to infer how the deficits affect school function, it is often administered in a clinic versus a school-based setting.

Informal Observation

In addition to completing a standardized assessment or inventory, occupational therapists should observe students in the classroom and other school settings (depending on the area of concern). It is always important to consult with a student's classroom or special education teacher to ensure that the observation occurs at the most opportune time to observe the teacher's or parent's concerns. For example, if a student is falling apart in the afternoon each day, an observation both in the morning and afternoon would be important to compare the student's behaviors. If he or she is having difficulty managing behavior in the general education classroom but thrives in the small group special education setting, an observation should be conducted in both areas to compare the differences in the student's behaviors. Specific subject areas may need to be observed (e.g., music, physical education class) if the student is having difficulty in these areas. The observation can provide vital information in determining if the problem is truly a sensory integration issue or strictly a behavioral issue. Aspects of the observation should include the areas described below.

Classroom Set-up and Structure. The occupational therapist should observe in which part of the classroom the student is seated (e.g., front or back, by the door, under the public announcement speaker). The therapist should note whether the student's desk and chair match his or her individual needs (e.g., chair depth not too large, whether the height of the chair and desk support the student's back and feet). The therapist also should observe any clutter or visual distractions in the classroom (e.g., mobiles hanging from the ceiling, posters on the wall, screen savers) as well as any auditory distractions (e.g., music, fans, toilet flushing, water running) and the volume of noise in the room. In addition, the therapist should notice how well the lessons and procedures of the classroom are structured (e.g., providing a consistent place to turn in assignments, organizing the classroom, hanging up a daily schedule in the classroom to provide students with expectations for the day, developing classroom management policies with clear expectations).

Length and Structure of Lessons. The length of time the student is expected to sit, attend to a lecture, and take notes should be noted by the occupational therapist. The therapist also should observe whether the teacher incorporates manipulatives or movement within the lessons and if students are expected to sit at their desks and attend to lecture-based instruction for 30–45 minutes at a time.

Student's Activity Level. The occupational therapist should observe the student's behavior in the classroom. Does he or she appear to be fidgeting or hyperactive? Is the student disruptive to others or to him- or herself? Does he or she fidget with objects or place objects in his or her mouth? Is the student attending to classroom tasks even when not facing the teacher? Does he or she appear to be lethargic? Does the student lean or lay on the desk? Does he or she become easily tired or fall asleep during class?

Student's Ability to Meet Demands of the Activity. The occupational therapist

should observe whether the student's attention or activity level affects his or her ability to follow the directions (e.g., does the student successfully complete morning routine, follow the instructions in a game in physical education class, or work collaboratively with peers to complete a group activity?).

Occupational therapists should note whether the student understands the provided content material or directions. Students with disabilities may present with varying schedules depending on their cognitive level and ability to manage the grade-level curriculum. Some students may remain in the general education classroom the entire school day and be pulled out only for reinforcement or may receive special education services within the general education classroom. Other students may be included in the general education classroom for selected subjects and be in a special education classroom only for subject areas in which the student needs major modifications to the general curriculum or a modified curriculum. Some students receive all of their academic instruction in a special education classroom.

It is important to remember that students need to be presented with "just-right challenges." If a student with cognitive impairments is placed in a situation in which material is above his or her cognitive abilities or developmental level, behaviors including fidgeting, acting out, becoming frustrated, or falling asleep may occur because the demands of the task are well above the student's cognitive level and not due to a sensory integration issue. The student's behavior may change once he or she uses materials that correspond to his or her cognitive level (which may not be at the student's grade level).

Finally, the occupational therapist should note how the student's sensory issues affect his or her ability to complete classroom tasks. Is the student unable to perform projects in art class because tactile defensiveness interferes with his or her ability to use the mediums needed to complete the project? Is the student unable to follow multistep directions due to poor attention to task, and does his or her hyperactivity affect his or her ability to follow a gross motor game in physical education class? It is important to define what is interfering with the student's ability to perform to plan interventions and modifications effectively in the school setting.

Determining If Sensory Intervention Strategies Would Benefit the Student

All students, regardless of age and ability level, benefit from being provided with sensory breaks during the school day, including having access to recess, free play time, bathroom and water breaks, and lunch. Students benefit from multisensory approaches to learning, including not only listening to lectures but also completing hands-on activities like using manipulatives to learn math concepts or completing experiments in science class. A student with sensory processing issues may need additional supports throughout the school day to assist with occupational performance.

After the sensory evaluation is completed, it needs to be determined if the student's sensory issues affect his or her ability to benefit from his or her education and if a sensory intervention plan needs to be developed. If the educational team determines that the student would benefit from sensory-based interventions during the school day, the interventions, the frequency and the context in which the interventions will occur, and the staff who will be involved in the implementation of the intervention plan need to be determined and stated. Smith Roley et al. (2003) defined five intervention approaches when using a sensory integration frame of reference in a school setting:

1. *To create and promote healthy sensory integration.* This strategy involves providing proactive strategies within the school and community to support sensory integration. This may include providing parent or teacher in-services regarding sensory processing skills and ways in which sensory strategies can be incorporated naturally into a school day or activities at home, supporting physical activities for students during the day, and supporting the installment of equipment available to students at the school or in the community to provide children with enriched sensory experiences.

2. *To establish or restore function.* This strategy involves structuring the environment (both in the classroom and at home) to meet the student's sensory processing needs. This includes designing specific activities to focus on developing the student's sensory processing or motor planning skills needed to engage in occupations. It also may include teaching the student self-regulation strategies to be able to perform optimally throughout the school day.

3. *To maintain a student's ability to function and cope at school.* This strategy involves designing specific interventions to assist the student in organizing his or her behavior to participate within the classroom setting and to maintain relationships with same-age peers. It also involves providing classroom modifications or accommodations within the school environment to assist the student with his or her productivity level at school.

4. *To modify an activity to help the student compensate for dysfunction in sensory processing and motor planning.* This approach supports consultation between the occupational therapist and the student's special education or general education teacher to design ways to modify the student's assignments or demands of the activities so that the student can be successful in the general education classroom as much as possible.

5. *To prevent injury and barriers to participation*. This strategy supports allowing a student to be able to participate in activities throughout the day by modifying the environment and providing interventions throughout the school day to meet the student's needs. The goal of incorporating these proactive strategies is to prevent social isolation, inappropriate behaviors, and injury to the student or to others.

Specific intervention strategies and modifications can be designed by the occupational therapist in collaboration with the team to meet the student's individual needs. Strategies may include designing alerting activities for a student who appears lethargic and has difficulty remaining alert during the day, designing calming activities for a student who becomes easily overstimulated and demonstrates hyperactive or aggressive behaviors, or combining alerting and calming activities into the plan for a student who demonstrates fluctuating behaviors. Modifications to the classroom or school environment also can be designed and implemented.

Considerations When Planning Interventions

There are many factors to consider when designing a student's sensory intervention plan, including determining the student's individualized needs, age-appropriate activity recommendations, equipment options, configuration of the student's school day (e.g., in general education classroom full day, split between general education and special education classrooms, or in special education classroom full day), and the accessibility of staff to help carry out the sensory plan.

When writing a sensory intervention plan, it is important to organize the activity recommendations and suggested modifications based on the student's needs. The sensory activities included in the intervention plan should be incorporated into the student's daily schedule at school. The organization of the sensory plan may depend on the individual assessment tool used by the occupational therapist. For example, if the Sensory Integration Inventory (Reisman & Hanschu, 1992) was used, the therapist may decide to organize the sensory plan and plot activities based on the student's profile in the four domains defined by the assessment. If the Sensory Profile (Dunn, 1999) was used, the therapist may decide to organize the sensory plan and provide activity recommendations based on the four profiles that Dunn defined. It is important to remember to write the student's assessment results, suggested activities, and modifications in easy-to-understand terms. Using complex sensory terminology or medical terms may result in the student's parents or teachers not being able to understand the information, which may affect the implementation of the plan.

When designing a sensory plan, the occupational therapist needs to remember the student's developmental level and chronological age. Sensory activities requiring multiple steps may be difficult for a student with a cognitive impairment to successfully complete independently. This student may initially benefit from simplified one- or two-step activities. Once the student demonstrates the ability to complete these activities, more complex activities can be designed. A student's chronological age also needs to be remembered. Would a teenage student be able to fit on a Sit-n-Spin™ to obtain vestibular sensory input, and is this an age-appropriate activity for a middle school or high school student? Perhaps more appropriate options could be recommended to provide vestibular input, including ball activities, reading a book in a rocking chair, or completing exercise movements requiring the student to frequently change body positions.

When writing a sensory intervention plan for a student in a school setting, it is important to understand how the student's day is structured, which often depends on the child's level of functioning or disability. A student in the general education classroom the entire school day may not have access to using large equipment housed in a sensory or gross motor room. The teacher may want to keep some sensory items in the general education classroom for the student to use. The student may benefit more from activities that could be conducted within the classroom setting. The classroom teacher may be open to incorporating sensory activities for the entire classroom into the school day. Diana Henry, OTR/L, has developed numerous sensory activities that can be conducted in the classroom setting, including instructional books (*Tool Chest: For Teachers, Parents, and Students*) and videos and DVDs (*Tools for Teachers* and *Tools for Students*) that can be shown to teachers who are receptive to incorporating these strategies.

Mary Sue Williams and Sherry Shellenberger (1996) developed the Alert Program to assist students in learning how to monitor, maintain, and change their level of alertness so that it is appropriate for a particular task or situation. The students are taught a variety of self-regulation strategies that they can use in a variety of settings to assist them in responding adaptively and efficiently to the demands of a task or situation. It was developed for children with learning disabilities between ages 8 and 12 years, but the program has been adapted by professionals to be used with students ranging from preschool to high school. Students can complete many of the activities in the classroom or school. The occupational therapist can consult with the student, parents, and teaching staff to monitor the effectiveness of the program in the school setting.

If the student shifts between a general education and special education classroom or is predominantly in a special education classroom during the school day, his or her schedule may be more flexible and provide more opportunities to access larger equipment. This student's sensory intervention plan may incorporate more activities that involve using equipment (e.g., scooter boards, swing, trampoline, tunnels).

When developing and writing up sensory strategies that the student can complete during the school day, the occupational therapist must ensure that the activities that are recommended can be realistically incorporated. It is unfair to write a sensory plan that looks great on paper but is unlikely to be implemented because there is either no time or no adult assistance.

For a student that is in the general education classroom the entire school day, it is important to coordinate with teaching staff to ensure that his or her needs are being met. If the student is able to remain on task by taking periodic breaks with activities that can be conducted in the classroom, he or she may not need adult assistance to facilitate the tasks. On the other hand, if a student is in the general education classroom the entire day but would benefit from using larger sensory equipment available in the building, then it is up to the educational team to determine when the student would have time and what personnel are available to assist that student. Students who spend time in a special education classroom during the school day often have easier access to equipment or adult assistance (e.g., special education teacher or teacher assistant) to enforce the activities on a daily basis. An older student (e.g., middle school or high school) may be responsible enough to use equipment or complete the recommended activities on the plan independently after they are demonstrated by the occupational therapist. The therapist and special education staff need to ensure that the student can be alone and is safe in completing the activities without adult assistance (due to liability issues to the school district if the student gets hurt).

Finally, the occupational therapist must take into consideration the equipment available. A therapist would not want to recommend activities using certain pieces of equipment if that equipment is not available (or not able to be purchased by the district in the near future). The therapist needs to realistically determine what equipment is vital for the student when designing the sensory plan before making recommendations to the school district to purchase the equipment. If a student would benefit from certain sensory items to make an effective plan (e.g., the student would greatly benefit from access to a Movin' Sit cushion, mini-trampoline, and a therapy ball), then it is up to the therapist and educational team to advocate for purchasing the equipment.

It is important for school-based occupational therapists to keep track of sensory equipment that has previously been purchased by the school district and follow up on students using the equipment to ensure that students continue to benefit from using the equipment items and to monitor the conditions of the sensory items (e.g., the Movin' Sit cushion may need more air, the ropes on the platform swing may need to be adjusted, or new ropes may need to be ordered due to fraying). Safety rotational devices and safety snaps on swings require periodic maintenance to ensure the continued safety of students.

Sometimes students may refuse to use equipment, may no longer benefit from using the equipment, or may have outgrown the equipment (e.g., a weighted vest). If the student no longer needs the equipment, it could be used for another student in the district. If it appears that a student within a building would benefit from a piece of equipment that the building currently does not own (e.g., a platform swing or scooter board), it is up to the occupational therapist to talk to the principal or special education coordinator to see if the district could purchase the equipment. Equipment often also can be purchased through grants from local special education agencies or nonprofit organizations.

Reinforcing the Sensory Plan

After a sensory intervention plan has been designed, the occupational therapist should meet with the team members who will be involved in its implementation, including the occupational therapist, student, parents, regular education teacher, special education teacher, and teacher assistant. During the meeting, the therapist should review the results of the assessment and describe the student's specific sensory needs and explain the activity recommendations (including how to conduct the activities, frequency of the activities, and any safety precautions that need to be taken). Any additional questions can be answered at this time. The educational team also needs to determine what type of assistance will be needed by the occupational therapist to support the student's sensory plan.

The occupational therapist often needs to be involved as a resource for continued consultation and collaboration to ensure that the sensory plan is being reinforced. Through ongoing collaboration, the therapist can determine if the activities are beneficial for the student or if the sensory intervention plan needs to be revised and new activities need to be developed to meet the student's needs. If the therapist provides intervention to the student through a direct service model, the sensory strategies from the student's plan also can be incorporated into the intervention session.

Determining Plan Effectiveness

It is critical that the student's sensory intervention plan is implemented daily. If the strategies are conducted inconsistently, the team will be unable to determine if the sensory interventions are aiding the student. Additionally, it will be difficult to discontinue the sensory intervention plan (if determined that the sensory interventions are not assisting the student's needs) if there is no information to support why the interventions did not work.

It is at times difficult to collect data on the effectiveness of sensory interventions. If specific data are going to be collected, then the team should define a specific behavior to be targeted by using sensory intervention strategies. Specific and consistent terms should be developed by team members to describe or quantify the student's behavior so that team members record the data consistently. For example, Brian, a preschooler, becomes overstimulated and often throws himself on the floor and refuses to transition to circle time. He also has difficulty attending during circle time, fidgeting while seated on the floor or getting up and running away from the circle. The educational team decided that that they would have Brian wear a weighted vest 5 minutes prior to the transition to circle time and during the 15-minute activity. The team then collected data on Brian's behavior during the transition when wearing the weighted vest and his ability to attend to circle time tasks. An example data sheet is provided in Figure 8.1.

It may be helpful to the occupational therapist and student's parents to chart which sensory interventions are being conducted during the school day. This is an effective method of documenting that the activities are being implemented on a daily basis and may provide data on what sensory activities are beneficial to the student based on the student's behavior after the sensory activities have been completed. The therapist can send a copy of the data sheet home to the

Date	Duration Vest Was Worn	Did Brian Transition to Circle Time (+/−)?	Brian's Attention During Circle Time
3-1-04	On: 10:00 a.m. Off: 10:20 a.m.	+	Remained at circle for 5 minutes before getting up and running away from group
3-2-04	On: 10:00 a.m. Off: 10:20 a.m.	+	Remained seated for 2 minutes before getting up and running away
3-3-04	On: 10:00 a.m. Off: 10:20 a.m.	+	Remained at circle for entire activity, actively participated in all tasks
3-4-04	On: 10:00 a.m. Off: 10:20 a.m.	+	Remained at circle for entire activity, actively participated in all tasks

Figure 8.1. Brian's Weighted Vest Sensory Data Sheet

Week of _____

Please place a ✓ in the box to indicate if the selected activity was conducted.

Sensory Activity	Monday	Tuesday	Wednesday	Thursday	Friday
Vertical bouncing on therapy ball	✓		✓		
Vertical jumping on mini-trampoline		✓			✓
Wall/chair push-ups	✓		✓		
Heavy work activity		✓		✓	
Linear swinging				✓	
Weight bearing on arms over ball			✓		✓
Crab/wheelbarrow walking	✓				
Scooter board activity		✓			✓
Other				✓	

Figure 8.2. Sensory Checklist for Matthew

student's parents and keep the original to review at scheduled consultations or if concerns arise between consultations.

Two examples of informational data sheets are provided here. The first data sheet (Figure 8.2, for Matthew) acts as a checks-and-balances sheet. This type of data sheet is used to prove that the sensory strategies are being incorporated into the student's school day. The sheet could be attached to the student's daily communication notebook with the parent (if applicable) or to the assignment notepad that goes home daily so that the parent can see what activities have been con-

ducted each day. In this type of data sheet, the person completing the form simply checks which sensory activities were conducted.

The second data sheet (Figure 8.3, for Ethan) requires the person completing the form to list the sensory activity that was conducted, including the date and time; list the academic task that followed the sensory activity; and define the student's behavioral response to the activity after the sensory input has been given. In the example, the team is looking at Ethan's attention to task by tracking the amount of time he is able to remain in his seat before getting up after the sensory

Date	Time of Day	Sensory Activity Completed	Academic Task Following Sensory Activity	Time Ethan Remained Seated During Academic Task
3-1-03	9:30 a.m.	Vertical bouncing on therapy ball	Math	6 minutes
3-1-03	1:00 p.m.	Vertical jumping on mini-trampoline	Science	9 minutes
3-2-03	8:00 a.m.	Linear swinging on platform swing	Language Arts	5 minutes
3-2-03	1:30 p.m.	Prone on scooter board to complete obstacle course	Social Studies	13 minutes

Figure 8.3. Sensory Checklist for Ethan

input has been given. This form differs from Matthew's data sheet in that the team is not measuring just one sensory strategy (as in the weighted vest) but a variety of sensory strategies providing Ethan with movement activity. The data sheets should be completed by the person who is with the student while completing the sensory activities (e.g., regular or special education teacher, teacher assistant) and who follows the student to the next academic task. The list can be attached to a clipboard and kept in a consistent place if there is more than one person involved in collecting the data.

It is important for occupational therapists to remain involved in a student's sensory intervention plan and revise the plan as needed. If the therapist determines that the student no longer needs or benefits from a structured sensory intervention plan, he or she needs to communicate with the student's teachers and parents before discontinuing the plan. The student may continue to benefit from having structured breaks during the

school day but may not need specifically designed sensory strategies to be conducted that target deficit areas.

Examples of Sensory Activities

Following are some sensory strategies that can be incorporated into the sensory plan. The strategies are categorized by whether they provide proprioceptive, vestibular, and tactile input to the student. The list includes suggested modifications for a student who demonstrates defensive behaviors to oral, visual, tactile, or auditory input. General organizational and behavioral strategies also are listed that may assist with further structuring the student's school day.

Proprioceptive Sensory Activities

The following activities and modifications provide proprioceptive input to students:
• *Vertical bouncing on a therapy ball:* Allow the student to sit on a therapy ball with his or her feet touching the floor and bounce up and down.

- *Vertical jumping on a mini-trampoline:* Allow the student to jump up and down on mini-trampoline. The student may need to hold on to an adult's hand or attached bar while jumping.
- *Hippity-hop (therapy ball with handles):* Allow the student to sit on the Hippity-hop and hold on to the handle. Allow student to bounce up and down.
- *Weight bearing on hands-on ball:* Have the student lay on his or her stomach on a large therapy ball, extend his or her arms, and walk out on his or her hands, ensuring that palms have contact with the ground. An adult will need to support the legs and pelvic region on the ball to ensure that the student is stable and will not fall off the ball. This activity can be easily incorporated into a game requiring the student to cross midline, reach against gravity, or complete a bilateral task (e.g., crossing midline to pick up a bean bag and make a basket through a hoop, reaching above the head to place a flashcard into a container positioned on a chair, or laying over the ball while the body is stabilized by the therapist and pulling apart pop beads or pop tubes to work on bilateral skills).
- *Steamroller:* Using a large therapy ball, roll the ball over the student while he or she is lying prone on the carpet. Provide downward pressure through the ball as it is being rolled over student. *Do not roll the ball over the student's head.*
- *Hand pushes with small playground ball:* Using a slightly deflated small playground ball, have the student press his or her hands into the ball, ensuring that the entire palm of the hand is receiving the deep-pressure input.
- *Wall/chair push-ups:* Have the student do push-ups against the wall or while sitting in a chair. When the student is seated in a chair, have the student place his or her hands against the seat and push his or her body off of the seat.

- *Animal walking and wheelbarrow walking:* Special walks can include
  - *Bear walking:* The student is in a four-point posture on the ground and moves forward using the arms and legs on the same side of the body.
  - *Crab crawling:* The student initially is in a squatting position and reaches back to place hands on the floor. The student lifts his or her bottom off of the floor and moves forward and backward using the hands and feet.
  - *Wheelbarrow walking:* The student walks on extended arms while an adult/peer holds his or her feet. This can be incorporated into a game by having the student retrieve items and reach (either on the same side as an object or crossing midline of the body) to place items into a container.
- *BodySox™:* BodySox™ are made of stretchable Lycra™. The student places his or her feet into the BodySox and then pulls it up over his or her head, hiding his or her arms inside. The child can then move around and press against the BodySox, thus providing deep-pressure to the student's body. BodySox can be purchased from a variety of catalogs, including Sportime Abilitations, Achievement Products for Children, Therapro, and Sammons Preston (see Appendix 8.1).
- *Heavy work activities:* Provide student with opportunities throughout the school day to engage in heavy work activities, including carrying heavy items or pulling/pushing items. Activities might include carrying a book bag loaded with heavy materials when transitioning between classes, carrying/pushing a cart with the class's lunches to the lunch room, returning a stack of library books, washing or erasing the chalkboard in the room, carrying a heavy box to the office, and putting chairs on or taking chairs off of the desks at the beginning or end of the school day. Heavy

work activities provide the student with added deep-pressure input during the school day. The therapist needs to ensure that the weight of the objects the student is encouraged to hold is appropriate for his or her size.

- *Theraband pulls:* Allow the student to pull at a Theraband with in horizontal, vertical, and diagonal directions. This activity provides resistance and additional deep-pressure input.
- *Playground equipment:* Running, swinging, going down the slide, and climbing all provide movement input. Encourage the student to be active on the playground. Monitor the student to ensure that he or she is active. Many times students simply stand around or sit and talk to peers. Ensure that the student is utilizing this time to gain additional sensory input by using the playground equipment.
- *Movement in instruction:* Incorporate movement throughout the day by including "wake-up" activities or movement-oriented activities while transitioning between tasks. Simple movement activities, including hopping, jumping, bear walks, crab crawls, wall push-ups, jumping jacks, and Simon Says, could be incorporated into circle time or into the free play center. These are natural times during the school day when the student and other classmates could receive movement breaks.

Proprioceptive Input Modifications

- *Weighted vest:* Allow the student to wear a weighted vest (which needs to be calibrated by the occupational therapist to 5% of the child's body) during high-demand activities in the classroom. The vest provides the student with added deep-pressure input and may assist in calming the student so that he or she can attend to a given classroom task. The vest should be left on for no longer than 20 minutes and should be used only if the student attends better during the activity or for a time period after taking the vest off.
- *Compression vest:* A compression vest provides similar input as a weighted vest without using the weight. The compression vest is fitted over the student's chest and provides added deep-pressure input through the shoulders and chest to provide a calming and organizing effect on the body.
- *Weighted sock/lap pad:* Fill a tube sock with beans or lentils and have the student place the sock over his or her shoulders or in his or her lap while seated at the desk or on the floor. This sock provides deep-pressure input and may help the student to attend to a classroom task. Weighted lap pads that can rest on the student's lap while seated on the floor or when at a desk are available commercially.
- *Weighted blanket:* The student can place a weighted blanket over his or her body. The blanket provides deep-pressure input and can help calm a student when agitated.
- *Movin' Sit cushion/Disc'O'Sit cushion:* Place the cushion on the student's chair or on the floor during floor activities. The cushion provides added movement and deep-pressure input that should assist the student in maintaining attention to a given classroom task. These cushions can be purchased from the same catalogs as mentioned earlier for the BodySox.
- *Beanbag chair:* Allow the student to sit in a beanbag chair to provide additional deep-pressure input and to further define the student's space while seated.
- *Theraband at desk/chair:* Tie a piece of Theraband around the legs of the student's desk or chair. The student can push his or her legs/feet against the Theraband for added resistance while completing work.

Vestibular Input

- *Linear swinging:* Swing the student in a linear direction on a platform, net, or bolster swing. Encourage the student to propel himself or herself while on the swing. (If on a platform or bolster swing, ensure that the student holds on to the ropes for safety.)

- *Rocking chair:* Have the student sit and slowly rock in a rocking chair. Allowing the student to sit in a rocking chair during classroom group activities when students are seated on the floor or during classroom lessons may assist the student in attending better.

- *Sit-n-spin:* Allow the student to sit with legs crossed (pretzel style) on a Sit-n-spin and spin himself or herself in both directions.

- *Playground equipment:* Running, swinging, going down the slide, and climbing all provide movement input. Encourage the student to be active on the playground. Monitor the student to ensure that he or she is active on the playground and does not simply stand around or sit and talk to peers.

Tactile Input

- *Brushing:* Follow the procedures as outlined by the Wilbarger Brushing Protocol, using the brush recommended by the approach and provided to school staff by the occupational therapist. (This technique should be demonstrated by the therapist to all staff members who will be brushing the student.) Specialized training is required by the therapist recommending this sensory technique. Courses that provide training are offered from Julia and Patricia Wilbarger across the United States and are sponsored by Avanti Educational Programs. If this technique is going to be recommended, it needs to be discussed with the student's parents, as it is conducted every 2 hours. Doing this technique once or twice a day without consistent followthrough can interfere with its effectiveness.

- *Lotion rubs:* Apply lotion to the student's arms and hands. A teacher or assistant can provide deep-pressure input to the student's arms and hands as they rub in the lotion. After the lotion is applied, dry off the arm and hand by completing the towel rub (described below).

- *Towel rubs:* While an adult holds an open hand or bath towel, have the student place his or her arm on the towel. Wrap the towel around the upper arm and provide downward deep-pressure input to the arm while moving the towel toward the hand. Have the student actively pull his or her arm out of the towel as the adult pulls the towel down the arm or hand. *Be sure to provide added input to the palm.* Perform on both arms two to three times as demonstrated by the occupational therapist. This also can be completed on student's feet if they are defensive. Unlike the brushing protocol, the student is an active participant in the process and is in control of how many times he or she would like to engage in the towel rub by either pulling his or her arm away to indicate wanting to finish the activity or by placing his or her arm out to the therapist to have it performed again. Due to hygiene issues, use different towels for each student engaging in the technique. The towels should be washed after each use. Due to skin allergies, always consult with the student's parents regarding lotions that the student can tolerate.

- *Tactile activities in bins:* Have the student complete tactile-related activities, including filling small bins with dried beans, lentils, or rice and exploring the bins with both hands. Small toys or objects can be hidden within the bins for the student to reach in' and find.

- *Deep-pressure activities:* Another calming activity is playing in a ball pit, which provides deep-pressure input to a student with tactile defensiveness.

Modifications That Provide Tactile Input.

- *Velcro under desk:* Attach a piece of Velcro™ (coarse side) under the student's desk. The student can use the strip when he or she needs to fidget with his or her hands. The student can rub his or her fingers along the Velcro™ for added sensory input.

- *Fidget toys:* Provide the student with a fidget toy to squeeze or manipulate during a high-demand activity. Squeezing the fidget toy may assist the student with sustaining attention to the given classroom task. Fidget toys can include fidget pencils, squeezable animals, Koosh™ balls, Tangle, Theraputty, Pop Tubes, and Bend Band (all items can be found in the Therapro catalog). The therapist and teacher will need to monitor the student to ensure that he or she is not distracted by the toy or focusing more on the fidget toy than on the classroom activity.

Modifications for a Student With Tactile Defensiveness.

- *Preferential seating:* If the close proximity of classmates bothers the student, position him or her in a spot where he or she feels safe (e.g., seated at head of the table, edge of the rug, end of the line, corner of the classroom, or front/back of the class).
- *Define the student's personal space:* Help to define the student's space by using tape around the student's desk or on the floor, or use a carpet square when seated on the floor. Verbally warn the student when entering this personal space, especially when he or she cannot see you.

Oral Defensiveness/Oral Sensory Seeking Input

- *Nuk Brush:* Provide downward strokes to the inside of the student's cheeks and tongue to provide deep-pressure input to the mouth prior to an oral activity or feeding.
- *Water bottle:* Allow the student to have a water bottle at his or her desk that requires the student to drink from a straw. This provides student with added oral

input and can help him or her remain alert during a high-demand task.

- *Vibrating toothbrush:* Allow the student to use a vibrating toothbrush to provide added oral input. Guide the toothbrush to the mouth while the student holds it, making sure it contacts his or her cheeks, tongue, and top of mouth as tolerated by the student.
- *Crunchy/chewy foods:* Allow the student to have access to crunchy or chewy foods throughout the school day (at lunch, snack, or breaks during the day). Items can include chewing gum, hard candy, Starburst, Skittles, Twizzlers, or hard pretzels. This provides the student with increased oral input and may improve his or her attention to task during a high-demand activity.
- *Oral motor toy:* There are many "chew toys" now commercially available to assist students who seek oral input. This includes attaching Theratubing to the student's pencil or providing an oral motor toy such as Chewy Tubes (designed by Speech Pathology Associates, LLC) or the Ark's Grabber (designed by ARK Therapeutic Services). See Appendix 8.1 for ordering information.

Modifications for Students With Auditory Defensiveness

- *Provide adequate warning:* Warn the student when there is going to be a tornado drill, fire alarm, or another event that is very loud (e.g., gym class, lunch, an assembly).
- *Listen to music:* Allow the student to wear headphones playing soft music to assist in calming him or her or when in a loud environment.
- *Using pilot headphones:* Use this type of headphone to block out/decrease the amount of noise.
- *Using preferential seating:* Seat the student away from noisy or heavily trafficked areas (e.g., by a doorway or speaker).

- *Covering public announcement speaker:* In some classrooms (especially smaller classrooms), the public announcement system can be overwhelmingly loud. Covering the speaker with a box padded with foam may assist in muffling the sound without removing the ability to hear the speaker.
- *Writing social stories:* Write social stories that describe a noise that will occur (e.g., fire drill, lawn mower, assembly) and describe appropriate behavioral choices of how the student can respond to the situation. The teacher can read these to the student prior to a loud sound to ease his or her anxiety and help prepare him or her with options for how to handle the situation.
- *Placing tennis balls on classroom chairs:* Poking holes in tennis balls and placing them on the legs of chairs in the classroom can greatly reduce the amount of noise in an uncarpeted classroom. Teachers can get old tennis balls at racquetball clubs or country clubs or ask a sporting goods store to donate tennis balls to the school for this purpose.

Modifications to Reduce Visual Stimulation

- *Dim classroom lighting:* If the lighting is very bright (as is usual with fluorescent lighting), covering certain lights or dimming a section of the lights during certain activities may calm the students. When fluorescent lights are about to burn out they often flicker, which can be distracting to a student. When this is detected, have the custodian install a new light in the room.
- *Reduce clutter and distractions on necessary work surfaces:* Surfaces may include the chalkboard, assignment board, or the table where students turn in assignments. This assists the student in better seeing necessary information without having to try to ignore the irrelevant visual information.

- *Avoid hanging objects from ceiling:* If the student is very easily distracted or overstimulated by visual information, request that the teacher take down items hanging from classroom ceilings (e.g., mobiles, art projects).
- *Allow the student to wear a hat:* If the lighting in the classroom bothers or distracts the student, allowing him or her to wear a hat that has a brim (e.g., baseball hat) may assist in dimming the light for the student and allow for him or her to better tolerate the classroom's lighting.

Modifications to the Classroom

- *Use a picture/printed schedule:* The student may benefit from using a picture or printed schedule (if the student is a reader) to assist with transitioning from one task to the next. This allows the student to know what the expectations are during the school day and limits surprises during transitions. The student may initially need to have actual photographs of him or her engaging in the tasks used. Boardmaker symbols are also effective.
- *Define the student's personal space:* Assist in defining the student's personal space so that he or she has a visual reminder of what space he or she has to move around in. Define the student's personal space by taping a square around his or her desk or by providing a cushion, carpet square, or chair to sit on while engaged in floor activities.
- *Use social stories:* The student may benefit from using social stories to prepare for new activities or transitions during the school day (e.g., for an assembly, class party, speaker, field trip, or unexpected classroom task).
- *Provide the student with warning before an activity is beginning/ending:* In addition to using a picture schedule, the student may

benefit from being given a verbal warning a few minutes before an activity occurs or warned a few minutes before an activity ends (e.g., telling the student that he or she can go down a slide twice more before going to art class). This may assist in further defining the expectations of the day for the student and may help ease transitions (especially from high-interest or low-interest activities).

- *Use a timer:* The student may benefit from using a timer to count the number of minutes he or she has left in an activity.

- *Set limits/encourage the student to try task:* When the student is choosing not to participate in a given activity, it is important to set a limit and have him or her complete a portion of the task before allowing him or her to take a break.

- *Encourage the student to work for a reinforcer:* Talk to the student's parents and teachers to determine what activities or items are highly motivating to the student (e.g., receiving stickers, blowing bubbles, playing with playdough). The student can be encouraged to complete a given classroom task to receive a reinforcer. Over time, as the student gains success and confidence with completing the task, the reinforcer can be given less frequently, as the student is able to complete the task independently.

- *Encourage changes in position while completing seat work:* When the student is expected to sit and complete tasks for a period of time, he or she may benefit from being given the option to stand or lay prone on the floor to complete the work. Providing the student with these opportunities incorporates more movement into the school day and helps him or her sustain attention to a task.

- *Provide a "quiet corner" in the classroom:* When the student appears to be tense or overwhelmed or appears to need a break, creating a quiet spot in the room may help him or her be able to calm him- or herself down to transition to the next task and attend to the activity. The student could draw a picture, work on the computer, or look at a book before returning to work. Providing this alternative in the classroom may prevent having to remove the student from the classroom (when possible) when he or she appears overwhelmed or has an emotional outburst.

Summary and Conclusion

Educators must meet the needs of students with sensory processing issues within school settings. As experts, it is up to occupational therapists to stay current on sensory integration theory, applications of sensory integration theory to a variety of diagnosis and ability levels, the *Occupational Therapy Practice Framework* (AOTA, 2002), and activity suggestions and modifications that are relevant to schools. Therapists need to observe students in their school and conduct multifaceted evaluations that include receiving input from parents, teachers, and other service providers regarding how a student's sensory processing issues affect his or her education. Based on assessment results, occupational therapists can design intervention plans in conjunction with the educational team to meet the individualized needs of students.

The sensory interventions listed on the plan should be incorporated into a student's school day and carried out daily. Informational data can be taken to determine the effectiveness of sensory intervention strategies. Occupational therapists can incorporate sensory activities into an intervention session with students or can act as resources to teachers and staff who implement the plan to determine the overall effectiveness of that plan.

References

American Occupational Therapy Association. (2002). Occupational therapy practice framework: Domain and process. *American Journal of Occupational Therapy, 56,* 609–639.

Ayres, A. J. (1979). *Sensory integration and the child.* Los Angeles: Western Psychological Services.

Ayres, A. J., & Marr, D. B. (1991). Sensory integration and praxis tests. In A. G. Fisher, E. A. Murray, & A. C. Bundy (Eds.), *Sensory integration: Theory and practice* (pp. 203–229). Philadelphia: F. A. Davis.

Berk, R. A., & DeGangi, G. A. (1983). *DeGangi–Berk Test of Sensory Integration.* Los Angeles: Western Psychological Services.

Blanche, E. I., & Schaaf, R. C. (2001). Proprioception: A cornerstone of sensory integrative intervention. In S. Smith Roley, E. I. Blanche, & R. C. Schaaf (Eds.), *Sensory integration with diverse populations* (pp. 109–124). San Antonio, TX: Therapy SkillBuilders.

Dunn, W. (1999). *Sensory profile.* San Antonio, TX: Psychological Corporation.

Fisher, A. G., & Murray, E. A. (1991). Introduction to sensory integration theory. In A. G. Fisher, E. A. Murray, & A. C. Bundy (Eds.), *Sensory integration: Theory and practice* (pp. 3–26). Philadelphia: F. A. Davis.

Haack, L., & Haldy, M. (1998). Adaptations and accommodations for sensory processing problems. In J. Case-Smith (Ed.), *Making a difference in school system practice* (pp. 1–38). Bethesda, MD: American Occupational Therapy Association.

Hanschu, B. (2003, August). *Evaluation and treatment of sensory processing disorders from the perspective of the Ready Approach.* Course presented by Developmental Concepts, Hudson, OH.

Knickerbocker, B. M. (1980). *A holistic approach to learning disabilities.* Thorofare, NJ: Slack.

Martin, J. (1996). *Neuroanatomy text and atlas* (2nd ed.). Stamford, CT: Appleton & Lange.

Miller, L. J., Reisman, J. E., McIntosh, F. N., & Simon, J. (2001). An ecological model of sensory modulation: Performance of children with fragile x syndrome, autistic disorder, attention-deficit/hyperactivity disorder, and sensory modulation dysfunction. In S. Smith Roley, E. I. Blanche, & R. C. Schaaf (Eds.), *Sensory integration with diverse populations* (pp. 57–82). San Antonio, TX: Therapy SkillBuilders.

Murray-Slutsky, C., & Paris, B. A. (2000). *Exploring the spectrum of autism and pervasive developmental disorders.* San Antonio, TX: Therapy SkillBuilders.

Neisworth, J. T., Bagnato, S. J., Salvia, J., & Hunt, F. M. (1999). *Temperament and Atypical Behavior Scale.* Baltimore, MD: Paul H. Brookes.

Reeves, G. D. (2001). From neuron to behavior: Regulation, arousal, and attention as important substrates for the process of sensory integration. In S. Smith Roley, E. I. Blanche, & R. C. Schaaf (Eds.), *Sensory integration with diverse populations* (pp. 89–108). San Antonio, TX: Therapy SkillBuilders.

Reisman, J. E., & Hanschu, B. (1992). *Sensory Integration Inventory—Revised for individuals with developmental disabilities.* Hugo, MN: PDP Press.

Royeen, C. B., & Lane, S. J. (1991). Tactile processing and sensory defensiveness. In A. G. Fisher, E. A., Murray, & A. C. Bundy (Eds.), *Sensory integration: Theory and practice* (pp. 108–133). Philadelphia: F. A. Davis.

Smith Roley, S., Clark, G. F., & Bissel, J. (2003). Applying sensory integration framework in educationally related occupational therapy practice—2003 statement. *American Journal of Occupational Therapy, 57,* 652–659.

Wilbarger, P., & Wilbarger, J. L. (1991). *Sensory defensiveness in children aged 2–12: An intervention guide for parents and other caretakers.* Santa Barbara, CA: Avanti Educational Programs.

Williams, M. S., & Shellenberger, S. (1996). *How does your engine run: A leader's guide to the alert program for self-regulation.* Albuquerque, NM: TherapyWorks.

Appendix 8.1.
Sensory Catalogs and Ordering Information

Achievement Products for Children
P.O. Box 9033
Canton, OH 44711
800-373-4699
Fax: 800-766-4303

ARK's Grabber
ARK Therapeutic Services, Inc.
800-899-8055

Boardmaker
Mayer-Johnson, Inc.
P.O. Box 1579
Solana Beach, CA 92075
800-588-4548
www.mayer-johnson.com

Chewy Tubes
Speech Pathology Associates, LLC
P.O. Box 2289
South Portland, ME 04116
297-741-2443
Fax: 207-799-2289
www.chewytubes.com

Flaghouse
601 FlagHouse Drive
Hasbrouck Heights, NJ 07604-3116
800-793-7900
Fax: 800-793-7922

Movin' Sit
BodyTrends
304 Tequesta Drive
Tequesta, FL 33469
800-549-1667
www.bodytrends.com

Sammons Preston Roylan
An AbilityOne Company
P.O. Box 5071
Bolingbrook, IL 60440-5071
800-323-5547
Fax: 800-547-4333
www.sammonsprestonroylan.com

Sportime Abilitations
P.O. Box 620857
Atlanta, GA 30362
800-850-8602
Fax: 800-850-8602
www.abilitations.com

Therapro
225 Arlington Street
Framingham, MA 01702-8723
800-257-5376
Fax: 800-268-6624
www.theraproducts.com

Tool Chest: For Teachers, Parents, and Students
Tools for Parents
Tools for Students
AOTA Products
P.O. Box 0151
Annapolis Junction, MD 20701-0151
877-404-AOTA
Fax: 301-206-9789
www.aota.org

Information accurate as of October 2004.

Index

Page numbers in *italics* refer to tables, figures, and exhibits.

A

Activities of daily living
  determinants of capability, 101
  evaluation, 106–108, 125–127
  intervention approaches, 111–113
  intervention methods, 113–115
  intervention planning, 110–111
  needs determination, 108–110
  in school environment, 101, 124–125
  skills development for, 102–106
  task-specific interventions, 115–125
Adaptive responding, 250
Alert Program, 267
Americans with Disabilities Act, 22
Amygdala, 256
Annual goals, 17–18
Assessment. *See* Evaluation
Assistants, occupational therapy
  roles, 26–27
  supervision, 27
Assistive technology
  activities of daily living interventions,
    112–113
  definition, 19, 112
  devices, 19
  handwriting intervention, 192–193, 195–198
  IDEA evaluation, 18–19
  services, 19
Attention skills
  dyspraxia intervention, 85
  for fine motor tasks, 136
  sensory processing, 251
Auditory sensation, 275–276
Autism, 239–240

B

Batelle Developmental Inventory, 107, 152, 219
Beery Developmental Test of Visual–Motor
  Integration, 82, 220

Best practices
  definition, 19
  guidelines, 19–21
  IEP development, 14–15
Body awareness, 177–178
Brain stem, 253
Brain structure and function, 253–254
Brigance Diagnostic Inventory of Early
  Development, 107, 219–220
Bruininks–Oseretsky Test of Motor Proficiency,
  153, 220–221

C

Callirobics, 192
Cerebellum, 254
Cerebral hemispheres, 254
Chaining techniques, 113–114
Children's Handwriting Evaluation Scale, 181
Children's Handwriting Evaluation Scale for
  Manuscript Writing, 181
Clients, 20
Code. *See* Federal law
Cognitive functioning
  assessment, 179
  brain structure and, 254
  in dyspraxia, 79–80
  for fine motor tasks, 135–137
  handwriting and, 178–179
  preschool intervention, 239–240
Collaborative service delivery, 15, 20, 24, 25
  in developing goals and objectives, 33
  in handwriting intervention, 191
  in preschool intervention, 212
  self-care interventions, 110
Consultation, 23–25
  combined with direct service, 233–234
  performance evaluation, 41
  preschool services, 212, 226–229
  self-care interventions, 110

About the Authors

Lynne Pape, MEd, OTR/L, received her bachelor's degree in occupational therapy at The Ohio State University and her master's degree in education at Cleveland State University. She has been providing occupational therapy services in pediatric and school settings for 30 years and has taught at the college level. She has training in sensory integration and is SIPT and NDT certified. Lynne is the president of North Coast Therapy Associates, Inc., LLC, a private practice that has provided occupational and physical therapy services to school districts for over 15 years. Lynne has developed approaches, specific referral processes, guidelines, and checklists and questionnaires to deal with a variety of topics related to school-based practice, including evaluation and treatment of handwriting issues, functional activities of daily living, fine motor skill development, and alternate assessments. She shares this information with her staff, teachers, administrators, and fellow practitioners at conferences around the state.

Kelly Ryba, OTR/L, is a graduate of The Ohio State University and has been a pediatric occupational therapist since 1999, working in school-based settings. Kelly is Vice President of North Coast Therapy Associates, Inc., LLC, where she manages occupational therapists working in school districts and provides direct service and consultation services to students. She also is involved in program development for handwriting, motor planning, and data collection. Kelly developed the data collection procedure used at North Coast Therapy. Kelly has presented to parent groups, teachers, staff members, and colleagues at the Ohio Occupational Therapy Association state conference and the OT/PT Institute held in Columbus on a variety of topics related to school-based practice, including data collection, academic content standards, evidence-based practice, providing services to children with dyspraxia, and sensory integration.